CULTURAL HEALING
AND BELIEF SYSTEMS

Edited by

JAMES D. PAPPAS
WILLIAM E. SMYTHE
ANGELINA BAYDALA

DETSELIG
ENTERPRISES LTD

Cultural Healing and Belief Systems

Library and Archives Canada Cataloguing in Publication

Cultural healing and belief systems / [edited by] James D. Pappas, William E. Smythe, Angelina Baydala.

Includes bibliographical references.
ISBN 978-1-55059-334-1

1. Traditional medicine. 2. Mental healing. 3. Spiritual healing.
I. Pappas, James D. II. Smythe, William E. (William Ernest), 1953-
III. Baydala, Angelina

RC455.4.E8C824   2007   615.8'8   C2007-904631-2

Detselig Enterprises Ltd.
210, 1220 Kensington Road NW
Calgary, Alberta
T2N 3P5

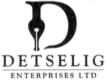

DETSELIG
ENTERPRISES LTD

www.temerondetselig.com
temeron@telusplanet.net
Phone: (403) 283-0900
Fax: (403) 283-6947

We acknowledge the support of the Government of Canada through the Book Publishing Industry Development Program (BPIDP) for our publishing program.

We also acknowledge the support of the Alberta Foundation for the Arts for our publishing program.

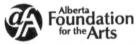

COMMITTED TO THE DEVELOPMENT OF CULTURE AND THE ARTS

SAN 113-0234
ISBN 978-1-55059-334-1
Printed in Canada on 100% recycled paper   Cover Design by Alvin Choong

CONTENTS

CLINICAL ISSUES IN CULTURAL HEALING

ABOUT THE AUTHORS

Angelina Baydala, Ph.D., is a registered Clinical Psychologist and Associate Professor in the Department of Psychology at the University of Regina. Her research focuses on histories, cultures, and theories of psychological healing. Dr. Baydala regularly teaches undergraduate courses on the history of psychology, systems of psychology, theories of personality, and yoga psychology, as well as a graduate course on theories and practices of psychotherapy. She can be contacted at angelina.baydala@uregina.ca.

Goffredo Bartocci, M.D., is a psychiatrist and psychoanalyst whose work includes field research conducted with Bantu people in South Africa and Desert Aborigines in Central Australia. He was Clinical Professor at the University of Turin and Head of the Transcultural Psychiatry Unit in Rome. Currently, he is Honorary Advisor and Past-President of the Transcultural Psychiatry Section of World Psychiatric Association, and sits as President-Elect and Founder of the World Association of Cultural Psychiatry (www.waculturalpsy.org). Dr. Bartocci has three books to his credit and several papers about the influence of magic and the sacred on psychopathological expression. He can be contacted at tpsection@quipo.it.

Norma-Jean Byrd currently serves as the Resident Elder at the University of Regina, Saskatchewan Institute of Applied Technology, and the Regina Public School Division. As part of her duties, she counsels students, staff, and faculty. She offers workshops on the Medicine Wheel Teachings as well as hosting regular community Talking Circles. Born of Cree ancestry, Ms. Byrd is recognized as an Elder throughout Saskatchewan. Her extensive understanding of the Aboriginal cultures and issues is bolstered by the wisdom she has gleaned from over forty years of experience in the workforce. In recognition of her outstanding contributions to Saskatchewan's communities, the Governor-General of Canada awarded her the 125 Canada Medal. Some of Ms. Bird's other awards include the Woman of Distinction award from the Y.W.C.A. for work with children, youth and families in Regina and a Community Work and Service award presented by the First Nations group, Women of the Dawn of Regina. She can be contacted at nbyrd@accesscomm.ca.

Nancy Clark, Ph.D. Candidate, is currently an adjunct professor at the University of British Columbia, School Of Nursing. Ms. Clark has worked in community mental health services in Vancouver BC for 15 years as a clinical nurse educator and community mental health practitioner. Her research interests and experience are focused in the following categories

 caregiver efficacy, spirituality, and mental health practice; the integration and exploration of the utilization of spirituality in psychiatric assessment; and the development of cultural understandings of Indigenous perspectives on spirituality and mental health in the context of the current Canadian Mental health system. Ms. Clark is currently working on her dissertation on the spiritual roots of resilience and the mental health of Canadian Indigenous people at McGill University. Contacted her at n.clark@shaw.ca.

Simon Dein, Ph.D., is a senior lecturer in Anthropology and Medicine at University College London, England. He has worked extensively on millennialism and religion and healing and has authored three books. Dr. Dein also serves as the joint editor of the Journal of Mental Health, Religion, and Culture and an Honorary Consultant Psychiatrist in Essex, England. He can be contacted at rmhasde@ucl.ac.uk.

Jonathan H. Ellerby, Ph.D., is an ordained Interfaith minister whose academic training addressed the understanding and articulation of holistic healing systems with a focus on cross-cultural models of spiritual well-being. Over his twenty years of global travel and extensive study, Dr. Ellerby has explored healing systems from holistic healers from more than 35 different cultures. He has published in the fields of holistic health, spirituality and health, and organizational wellness and has years of experience as a consultant, speaker, and facilitator. He has also worked as a spiritual counselor and integrative healing practitioner, utilizing a variety of therapeutic traditions in private, resort, and hospital settings. Currently, Dr. Ellerby works as the Spiritual Program Coordinator for Canyon Ranch, one of the world's leading holistic health resorts. He can be contacted at jellerby@canyonranch.com.

Lyn Freeman, Ph.D., is Executive Faculty and Chair of Integrative Health Studies at Saybrook Graduate School and Research Center in San Francisco. She is also President of Mind Matters Research, an Alaskan organization performing research on imagery as treatment for chronic disease. She is author of *Mosby's Complementary and Alternative Medicine: A Research-Based Approach and other texts and CMEs* by Aspen and Thomson-Delmar. In 2005 and 2006, she served as principal investigator for a Phase I National Cancer Institute-funded clinical trial on imagery as treatment for breast cancer survivors, a study that produced statistical and clinically significant outcomes. She co-founded a non-profit mind-body research organization in Alaska called Envision Innovative Health. Dr. Freeman is currently working on the third edition of the Mosby textbook, which will publish in 2008. She can be contacted at lfreeman@gci.net.

Harris L. Friedman, Ph.D., is Research Professor of Psychology at University of Florida, as well as a Florida licensed psychologist. He is interested in scientific approaches to transpersonal psychology, as well as in transpersonal applications in clinical and environmental psychology. He has written or edited more than sixty publications, including books, book chapters, and professional articles. Currently, Dr. Friedman serves as the Editor of the *International Journal of Transpersonal Studies* and the Associate Editor of *The Humanistic Psychologist*. He can be contacted at harrisfriedman@floraglades.org.

Amanda L. Gorchynski received a Bachelor of Arts Honors degree in Psychology from the University of Regina in the fall of 2006. Her undergraduate thesis, entitled Yoga and Addictions: A Feasibility Study, is a qualitative examination of community attitudes towards the use of Yoga in addiction treatment programs. She is interested in continuing her research and counselling work in the field of psychology. Currently, Ms. Gorchynski conducts inpatient substance abuse counselling in Regina, Saskatchewan. She can be contacted at a.gorchynski@sasktel.net.

Andrea Grabovac, M.D., obtained her specialization in psychiatry at the University of British Columbia in 2002. As Clinical Assistant Professor in the Department of Psychiatry at the University of British Columbia, she directs the Interface between Religion, Spirituality and Psychiatry course for psychiatry residents. To her credit, the course received a $30,000 US grant from the George Washington Institute for Spirituality and Health for further course development. She works as a consultant psychiatrist on the inpatient Brief Intervention Unit at Vancouver Hospital and at the BC Cancer Agency. Dr. Grabovac sees patients referred for psychiatric assessment of religious and spiritual issues at the Cross Cultural Psychiatry Outpatient Clinic at Vancouver Hospital. She can be contacted at nickandandrea@shaw.ca.

Mary Rucklos Hampton, Ph.D., is a Professor of Psychology at Luther College, University of Regina and Research Faculty Member at the Saskatchewan Population Health Evaluation Research Unit. She is a registered doctoral clinical psychologist in the province of Saskatchewan. Her research interests include women's health, cross-cultural psychology, and end-of-life care. Her work is inspired by her strong family ties to Aboriginal communities. She can be contacted at Mary.Hampton@uregina.ca.

Marcia Hermansen, Ph.D., is Professor of Theology and Director of the Islamic World Studies program at Loyola University Chicago where she teaches courses in Islamic Studies and Religious Studies. She received her Ph.D. from the University of Chicago in Arabic and Islamic Studies. In the course of her research and language training she lived for extended periods in Egypt, Jordan, India, Iran, Turkey, and Pakistan. Remarkably, her broad field of studies requires her to conduct research in Arabic, Persian, Urdu, and Turkish in addition to the major European languages. Her book, *The Conclusive Argument from God*, a study and translation (from Arabic) of Shah Wali Allah of Delhi's, Hujjat Allah al-Baligha was published in 1996. She is co-editor of the Encyclopedia of Islam and the Muslim World (2003). Dr. Hermansen has contributed numerous academic articles in the fields of Islamic Thought, Sufism, Islam and Muslims in South Asia, Muslims in America, and Women and Gender in Islam. She can be contacted at mherman@luc.edu.

Stanley Krippner, Ph.D., is the Alan Watts Professor of Psychology and Chair of the Study of Consciousness at Saybrook Graduate School, San Francisco. He is a Fellow in four APA divisions, and former president of the thirtieth and thirty-first divisions. He has written over five hundred articles and has co-authored several books, including *Haunted by Combat,* which focuses on Posttraumatic Stress Disorder among U.S. combat veterans,. and has conducted workshops and seminars on dreams and hypnosis throughout the world. Dr. Krippner is a member of the editorial board for the Journal of Indian Psychology and Revista Argentina de Psicologia Paranormal, and serves on the advisory board for the International School for Psychotherapy, Counseling, and Group Leadership (St. Petersburg) and the Czech Unitaria (Prague). He holds faculty appointments at the Universidade Holistica Internacional (Brasilia) and the Instituto de Medicina y Tecnologia Avanzada de la Conducta (Ciudad Juarez). His academic interests include educational, cross-cultural, and health issues. He can be contacted at skrippner@saybrook.edu.

Charles Mather, Ph.D., is an Assistant Professor in the Department of Anthropology at the University of Calgary. His research in medical anthropology brought him from Calgary to Africa to conduct fieldwork. He is currently engaged in research on the role of pharmaceuticals in the medical systems of Northern Ghana. His other work includes researching the cultural and social determinants behind patient decisions in managing cardiovascular disease risk in Calgary. Dr. Mather's subjects of interest include pharmaceuticals, shrines, divination, disease etiology, and ethnomedicine. He can be contacted at cmmather@ucalgary.ca.

Kim McKay-McNabb, M.A., is a Cree woman originally from Sakimay First Nation. She is currently an Assistant Professor at the First Nations University of Canada in the Department of Science. She is in the process of completing her Ph.D. in the Clinical Psychology program at the University of Regina. Her research interests are community-based and include: end of life health care, HIV/AIDS in Aboriginal communities, and sexual health with Aboriginal youth. Her interests always tie back to her Aboriginal community to assist with the journey to healing. Contact her at kmckaymcnabb@firstnationsuniversity.ca.

Bob Morgan, Ph.D., has four decades of experience with clinical, educational, and community development programs related to the health service needs of American Indians and Alaska Natives. His life training occurred in indigenous communities around the world as he participated in ceremony and prayer with tribal leaders, traditional healers, and other individuals from the Four Directions. He has lectured and developed programs at all academic levels for a variety of universities and public schools. He has come to appreciate the vast amount of past wisdom that is available to all who seek to heal both other people and Mother Earth. Currently, Dr. Morgan is teaching and organizing a traditional healing conference for the psychology department at the University of Alaska, Anchorage. He can be contacted at garden1530@webtv.net.

James D. Pappas, Ph.D., is in group practice at PAR Consultants and Counselors and also teaches psychology at the University of Regina's Luther College, Department of Psychology and Faculty of Education. His clinical research explores efficacy of mindfulness used in conjunction with conventional psychotherapies, while his academic research lies in the application of quantitative and qualitative approaches to the study of trauma, stress, depression, and personality as it relates to spirituality and transpersonality. Courses that pertain to his research include Psychology of Belief Systems and Consciousness Studies. Dr. Pappas is also the recipient of the Sidney Jourard Award by the American Psychological Association and the William James Award by the Council on Spiritual Practices for distinguished dissertation research and has received a Certificate of Recognition for outstanding contributions in teaching by the University of Regina. He can be contacted at pappas1j@uregina.ca.

Sherry Farrell Racette, Ph.D., is an interdisciplinary scholar who is actively involved with the Arts. She has worked in the fields of Aboriginal teacher education, curriculum development, and Indigenous Studies with the Gabriel Dumont Institute, the University of Regina and First Nations University of Canada. She has a B.F.A. from the University of Manitoba, an M.Ed. in Curriculum and Instruction from the University of Regina and an Interdisciplinary Ph.D. (Native Studies, Anthropology, History) from the University of Manitoba. Her broad research focus is on Métis and First Nations women's history, particularly reconstructing indigenous art histories that recontextualize museum collections, and reclaiming women's voices and lives. Some of her publications include: *Sewing for a Living: The Commodification of Métis Women's Artistic Production in Contact Zones: Aboriginal and Settler Women in Canada's Colonial Past* (2005), *Métis Man or Canadian Icon: Who Owns Louis Riel in Rielisms* (2001), *Beads, Silk and Quills: the Clothing and Decorative Arts of the Métis in Metis Legacy* (2001) and *Sex, Fear, Women, Travel and Work: Five Persistent Triggers of Eurocentric Negativity in Pushing the Margins* (2001). Dr. Racette currently teaches in the Department of Art History, Concordia University, on leave from First Nations University of Canada. She can be contacted at SFarrell-Racette@firstnationsuniversity.ca.

Ruth Richards, M.D., Ph.D., is a Board Certified psychiatrist and educational psychologist. She is a professor of psychology at Saybrook Graduate School in San Francisco, in the areas of Consciousness and Spirituality, and Integrative Health. She is a psychiatric affiliate of Massachusetts General Hospital, a research affiliate at McLean Hospital, Belmont, Massachusetts, and a lecturer in the Department of Psychiatry, Harvard Medical School. For many years, Dr. Richards has studied creativity as expressed through everyday life in clinical and educational settings. She also published on creativity and spiritual development as well as creativity and social action. With Mark Runco, Dr. Richards co-edited *Eminent Creativity, Everyday Creativity, and Health* (Ablex, 1998), and is editor of *Everyday Creativity and New Views of Human Nature: Psychological, Social, and Spiritual Perspectives* (American Psychological Association, 2007). She served on the executive advisory board for the *Encyclopedia of Creativity*, and is also on the editorial boards of three journals: *The Creativity Research Journal*; *The Journal of Humanistic Psychology*; and *Psychology of Aesthetics, Creativity, and the Arts*, the journal for the tenth division of the American Psychological Association where she also holds elective office. Furthermore, Dr. Richards is on the associate board of AHIMSA (meaning non-violence in Sanskrit, www.ahimsaberkeley.org), a non-profit interfaith organization that works to encourage dialogues and public forums on issues that bridge spirituality, science, and society, toward greater mutual understanding and a better world. She can be contacted at rrichards@saybrook.edu.

Bruce, W. Scotton, M.D., D.F.A.P.A., is Clinical Professor of Psychiatry, School of Medicine, University of California San Francisco, and a certified Jungian analyst at the C. G. Jung Institute of San Francisco. He is the recipient of the Will Solimene Award for Excellence in Medical Communication as the senior editor of the Textbook of Transpersonal Psychiatry and Psychology. Due to his desire to learn how cultural mindsets affect disease and healing, he has studied Hinduism and Buddhism for thirty years and Huichol shamanism for seventeen. Dr. Scotton maintains a private practice incorporating those lessons learned from other cultures. He can be contacted at bruce.scotton@ucsf.edu.

Rebecca Shaw, Ph.D., is a licensed professional counselor and has experience working with various cultures within clinical, educational, and training settings. A great deal of her experience has focused on enhancing resiliency by helping those exposed to traumatic experiences weave a tapestry of life based on personal strengths and skills. She co-developed and co-facilitated a multicultural Family Circle of Healing program for women and children exposed to severe traumatic experiences utilizing a blend of traditional and contemporary healing strategies.

She also uses a modified version of the Circle of Healing approach to facilitate growth and learning in children and adolescents from multicultural backgrounds who are challenged with neurological disorders and living in a residential setting. Moreover, she utilizes a similar strategy to help women in her local church to further develop their spiritual growth. For Dr. Shaw, there are no failures in life when challenges are seen as opportunities to learn and grow by drawing from our inner strengths. She can be contacted at rmshaw@mtaonline.net.

William E. Smythe, Ph.D., is currently Professor and Head of the Psychology Department at the University of Regina, where he has taught since 1995. He has held prior academic appointments at the University of Alberta, where he was a Killam Scholar and Canada Research Fellow, and at Okanagan University College. Formerly a member of the Center for Advanced Study in Theoretical Psychology at the University of Alberta and currently active in the International Society for Theoretical Psychology. Dr. Smythe has published extensively in theoretical psychology and human cognition. He can be contacted at smythew@uregina.ca.

Louise Sundararajan received her Ph.D. in History of Religions from Harvard University, and her Ed.D. in Counseling Psychology from Boston University. Currently a forensic psychologist, she was president of the International Society for the Study of Human Ideas on Ultimate Reality and Meaning. A member of American Psychological Association, and the International Society for Research on Emotions, Dr. Sundararajan has authored over forty articles in refereed journals and books, on topics ranging from Chinese poetics to alexithymia. She can be contacted at louiselu@frontiernet.net.

Tobi Zausner, Ph.D., has an interdisciplinary doctorate in Art and Psychology. She is also an art historian and an award-winning visual artist, with works in major museums and in private collections around the world. Dr. Zausner writes and lectures widely on the psychology of art, teaches at the C. G. Jung Foundation in New York, and is an officer on the Board of A.C.T.S. (Arts, Crafts, and Theatre Safety), a non-profit organization investigating health hazards in the arts. A native New Yorker and an avid reader, walker, and hiker, she wishes there were more trees, grass, and hills in New York City. Her recently published book *When Walls Become Doorways: Creativity and the Transforming Illness* (2007) is about the influence of physical illness on the creative process of visual artists. It shows that instead of stopping artists, physical difficulties transform them, enhancing both their life and their work. She can be contacted at tzausner@earthlink.net.

INTRODUCTION

The inception of this volume stemmed from the need for an integrated teaching resource that would bring together cultural and clinical perspectives on healing in a novel and thematically coherent way. Addressing a wide range of belief systems and healing practices with a variety of approaches became, for us, a necessity. We intended to create a text that could be accessible to the general reader interested in a range of topics from psychological theory, cultural and anthropological psychology, and psychiatric studies, to alternative medicine and religious studies. Nonetheless, we believe that this volume will be a useful resource for scholars, researchers, and clinicians and, most specifically, for graduate and senior undergraduate students. The wide range of fields covered in this publication make it applicable to coursework in belief systems, consciousness and health studies, psychology of religion, cultural and anthropological studies, as well as medical studies, specifically psychiatry.

This volume considers the nature of culturally organized belief systems and traditional healing practices from psychological, religious, spiritual, and cultural perspectives. The contributors to this volume address diverse belief systems that shape and mediate healing. Belief systems may be expressed in ritual, folklore, metaphors, symbols, and various communal practices that facilitate healing. Our aim is to encourage mutual understanding and respect among different traditions of scientific, religious, spiritual, and psychological knowledge, as well as to provide resources for enhancing personal growth and mental health. In an increasingly multicultural world, we believe that it is important to understand culturally situated practices and modes of healing as they relate to science, religion, philosophy, psychology, and medicine. The chapters in this volume discuss the development and diversity of cultural healing and belief systems and how they affect human life: psychological health, relationships, ethical and moral behavior, and wholeness.[1]

The first two chapters of this book lay the theoretical groundwork for examining belief systems and healing. James D. Pappas and Harris L. Friedman undertake in chapter one a conceptual clarification of the terms *religious*, *spiritual*, and *transpersonal*, in the context of empirical approaches to transpersonal phenomena. Following a review of the conceptual status of these terms, they go on to review the theoretical contributions of a number of prominent theorists in this area. The authors follow with their own transpersonal perspective, based on an integrative psychometric approach to *self-expansive* phenomenon, before they conclude by noting some implications of their approach for empirical inquiry into the realm of the transpersonal.

In chapter two, William E. Smythe examines shamanism as a healing motif that manifests in several cultural contexts. Specifically, he compares themes of sickness and healing from traditional, indigenous shamanistic practices with modern parallels in psychoanalysis and personal mythology. Noting some significant similarities and differences among these variants of the shamanic motif, he concludes with some implications of understanding shamanic healing as myth.

The second section of this publication focuses on cultural systems of healing and illustrates diverse cultural belief systems and practices with significant healing potential. Stanley Krippner describes in chapter three ethnomedical aspects of the North American Navajo and South American Peruvian traditions. He compares a shamanic medical model, an eclectic folk healing model, and the allopathic biomedical model, using critical factors to systematically describe each system. The intention of this work is to demonstrate possible points of collaboration between allopathic biomedicine and various indigenous systems of healing.

In chapter four, Charles Mather examines the ethnomedical tradition of the Kusasi in Northern Ghana. Kusasi medicine is depicted as simultaneously natural, supernatural, and social, such that healing extends beyond physical well-being. Health is understood in terms of interpersonal relations that determine personal identity, status, and role. As such, the Kusasi cultural system of healing seeks to address social, psychological, and cultural needs.

The fifth chapter presents the beliefs of the Huichol shamans of the Sierra Madre as described by Bruce Scotton. He considers their world-view – humanity's place in the world, human nature and behavior, and the basis of healing – and examines why Western science does not typically recognize the knowledge that underlies the shamanistic healing system. Scotton's intention is to illustrate the importance of cross-cultural study and travel to understand what is possible for the human psyche.

Tobi Zausner discusses how artistic expression brings healing through elevated awareness in the sixth chapter. She discusses the healing capacity of religious and secular archetypal symbols from prehistoric times to the present day in both non-industrialized and technologically advanced cultures. The chapter describes viewing and creating art as a multicultural and historical phenomenon that enables traumatic recovery and good health.

Louise Sundararajan's chapter on second-order desires, or the power to evaluate the desirousness of our desires, closes this section. She examines the second-order desire in the Chinese Buddhist tradition known as kong (emptiness) and its implications for healing. She situates kong in its cultural and historical context, examines the cognitive processes involved in its realization, and contrasts kong with the Western concept of hope as a first-order desire. Finally, the therapeutic implications of kong are compared with Gendlin's formulations of Focusing.

Section three of the text considers healing practices from the perspectives of traditional religious belief systems. Chapter eight, by Andrea Grabovac and Nancy Clark, examines the interface of spirituality and religion with modern psychiatry. In particular, they discuss research in biomedicine and cultural psychiatry that supports the integration of spirituality and religious belief systems with psychiatric clinical practice, citing research that shows a positive correlations between religious and spiritual practices and mental health, even at the level of neurobiology. The authors then explore an alternative epistemology that addresses the relationships among religion, spirituality, mental health, and illness. They go on to provide clinical examples of ways to bridge the gap between the Western medical model and beliefs about healing and wellness from other cultures, concluding with a review of several clinical assessment tools and suggestions aimed at helping to integrate spiritual and religious domains with clinical practice.

In chapter nine, Marcia Hermansen discusses some common elements of the Islamic religion that underlie healing practices in Muslim cultures with specific focus on Sufi healing practices. Sufism, the mystical or esoteric aspect of Islam, is an especially useful context from which to illustrate the religious and cultural aspect of Islamic belief systems and healing. Hermansen concludes with some reflections on historical change, cultural differences, contemporary healing practices, and the role of class and gender within Muslim healing systems.

Simon Dein and Goffredo Bartocci discuss various forms of healing in the Christian tradition in the tenth chapter. Following a brief historical overview, they survey a variety of examples of Christian healing from contemporary Catholicism to Pentecostal healing to Christian Science. They proceed to examine evidence for the efficacy of Christian healing, concluding that there is no empirical evidence that such healing has ever cured an organic disease. They conclude by advocating more rigorous assessment criteria for evaluating claims of Christian healing and then offer some reflections on cultural and ontological issues.

In the last section of the volume, clinical issues in cultural healing are addressed. Jonathan H. Ellerby argues, in chapter eleven, that credentialing is a central issue in collaboration between Western and traditional Indigenous healers. Therapeutic programs that draw upon Indigenous healers and healing approaches must be developed with cultural integrity, making appropriate credentialing critical. Ellerby shows that both Western and Indigenous medical communities have systems of credentialing; however, because these are very different models, collaborative work often proceeds upon misunderstandings or misrepresentation. His purpose is to reveal the ways in which Indigenous communities distinguish genuine healers from charlatans. Ellerby develops a four-fold model, based on Indigenous traditions, that identifies criteria for distinguishing between legitimate and illegitimate healers, which can be used to guide professional collaboration and consultation.

In chapter twelve, Mary R. Hampton, Kim McKay-McNabb, Sherry Farrell Racette, and Elder Norma Jean Byrd report on a qualitative research study that used grounded theory methodology to investigate how sexual health and healing is viewed by Elders. Their findings offer significant and novel insight regarding issues that Aboriginal youth have to face as a result of the deleterious effects of colonization. The impact of forced acculturation on First Nations People involving residential schools and sexual abuse, for example, has contributed to present-day health-related problems for Aboriginal youth. They propose that Elders in their traditional ways can help improve these circumstances through their involvement in the Aboriginal community.

Robert Morgan, Lyn Freeman, and Rebecca Shaw discuss in the thirteenth chapter a tri-disciplinary approach called the *Circle of Healing* that creates a partnership amongst allopathic, integrative, and tribal medicine. This model presents various options for healing, provides support through a Pathfinder or a guide that acts as the interpreter, implements a client-driven health plan or path, and provides follow-up treatment for client care. Their chapter discusses the operational utility of their model and its applications to a multicultural society, in addition to Native communities, as a holistic approach towards treatment and healing beyond the limitations posed by allopathic medicine.

The fourteen chapter examines the healing power of empathetic and authentic relationships by drawing upon Buddhist psychology and paralleling it to artistic creativity.   Ruth Richards writes about the qualities of immediacy, presence, richness, deep engagement, and openness to greater truths found in the creative process. She illustrates how Eastern wisdom can be infused into Western clinical practice in the context of a Relational Model developed by scholar-practitioners at the Stone Center at Wellesley College and Harvard Medical School. Richards presents a series of vignettes based on her clinical experiences in an inpatient psychiatric unit and discusses fundamental changes that occurred through creative involvement and empathetic connections between clinician and patient. The clinical applications and implications of the five key qualities of the relational model are discussed with emphasis on empathy and mutuality. In their fullest promise, such relational qualities even point us toward the Four Immeasureables of Buddhism: loving-kindness, compassion, sympathetic joy and equanimity.

The closing chapter in this section, by Angelina Baydala and Amanda Gorchynski, explores how yoga therapy, in combination with the Twelve-Step program of Alcoholics Anonymous, can be used to treat alcoholism. Comparing the similarities and differences between these two approaches, they argue for a blend of both to form a holistic treatment program. Paramount to this integration is the Caring Model based on a grounded theory analysis of interview data from Father Joe and four thematic areas for recovery from alcohol-use disorders. The authors' intent is to show how this play across culturally distinct belief systems can foster an approach to restoring psychological, emotional, physical, and spiritual health.

The apparent hegemony of allopathic practices notwithstanding, traditional spiritual approaches to healing remain powerful in many cultures around the world. Our purpose in this publication is to inspire consideration of the profound significance of cultural and spiritual dimensions of healing. These dimensions include aspects of health and healing that tend to be occluded by allopathic medicine. As illustrated by the chapters in this volume, there is wide diversity among these culturally and spiritually based approaches. Yet, a common thread runs through them all, namely that healing, in the broadest sense, is fundamentally culturally bound and spiritually informed. Many of the contributors clarify how these approaches can be successfully integrated with Western allopathic systems. Thus, our hope is that this volume will be a useful resource and a stimulus of new thought for students, scholars, and practitioners interested in alternative approaches to healing.

James D. Pappas, William E. Smythe, & Angelina Baydala
Regina, Saskatchewan

NOTES

[1] As a quick note, some authors use the term *patient* and others use the term *client*. We find that in psychiatric or medical care the term patient is preferred over client whereas in psychological practice the term client is commonly used.

THEORETICAL GROUNDWORK

CHAPTER ONE

TOWARD A CONCEPTUAL CLARIFICATION OF THE TERMS
RELIGIOUS, SPIRITUAL, AND TRANSPERSONAL
AS PSYCHOLOGICAL CONSTRUCTS

James D. Pappas
&
Harris L. Friedman

Increasingly, the terms *religious*, *spiritual*, and *transpersonal* are being used imprecisely in the psychological literature. In particular, they are seldom adequately delineated as distinct concepts and are even frequently used interchangeably as synonyms. However, we consider it important to distinguish these terms in order to increase their efficacy in psychological theory and provide a solid operational base for their use in empirical research and pragmatic application. We begin with a review of the conceptual status of each of these terms in order to reveal some of the latent problems that have caused theoretical and operational confusion. Next, we contextualize these terms within a number of classical and contemporary theories. Then, we present an overarching transpersonal perspective that we propose can integrate these terms in a meaningful way. Last, we conclude with a preview of some considerations that stem from our perspective.

CONCEPTUAL STATUS OF TERMS

THE RELIGIOUS CONCEPTUAL DIMENSION

Religion can be understood as a means for publicly and privately expressing a set of beliefs, values, symbols, behaviors, and/or practices related to what the practitioner considers sacred. Religious expressions are typically culturally based and commonly institutionalized. Even when only held privately, they are based on shared social understandings that have been internalized. Richards and Bergin (2000) suggested that being religious is consistent with beliefs, feelings, and practices that are most commonly expressed "institutionally and denominationally as well as personally" and religious expressions are inclined to be "denominational, external, cognitive, behavioral, ritualistic, and public" (p. 5).

In regard to cultural ascriptions of religion, these expressions involve procedures and techniques by which individuals express their relation to the sacred. In the major world religions, they are usually guided by ideologies expressed by supposed charismatic founders, such as in Four Noble Truths of Buddhism, attributed to Siddhartha Gautama, and the Christian Gospels, attributed to the teachings of Jesus Christ. The instrumental element of religion in such contexts is a *bond* or *connection* that exists between an individual and the sacred through some form of expression, whether an external practice such as a prayer or an internal, but socially shared, belief system. Moreover, it is often a source that unites individuals through community and, in this sense, binds individuals to each other as well as to the sacred, such as in Buddhism's sangha and Christianity's church. This is consistent with the etymology of *religion* from the Latin *religio*, which is based on the term *ligo* meaning to bind and connotes a "bond between humanity and some greater-than-human-power" (National Institute of Health Research, 1998, p. 15). Moreover, the similar expression in Sanskrit, yoga, which also means "to bind" or, more precisely, "to yoke," remains consistent with this sentiment.

Contemporary views of religion, such as those offered by Zinnbauer, Pargament, and Scott (1999), often divide the concept into substantive (i.e., what religion represents in terms of a motivational source) and functional aspects (i.e., what religion does in terms of a support system). The substantive quality is observed in religious activities, such as structured prayer, meditation, worship, chanting, or ritual, which constitute an individual's external religious expression (i.e., religiosity or religiousness) and is usually anchored in a shared cultural understanding. This concept of religion is congruent with Spiro (1966), who suggested that religion seen in this context is an "institution consisting of culturally patterned interaction with culturally postulated superhuman beings" (p. 96). However, in some cases such as Buddhism, the sacred can be seen alternatively as an individual's relatedness to a sacred, but impersonal, aspect that is typically not deified.[1] Religion in this sense is an institutional process whereby social rituals (e.g., attending an institutionalized place of worship and prayer) assign an individual a role inside a system of beliefs, attitudes, and practices. Nonetheless, these rituals do not directly represent the extent of an individual's internal devotion or indicate their level of religiousness; rather, such behaviors reveal an individual's involvement in a methodological and ideological consensus of religion. Wulff (2003) emphasized this point by arguing that religion is "nothing more than narrow, dogmatic beliefs and obligatory religious observances" (p. 47). This conceptualization of religion, in terms of an individual's devotion limited primarily to cultural-bound institutions, may be viewed as motivated by external factors, such as living up to community expectations and opportunities for personal gain, even when experienced or practiced in isolation.

　　Notions such as these have antecedents in the pioneering work of Allport (1950), who was the first to investigate religion from a psychometric perspective and to differentiate between religion as a means-to-an-end and as an end-in-itself. Although he initially used the terms immature religious sentiment and mature religious sentiment, he later changed them to extrinsic and intrinsic religious orientation, respectively, in studying the prevalence of religious bigotry and prejudice comparing churchgoers and non-churchgoers. An immature religious sentiment may be associated with magical thinking (e.g., how Christian children are often socialized to view Santa Claus in the West), the use of supplicatory prayer (e.g., to gain personal favors from a deity), or thinking of a tribal nature (e.g., ethnocentric religious beliefs leading to feelings of superiority of an in-group). In contrast, a mature religious sentiment may be motivated by a genuine purpose to serve an individual's religion, specifically as the "value underlying all things desirable for its own sake" (Allport, 1961, p. 301). For Allport, the major difference between immature religion and mature religion lies in the former's focus on an individual's self-centered motives – or other socially limited motives derived from family or tribal loyalty – in contrast to the latter's appeal to an individual's universal, or *master* motives. In other words, self-centered motives indicate a self-serving purpose, or the externalized aspects of religion, and master motives signify a faith-serving intention, or the internalized aspects of religion.

　　In regard to his later orientation, Allport (1960, 1961) differentiated between extrinsically and intrinsically oriented religious individuals, the former being religiously motivated as a means to achieving gain and the latter being religiously motivated for its own sake. According to Allport, much of religious sentiment is extrinsic and an extrinsic approach to religion may undermine the deeper meaning of religious expression, namely relatedness to the sacred. Consequently, extrinsically oriented religious individuals may not embrace the so-called intended function of religion (Allport, 1963, 1966). Moreover, they may even rigidly hold parochial and fundamentalist notions such that a given religion is the only true religion, since they may tend to pursue religion primarily for utilitarian concerns (Burris, 1994), such as personal or social rewards (Genia, 1993).

In contrast, intrinsically oriented religious individuals may emphasize the unifying character of religion, since it is based on authentic devotion to living a religion rather than using it instrumentally (Allport, 1966). The intrinsically oriented individual may also abandon aggrandizement, prejudice, and hatred to find deeper meanings through humility, compassion, and love (Allport, 1961, 1966; Allport & Ross, 1967). The master motive of such a person is to live religion according to its fullest by internalizing religious expressions as purpose and faith (Allport, 1963). However, intrinsically oriented individuals can also be fundamentalist in the sense that they may be so deeply devoted to their own religion that this excludes respecting other religions. It can even make them more susceptible to manipulating others to conform to their own religious orientation, perhaps even leading to deceptiveness (Burris, 1994). Yet, intrinsically oriented individuals may also be more optimistic than those who are extrinsically oriented since they may receive internal benefits, such as a basis for hope, from their devout dedication (Sethi & Seligman, 1993).

The functional quality of religion attempts to address the ontological and epistemological concerns of its practitioners.[2] It also deals with the various effects of religion on societies, such as increasing group cohesiveness, but these will not be further discussed here. Experiencing only externalized institutionalized expressions, such as beliefs and practices that do not connect deeply with their sense of the sacred, individuals can be frustrated in meeting their ontological and epistemological needs. Accordingly, Pargament (1997) argued that:

> This approach to religion [captures] the sense that religion is something more than a set of concepts and practices; rather, it has to do with life's most profound issues. It also opens up the study of religion to diverse traditions and innovative approaches, for no individual, group, or culture is spared the confrontations with ultimacy. (p. 27-28)

Unfortunately, religion alone often does not provide this feeling of deep connection, especially in the modern context where it may be devoid of inner aspects.

THE SPIRITUAL CONCEPTUAL DIMENSION

Greer and Roof (1992) discussed how some people become their own religious authorities by listening to their "own little voice" instead of only following "institutional authorities" (p. 346). This type of religion veers into what we call spirituality. This expression of spirituality may form a synthesis of organized and personal contemplations that expand an individual's unique religious worldview beyond any parochial religious orientation. In other words, though individuals may be affiliated with some particular religion, they are not necessarily limited to sanctioned methods and may instead develop their own way of living religiously. This unique religious expression may attempt to resolve what we refer to as *existential decay* – a lack of purpose, meaning, and hope that can impede coping with issues such as mortality and isolation – through forming personalized religious connections with a sense of the sacred. As such, the functional aspect represents a divergence from a methodical-religious way of living towards a non-methodical-religious way of living. This transition is evident where there is a detachment from institutionalism and adherence to functional matters of existence, meaning, purpose, morbidity, and suffering. In this sense, spirituality refers to a sense of connectedness with something sacred as well as to related practices without necessarily being vested in institutional or other predominantly culturally mediated practices or expressions of belief.

Historically, the term spiritual has antecedents in the ecclesiastical language of Judeo-Christian literature (e.g., *pneuma* in the context of the Greek New Testament) that describes an animating and supernatural force that has relevance to a divine figure, God. This has evolved from its etymological ascription in Latin, in which the term *spiritus* means "breath" or "life" or, perhaps better, "life breathing force." This prevailing understanding of spiritual has become intertwined with religion in Western psychology, as it is predominantly referenced within an exclusively Judeo-Christian context, namely as personalized religion or as the "subjective side of religious experience" in relationship to God (Hill & Pargament, 2003, p. 64). This theocentric approach reduces spirituality to a monocultural context, excluding those who declare themselves both spiritual and atheistic or agnostic (Smith, 2001). For example, Smith described four spiritual personality types as follows:

1. Atheists who think that there is no God
2. Polytheists who acknowledge many gods
3. Monotheists who believe in a single God
4. Mystics who say that there is only God. (p. 234)

It is more appropriate thus to refer to spirituality as idiosyncratically bound rather than culturally bound in that it is not exclusively tied to any religious expression, such as beliefs, feelings, or practices. In this sense, religious practice that once inextricably tied together both internal and external aspects is now *loosening* its tie with traditional religious communities while retaining the essence of spiritual connection to the sacred. Miller and Thorensen (2003) offered similar views, that religion is demarcated by boundaries (e.g., beliefs and practices that require social membership) as well as "nonspiritual concerns and goals (e.g., cultural, economic, political, social)," whereas spirituality is focused more on the individual rather than the social (p. 27). From another point of view, organized religion may be seen as one way of expressing an individual's spirituality (Spaeth,

2000) and in this sense religion is viewed a being a "subset of the spiritual" (Richards & Bergin, 2000, p. 5). That is, a spiritual experience suggests a connection with the transcendent as well as existential matters of purpose, meaning, and suffering; whereas, a religious experience does not necessarily entail this connection or this existential component (Richards & Bergin, 2000). Richards and Bergin summarize this relationship as follows:

> If a religious practice or experience (e.g., saying a prayer, engaging in ritual, reading a scripture) helps a person feel more closeness and connection with God or transcendent spiritual influences, then that practice or experience is also spiritual in nature. Without it, the practice or experience may be a religious one, but is not a spiritual one (p. 5).

Spirituality in this sense may replace traditional religion for people seeking transcendent connections that address existential and humanistic concerns, rather than religious concerns rooted in culturally determined theological, institutional, and/or scripturally based authority (e.g., relying on Biblical or other sacred texts). Individuals in North America increasingly self-identify as spiritual rather than religious, suggesting that the spiritual needs of individuals and society may be changing (Saucier & Skrzypinska, 2006). For example, Pappas (2003) found that, answering a question about being a religious and spiritual person, 99 of 201 undergraduate Canadian university/college participants responded "yes" and 102 responded "no" to indicate their status as a religious person, but 156 responded "yes" and 45 responded "no" to indicate their status as a spiritual person. Similarly, in another sample of 156 Canadian community participants who practiced Reiki, yoga, and meditation, 63 responded "yes" and 92 responded "no" to indicate their status as a religious person (one did not respond), but 153 responded "yes" and one responded "no" to indicate their status as a spiritual person (two did not respond). These numbers indicate of a change in how people see themselves in terms of religious and spiritual concepts.

Futhermore, Clark and Schellenberg (2006) reported on data from the General Social Survey and 2002 Ethnic Diversity Survey and found that reporting no religious affiliation increased 7% during the period from 1985 to 2004 for Canadians over the age of fifteen; when coupled with no attendance at religious services, there was an increase of 12%. The degree of religiosity in Canada is showing the following trend: 40% have a low degree, 31% are moderate, and 29% are highly religious, with religiosity being highest among the elderly and lowest among younger age groups (Clark & Schellenberg, 2006). These authors claim that, despite this decline in religious institutionalism, Canadians are more apt to practice religion on their own or in private, which constitutes a *privatized religion* congruent with the notion of increasing spirituality over religious adherence. Hout and Fisher (2002) also reported on a national General Social Survey that found that Americans who did not ascribe to a religious preference doubled from

1990 to 1991 and increased from 7% to 14% from 1998 to 2000. Similarly, the National Election Study also showed an increase in no religious affiliation from 8% to 13% from 1992 to 2000. However, a Gallup poll indicated that, for the first quarter of 2001, 8% of Americans reported no religious affiliation. Yet, reporting "no religion" does not necessarily mean loss of faith but, instead, may indicate a lack of adherence to religious institutionalism. According to Hout and Fisher, the most distinguishing feature is "avoidance of churches" and that most are "believers of some sort" (p. 175); most pray, believe in God, as well as an afterlife, and "many reject the 'religious' label, but they think of themselves as 'spiritual'" (p. 188). They further argue that one of the major reasons for choosing "no religion" is that political conservatives in the 1990s allied themselves with organized religion.

This schism between religion and spirituality may reflect a growing disillusionment with religious institutions resulting from the rise of secularism, which casts religion negatively and spirituality positively (Hill, Pargament, Hood, McCullough, Swyers, Larson, & Zinnbauer, 2000).[3] Interestingly, Wink, Dillon, and Kristen (2005) found that spirituality, when understood as a search for sacred connection, however defined, and practiced through means of personalized prayer, meditation, centering, or journeying outside religious institutions, showed the same correlation to autonomous or healthy narcissism as the "personal independence, high self-aspirations, and resistance to social pressures" observed in mainline Protestants in late adulthood (p. 154). According to this study, spirituality tends to be a result of ego strength or autonomy rather than of ego fragility or hypersensitivity.

Although spirituality has traditionally overlapped with religion in Western society, possibly because religion has traditionally been seen as the sole means to spirituality, increasing numbers of people are divorcing themselves from religious parochialism while maintaining their sense of being spiritual. This new sense of spirituality may be devoid of any religious connection or it may syncretically embrace multiple religious connections that are not based on or extracted from any particular faith. For example, an individual may construct a unique spiritual approach that expresses an affinity with beliefs from Native American Spirituality: beliefs that everything is interconnected; everything is alive and has a purpose, even rocks; that a kinship exists between all things; and that this kinship demands respect for Mother Nature, animals, and other people (Garrett, 2007).[4] Although these beliefs may generally fall under animism, holding such beliefs does not define a person as being part of any specific belief system. Instead, this eclectic approach suggests that the individual might be embracing an orientation to the world that is not grounded in any specific religion. This orientation may be the result of a personal philosophy of life based on personal lived experiences or ideas gleaned from others (ie. spiritual literature, mentors, etc.). Moreover, people may ameliorate beliefs and practices from religious organizations they depart from into a personalized spirituality.

Thus, spirituality is not socially dependent on religious doctrine but, rather, derives from personally constructed philosophy grounded in experience. Smith (2001) similarly argued that spirituality is "no more than a human attribute, spirituality is not institutionalized, and this exempts it from the problems that inevitably attend institutions-notably (in religious institutions) the in-group/out-group tensions they tend to breed" (pp. 255-256). In light of Smith's view, atheists can be spiritual but not religious, adding to the claim that spirituality is not directly related to religion or religiosity. These sentiments echo Porter (1995) who wrote:

> Conventionally, spirituality has arisen in the context of organized religion, which has told people what their spiritual goals should be. For some people the thought of spirituality outside an organized, institutional religion is unthinkable. For others, the thought of spirituality within the confines of a religious setting is intolerable. For still others, the concept of spirituality itself is unthinkable. (p. 70)

Therefore, we believe that what constitutes spirituality as opposed to religiosity is the manner by which an individual discovers a way of being or living outside religious affiliations. Said differently, spirituality derives from introspection, not institution. Expressions of spirituality may include appreciating a transcendent dimension that involves a deepened connection with the cosmos, nature, and others without necessarily invoking any concept of God. Such spirituality may also involve existential quests: personal searches for meaning, purpose, and hope; questions about the nature of existence, suffering, and mortality; and also humanistic goals related to spirituality, such as authenticity, integrity and respect for others. Numerous authors have expressed similar notions, such as Gall, Charbonneau, Clarke, Grant, Joseph, and Shouldice (2005), MacDonald and Holland (2002a, 2002b), Speck, Higginson, and Addington-Hall (2006), World Health Organization Quality of Life Spirituality, Religiousness, and Personal Beliefs Group (2006), and Wink, Dillon, and Kristen (2005). Despite the variety of scientific literature on spirituality, most agree that it is multi-dimensional but refers predominantly to inner experiences, such as purpose in life and transcendence, rather than external behaviors that we consider better classified as religious.

THE TRANSPERSONAL CONCEPTUAL DIMENSION

The problems involved in delineating religion from spirituality are complex and require greater conceptual clarity, specifically for operational utility and scientific standardization of terminology. The utility of these constructs in scientific deliberation depends upon greater theoretically demarcated or the introduction of newer, more precise terms.

Unlike the terms religion and spirituality, transpersonal is a relatively new term that might help in this delineation. The term transpersonal became commonly used in 1969 with the founding of transpersonal psychology, a discipline pioneered by such people as Abraham Maslow, Viktor Frankl, Stanislav Grof, and James Fadiman, who used the title in developing the so-called *fourth force* in psychology (Sutich, 1969).However, William James first used the word in 1905 to distinguish between the *higher* or spiritual self from the *lower* or personal self (Taylor, 1996; Vich, 1988). Moreover, one of the first transpersonal practitioners, psychiatrist Carl Jung, used the term transpersonal in the context of the collective unconscious, an eternal vortex that he saw as timeless and spaceless that made allowances for the experience of spiritual and religious phenomena.

We believe that transpersonal concepts can be useful in clarifying the distinction between the terms religious and spiritual by offering another approach. To introduce the transpersonal, a brief overview of some of the main classical and contemporary transpersonal theories is necessary. We will focus specifically on the contributions of William James, Carl Jung, Robert Assagioli, Michael Washburn, Ken Wilber, and Stanislav Grof. We then propose that a proper understanding of the transpersonal and self-expansiveness may alleviate some of the difficulties posed by the changing usages of the terms religion and spiritual. Throughout this section, the capitalization of the term Self connotes a self that is not limited to the egoic self but also includes transegoic aspects of the self.

WILLIAM JAMES.

For James (1890), the transpersonal self-concept was understood in the context of a connection with a higher part of the self – be it the universe, spirit, God, or cosmic energy. Through what James called the spiritual Self, individuals can enter an inner communion to save themselves from suffering errors generated from the lower parts of the self. In other words, rather than attempting to strengthen the personal will to alleviate anguish, individuals can surrender their lower selves – both material and social – for the salvation of their higher spiritual sense of Self. This salvation occurs primarily when the individual has come to the realization that the choices of the personal will are not viable enough to further personal development and, as such, searches for other answers through forces that are beyond the realm of the personal will. James (1890) wrote that the individual:

> becomes conscious that this higher part is conterminous and continuous with a MORE of the same quality, which is operative in the universe outside of him, and he can keep in working touch with, and in a fashion get on board of and save himself when all his lower being has gone to pieces in the wreck. (p. 508)

In view of these notions, James recognized the spiritual, transpersonal Self as an element of the empirical self, specifically as a part of an individual's reflective process of her or his "inner or subjective being" and the "most enduring and intimate part of the self" (1890, p. 296). To hone James' concept further, he saw the transpersonal Self as constituted of the collectivity of consciousness, an extension of the self. Through the activity of feeling states of consciousness (James, 1892), people experience this extension of self as their most intimate and essential sense of being. Unlike the other constituents of the self, the transpersonal Self is experienced through feelings and senses, rather than simply through abstract thoughts. James (1892) wrote that the "more active-feeling states of consciousness are thus the more central portions of the spiritual Me . . . a direct revelation of the living substance of our Soul" (p. 181).

Accordingly, religious or spiritual experiences are known through a feeling or sensing of inner expansion and contraction, not through rational thought (Taylor, 1996). Most importantly, James (1908) spoke of the transpersonal Self, or that which is spiritual in individuals, as mostly subconscious and one with the Divine. This conjecture posits the possibility that a subliminal Self resides within the unconscious connected continuously to the Infinite Spirit or God, while its corporal counterpart needs to consciously come into contact with this "divine inflow" (James, 1908, p. 101). James (1908) believed that the experience of a luminous or mystical moment marks a time in which consciousness expands and enters into another plane of existence. This transpersonal consciousness may be brought about through religious experiences or even from inhaling nitrous oxide, which James experimented with to "simulate the mystical consciousness in an extraordinary degree," unveiling deep mystical revelations (James, 1908, p. 387). The transpersonal aspect of the Self seems to be the foundational source of religious, spiritual, or mystical experiences. Furthermore, it may be seen as the agent that expands consciousness beyond the ordinary realm of everyday experiences and, as such, constitutes a transpersonal aspect of human existence.

CARL JUNG.

The Self was considered by Jung (1971) to be the totality of being, and includes both conscious and unconscious dimensions of the psyche, specifically the transpersonal unconscious commonly referred to as the collective unconscious. The Self was seen as the central archetype, since it is at the center of both psychic systems. The transpersonal unconscious is the "unknown quality of the world" (Jung, 1973, p. 433) and the primordial and inherited "secondary psychic system" (Jung, 1971, p. 60) that consists of archetypes of all beings, civilizations, and cultures. Archetypes represent "transpersonal content" (Jung, 1971, p. 91) in the form of symbolizations, primordial images of one's ancestral past, whose energy is expressed through the Self.

Jung (1989) suggested that an inherent dialectic exists between unconscious and conscious archetypes that the Self reflects. As the intermediary of these two polarities and the ego, the Self seeks balance and harmony.among these opposing forces. According to Jung (1989), as the ego matures, specifically during mid-life, it becomes more open to the transpersonal unconscious of the Self. For this reason, the transpersonal unconscious reveals itself through the Self, for example, as mandalas or as a divine child to represent symbols, which are understood as conceptions and perceptions of transpersonal content (Jung, 1989). However, both psychic systems remain hidden from the ego (guardian of the psyche) and the persona (external identity/social mask), which form the conscious psychic system (i.e., the individual and collective conscious, respectively).

In other words, the ego is a fragile structure of the personal consciousness that constantly protects itself from the threat of surfacing unconscious energies. Personas form the masks of the collective conscious psyche that negotiate the appearance or self-concept of individuals in their relationship with the external world. Individuation and analysis removes personas to reveal transpersonal essences, such as the shadow archetype (Jung, 1971). Jung (1971) wrote that the "aim of individuation is nothing less than to divest the self of the false wrappings of the persona on the one hand, and of the suggestive power of primordial images on the other" (p. 123).

Jung (1964) further suggested that the Self is known indirectly through dreams, which express their primordial nature symbolically in the form of visions of God or mandalas. In addition, Jung called the unconscious development of the symbolic content of dreams a "transpersonal control-point" (1971, p. 79) of the emerging Self, a deepening of unconscious perception of the Self. Through the process of individuation and through dreams, the transpersonal essence of the Self materializes as symbolic themes. The content of these themes expresses universal experiences and an expanded sense of a collective identity, be it spiritual, mystical, or mythical. Thus, the emergence of the transpersonal Self reveals transpersonal content submerged within the collective unconscious and fashioned by archetypical energies.

ROBERTO ASSAGIOLI.

Assagioli (1971, 1973) also conceived the transpersonal Self in terms of a higher dimension of the psyche. Assagioli's based his theory of psychosynthesis on a model of the human psyche consisting of the lower unconscious, the middle unconscious, the higher unconscious, the field of consciousness, the *I* or personal self, the higher or transpersonal Self, and, finally, the collective unconscious. Using the metaphor of the egg, Assagioli viewed the lower unconscious as located near the bottom of the egg, similar in character to the Freudian unconscious, which is motivated by drives and impulses. This is followed by the middle unconscious that surrounds the field of consciousness of the personal self and contains memories, thoughts, and feelings, which are revealed through remembering or turning in towards the personal self (Whitmore, 1991). The personal self is the central reference point (the focus of the field of consciousness) of all psychological experiences (sensations, emotions, impulses, imagination, thought, and intuition), which are located in the field of consciousness. This field of consciousness, in turn, is viewed as surrounding the personal self.

Directly above the middle unconscious is the higher unconscious, or the superconscious, whose nature consists of illuminations, inspirations, and intuitions, all of which emanate a transpersonal quality that is consistent with the virtues of artistry, creativity, altruism, humanitarianism, or states of pure clarity and joy (Assagioli, 1971). This transpersonal quality is a representation, "a moment of superconscious experience when we felt most fully who we essentially are" (Whitmore, 1991, p.114). At the top of the egg, or at the pinnacle of superconsciousness, is the transpersonal Self. This transpersonal Self, as Assagioli referred to it, is the amalgamation, Gestalt, or synthesis of being that permeates a unification with all existence that fosters transcendence, expanded states of consciousness, blissful synthetic realization, and emergence of experiences of spontaneous illumination.

According to Whitmore (1991), Assagioli understood the Self as an "ontological reality which exists on its own level as a stable centre of life and the source of superconscious energies" (p. 115). Additionally, the personal self is a reflection, a projection, and a component of the transpersonal Self. Furthermore, the transpersonal Self also has a relationship with the transpersonal will, which motivates the need to search for meaning and understand the significance of life. This includes transcendence through transpersonal love ("relationship between the superconscious levels in both" individuals within a relationship [Assagioli, 1971, p. 116]), transpersonal action ("highest forms of humanitarian and social action" [p. 119]), beauty (aesthetic way of being), and self-realization of all human potentials. The transpersonal will differs from the personal will in that it transcends or goes beyond elementary or basic needs and drives. This difference grows as the call or pull from the transpersonal Self intensifies through unification with a divine force or higher power. This intensifying unity may take the form of experiences that range from spontaneous illuminations of a mystical or religious nature to temporary states of persecution.

Finally, the collective unconscious is the aggregate or collection of the psyche's energy that forms a boundary around the psyche, that is, everything outside the eggshell. At this peripheral dimension of the psyche, the transpersonal Self disidentifies with all subordinate levels of consciousness and extends or expands outward towards transcendent reality, which constitutes the universal Self or Being (Assagioli, 1971). According to Assagioli (1973), the extent to which the universal Self is revealed as the transpersonal Self depends upon the progress away from the descending direction of the personality and towards the ascending direction of the collective unconscious. Thus, the further the transpersonal Self expands into the transcendent reality, the more it becomes the universal Self, to the point where corporal identity enters an interim state of ebb and flow.

MICHAEL WASHBURN.

Washburn's (1988) transpersonal theory of human development, a dynamic-dialectical model involving a bimodal interplay between egoic and non-egoic poles, places the concept of self within a triphasic network of egoic progression: pre-egoic, egoic, and transegoic. Within this triphasic system, Washburn combined dialectics – thesis and antithesis leading to synthesis – with a spiral loop epigenetic approach, that is, a predetermined sequence of ego emergence, negation, and return integration, to formulate a transpersonal understanding of the ego's interaction with the dynamic life, the dynamic unconscious, and the spiritual realm. Through the unfolding of the ego with what Washburn called the dynamic life, three triphasic relationships are formed with the *Dynamic Ground*, namely the bodily self (pre-egoic stage), the subjective self (egoic stage), and spiritual Self (transegoic stage). Washburn suggested the term Dynamic Ground to indicate the source that the self transcends through the ego's interaction with dynamic life. Stated more precisely, the Dynamic Ground is the "seat of the psycho-dynamic pole . . . [that fuels] 'psychic energy' . . . [and acts as a] magnifier of all dimensions of psychic life" (Washburn, 1988, p. 110-111).

For Washburn (1988), the transpersonal Self develops when the transegoic or integration stage begins, during or after middle life. Washburn believed this stage occurred infrequently due to the gravity or pull of the mental ego away from the Dynamic Ground. This stage is marked by "regression in the service of transcendence" or of spirit whereby the ego withdraws from the external world and regresses to the "physico-dynamic strata of the psyche," thus submitting it to the Dynamic Ground (p. 155). In other words, the mental ego loses its dependence with the external world because it transitions to the dark night of the soul. Such transitions catalyze the opening of Dynamic Ground and leads to the ego's descent to the abyss of the prepersonal unconscious.

During the transegoic stage, the mental ego collapses and, as such, simultaneously dismantles the self-concept that stabilized the ego against the ontological uncertainty of the present moment, the *here-and-now*. Washburn (1988) referred to this process as the "deanimation of the self-concept" (p. 163) in that the ego's functionality is relative to the stage at which it exists, which renders the self-concept an equivalent reality. In other words, as the ego distances itself from the world of the mental egoic stage, so does the self-concept, which bounds the ego's ontological identity. However, when the ego regresses in the service of transcendence, the self-concept ceases to anchor the ego. It thus loses its ground and becomes a mask, a pretend facade for existence in a derealized world experienced with disbelief and lifelessness.

Paradoxically, the ego's ceaselessness and estrangement permits it to expand and observe itself for the first time without a predetermined self-concept Liberated and emancipated from the personal unconscious, the ego acquires knowledge of itself without the means of an ontological proxy, transcends its ontological insecurity, and becomes a self-knowing entity – a transpersonal self-concept.

KEN WILBER.

Wilber (1980a, 1980b, 1986) produced a massive amount of writing that will be loosely summarized as a unified work, even though it has evolved over the years and he has taken several different positions in regard to the issues summarized here. In general, Wilber posits that consciousness, from its inception at birth, progresses through three different stages of development: primarily the prepersonal, personal, and transpersonal self. The prepersonal self comprises the sensoriphysical stage (matter, sensation, and perception), the phantasmic-emotional stage (emotional and sexual level), and the representational mind (symbols and concepts). The personal self consists of the rule/role mind stage (concrete operational thinking), the formal-reflexive stage (propositional reasoning and introspection), and the vision-logic stage (higher-order synthesizing capacity). The transpersonal Self comprises the psychic stage (opening of transcendental, universal, perennial awakening), the subtle stage (archetypal illuminations and transcendental insights), and the causal stage (universal or formless self, cosmic perception, and ego abolishment). Wilber (1986) also proposed an ultimate nature of Self where consciousness re-awakens to its "prior and eternal abode as absolute Spirit, radiant and all-pervading, one and many, only and complete integration and identity of manifest Form with the unmanifest Formless" (p. 74).

In terms of these notions, Wilber (1980b) posited that the development of the transpersonal ensues from integrating, negating, and transcending the lower stages of the self, the prepersonal and personal self. The self contends with dichotomies at each stage of development through the process of personal growth by preserving itself verses negating itself, holding on versus letting go, continuing to live at that level or dying to that level, and identifying with itself versus disidentifying with itself (Wilber, 1980a). In order to progress to the transpersonal Self, the individual undergoes these phases involving a loss of self-identity and false appearances with the body ego or the centauric realm, which consists of the lower aspect of the integrated self. As the individual apprehends existential reality, she or he is consumed by the totality of her or his being and the self-concept or inner self begins to emerge as an authentic representation of the individual.

Although this last phase in not marked by transpersonal experiences, it is the period where the transpersonal Self begins to emerge, since it becomes dominated by transverbal and transcultural experiences (Wilber, 1980b). As the experiences from the personal realm move the individual into the highest state of existential awareness, the realization occurs that he or she is living within the realm of the body and, with such perception, the self-concept or ego begins to acknowledge the subtle realms (Wilber, 1980b). This awareness initiates spiritual development, where ego death allows access to higher levels of consciousness that are dominated by astral and psychic abilities, known as the lower subtle realm, that include: out-of-body experiences, seeing auras, clairvoyance, extrasensory perception, precognition, and psychokinesis, which are known as extrapersonal experiences (Wilber, 1980b).

Wilber (1980a) wrote that these experiences transcend the self into transverbal and transpersonal realms of consciousness. This higher subtle realm further extends the self-concept to include experiences of a deeper unification of transcendent consciousness, the realm of religious or spiritual intuition, and liberal inspiration through "high archetypal forms of one's own being" (Wilber, 1980a, p. 68). The Self now appears as the *over-self*, since the self-concept or mental-ego transcends corporal ground, feelings, sensations, and perceptions and identifies itself as divine. Wilber (1980a) indicates that "one dissolves into Deity, as Deity – that Deity which, from the beginning, has been one's own Self or highest Archetype" (p. 69).

Finally, the transpersonal Self or the higher Self emerges fully when the archetypal deity itself dissolves and becomes synonymous with what Wilber called the *final-God*, where all archetypes reveal their entire essence and form a unity with the God source. This stage is defined by Wilber as the lower-causal self, since it precedes the higher-causal self. Simply put, the lower-causal self suggests a final illumination of the self that embodies transcendent compassion, even as the self remains bounded within consciousness. The higher-causal self, however, transcends form to a Formless Consciousness where the self, God, and final-God dissolve into nothingness, that is, boundless consciousness in-and-of-itself (1980b).

STANISLAV GROF.

Grof (1992) explored the transpersonal self within the domain of a space-time-consciousness model where he mapped the territory and expanded boundaries of the psyche, specifically through the realms of transpersonal experiences. Grof (1985) maintained that transpersonal experiences expand the corporal boundaries of phenomenal existence, temporally and spatially, beyond a Cartesian and Newtonian reality that insists we are just a "skin-encapsulated ego existing in a world of separate beings and objects" (Grof, 1992, p. 91). In other words, during corporal bound experiences, the ego's sense of self remains within the confines of the physical body and materially grounded perception. The ego functions within non-expanded, spatial-temporal, awareness. Fundamental to this reality is the experience of (physical) separateness and sovereignty of the ego in a materialistic world coupled with a sense of dwelling within the province of scientific realism and worldly artifacts (Grof, 1985, 1992; Grof & Grof, 1990).

During transpersonal experiences, however, an all-consuming consciousness besets the spatial-temporal dimension and expands the sense of self to a boundlessness, dissolution of the ego that produces moments of non-ordinary perceptions, emotions, and understandings of space, time, and consciousness (Grof, 1992). This deepening and expansion of inner time and space bequeaths to the individual astounding insights and personal discovery, which can only be known and experienced in transcendent states (Grof & Grof, 1990). Grof and Grof (1990) suggest that a definition of the self needs to include these inner dimensions of the human psyche, specifically the "dissolution of ego structures," the loss of self, and the fading of "ordinary reality" into a mystical, spiritual, or "oceanic" realm of merging the self with cosmic reality (p. 67).

For Grof (1985) the transpersonal Self undergoes transpersonal experiences of expanded states of consciousness through an ordered progression. First, temporal expansion of consciousness suggests a transcendence of the boundaries of linear time and includes, for example, collective experiences. Second, spatial expansion of consciousness implies the extension of space-time reality and consists of experiences such as dual unity, "a sense of fusing with another organism into a unitive state without losing sense of identity" (Grof, 1985, p. 129). Third, spatial constriction of consciousness indicates a narrowing of consciousness to physical substrates such as organs, tissue, and cellular consciousness. Fourth, experiential extensions of consciousness such as encounters with spirit guides, mediumistic experiences, and mythological journeys point beyond the objective or consensus reality of space-time. Last, transpersonal experiences of an extrapersonal nature are expressed through synchronistic links between consciousness and matter, supernormal physical feats, and ceremonial magic.

Therefore, the transpersonal self is expressed in terms of a field of expanding consciousness to include a realm of transpersonal identity and themes of spiritual realizations, cosmic unity and, sometimes, unfortunate psychotic emergence. In this model, the ego transcends its corporal limits of ontological existence, enters into a cosmic portal or dimension where the ego loses its sense of identity, and becomes a unitary consciousness inhabited by numinous, celestial, mythological, or even pathological, satanic, or demonic encounters.

TRANSPERSPONAL SELF-EXPANSIVENESS

AND SELF-CONTRACTEDNESS

It is evident in light of the literature presented thus far that not only are the constructs of religious and spiritual not mutually exclusive, but they also overlap with the constructs proposed by transpersonal thinkers. We now want to present the approach developed by Friedman (1981, 1983), one of the authors, that we believe clarifies the relationship between the constructs of the religious and the spiritual by offering an integrative transpersonal mode. Beginning with a review of the construct of the transpersonal, we will outline the constructs of self-expansiveness and self-contractedness before applying Friedman's transpersonal model towards delineating the constructs of religious, spiritual, and transpersonal.

The impetus of transpersonal psychology came from acknowledging the importance of experiences beyond the ego, self, or personality, namely experiences not egoic-centered (i.e., not stemming from the personal self) but transegoic-centered (i.e., pertaining to the transpersonal Self). The difference between these two modes of self-concept becomes apparent at *the point of intercept* as indicated or experienced by the dissolution of the egoic self. The transpersonal overlaps at this point of intercept where the *here-and-now* meets the *beyond the here-and-now.* As dissolution progresses further within the transegoic self, so too does the expansion of physical and/or temporal boundaries grow; consequently, the transpersonal experience extends into transcendent experience. Here, transpersonal implies "expanded dimensions of the self-which are characterized by deepened and boundless perceptions of being and reality that extend or transcend ordinary conceptualizations of time and space" (Pappas, 2004, p. 171). To use a metaphor, our personal self has the capacity to expands much like a rubber band and, the more it expands, the closer it gets to stretching beyond itself and encompassing a larger aspect of self-identity, namely the transpersonal self. Similarly, Yogananda (1968) believed that our sense of self is like a rubber band that expands infinitely without breaking.

These notions are consistent with the etymological understanding of the term transpersonal, such that *trans* in Latin means "to go beyond" the here-and-now or, more profoundly, the personal or *persona.* Hence, the idea of transpersonal involves moving beyond our egoic or phenomenological identity. The significance for the transpersonalist lies in reifying transpersonal, religious, and spiritual experiences as phenomena of great value worth submitting to scientific study. Transpersonalist see a need to explore this *other side of the self.* According to Brown (2001), it is exploring the "awareness beyond or on the other side of the masks and patterns of personality" that is paramount to transpersonal inquiry (p. 104). It should be noted that transpersonal psychology and, more generally, other transpersonal studies (e.g., transpersonal psychiatry) do not sanction any specific or exclusionary type of religious belief or affiliation; rather, this approach is open to the study of practices found within various religious expressions, such as meditation, yoga, and prayer. Kasprow and Scotton (1999) endorse similar ideas in the context of transpersonal psychiatry by arguing that:

> Transpersonal psychiatry does not promote any particular belief system, but rather acknowledges that spiritual experiences and transcendent states characterized by altruism, creativity, and profound feelings of connectedness are universal human experiences widely reported across cultures, and therefore worthy of rigorous, scientific study. (p. 13)

For example, altered states of consciousness commonly occur in transpersonal experiences whether brought on by entheogens or psychedelic hallucinogens (e.g., psilocybin or muscimol), or cultural rituals and practices (e.g., shamanic rites of passage or healing, ceremonial dancing or drumming, meditation, prayer, or chanting, or sweats or vision quests). In this sense, we may understand transpersonal experiences as an epiphenomenon of cultural beliefs, practices, and rituals. Such experiences – experimental, introspective, and existential – give rise to expanded states of consciousness that take the individual beyond the here-and-now and, ultimately, beyond the personal self.

Given this, non-duality forms a central tenet of transpersonal inquiry. Under the persuasion that everything is interconnected, we are inextricably a part of a greater whole that binds everything together – going beyond the dualism that encompasses the egoic-self (Davis, 2003). The work of Koltko-Rivera (2004) registers this rejection of dualism by suggesting that the world is not only a "living being," but also "One thing" and not "many things;" we exist as an interconnected web with all things, which gives us the opportunity to transcend "cognitive contradictions" given that the "true essence" of being cannot be experienced within the confines of the personal ego (p. 14). Notwithstanding these principles, it should be noted that some transpersonal approaches do endorse dualistic notions, such as those advocating dualistic beliefs based on a perceived radical separation of God from humanity. It is our opinion that these doctrinal positions cannot be resolved empirically and fall outside of discernable knowledge. [4]

Nevertheless, we contend that perceiving the egoic self as fundamentally dualistic produces detachment from our identity, the world, the universe, and existence, ultimately leading to a fragmented or disrupted state of being. This line of speculation may possibly explain the prevalence of neurotic and psychotic behavior in Western society, for many who seek clinical support present themes of disconnection, isolation, and distortion. Maslow (1968) discerned the same predicament when he wrote that "without the transcendent and the transpersonal, we get sick, violent and nihilistic, or else hopeless and apathetic" (p. iv). Davis (2003) similarly offers two central insights based on non-duality:

The *intrinsic health* and basic goodness of the whole and each of its parts and the validity of *self-transcendence* from the conditional and conditioned personality to a sense of identity which is deeper, broader, and more unified with the whole. (p. 7)

Thus, transpersonalism challenges conventions that circumscribe mental corporality within physical boundaries where thought and emotions merely proceed from epiphenomenal conditions. The current scientific paradigm still relies on a Newtonian perspective of linearly ordered time and space that adheres to a Cartesian edifice of a mind-body split. This perspective limits knowledge of transpersonal experiences or dismisses them as outside materialistic, mechanistic, reductionistic, and deterministic forms of objective or consensual reality.[6] Within a post-Newtonian worldview, however, an appreciation exists for non-local objectivity where there are no definite boundaries between space and time: i.e., phenomena are ethereal, transient, and without specific location in space-time, since our experiences are a function of an interconnected web of being, which allows for multi-dimensional participation. In such a belief system, space and time form a fourth dimension known as space-time where mass becomes interchangeable with energy and its appearance as matter at the three-dimensional level becomes challenged. Bohm (1980), Grof (1990), Strohl (1998), and Talbot (1999) also argued for such an undivided wholeness of all things, that everything is part of an infinite continuum despite the duality or separateness that exists in Newtonian perception. In the words of physicist David Bohm (1980):

Mind and matter are not separate substances. Rather, they are different aspects of one whole and unbroken movement. In this way, we are able to look on all aspects of existence as not divided from each other, and thus we can bring to an end the fragmentation implicit in the current attitude toward the atomic point of view, which leads us to divide everything from everything in a thoroughgoing way. (p. 14)

SELF-EXPANSIVENESS AND SELF-CONTRACTEDNESS

In Friedman's model, the self cannot be known in its entirety; however, conceptual understandings of "who I am" can be understood by virtue of the self-concept. Friedman uses the notion of self-expansiveness to indicate the extent to which the self-concept can expand its sense of identity both temporally and spatially. The temporal aspect of the self-concept signifies the degree to which an individual's identity expands beyond the present to identify with the past and the future. The spatial portion of the self-concept denotes the extent to which an individual's identity expands to enlarged and contracted conceptualizations of identity. In his original work, Friedman (1983) postulated that self-expansiveness suggests an "expanded nature of the self," such that the "relationship between self and nonself [is] inherently unlimited to such an extent that all absolute distinctions between the two are untenable" (p. 3). Simply, self-expansiveness is suggestive of a cognitive process of identity expansion at the temporal and spatial level to denote the boundaries that demarcate the *here-and-now* to the *beyond-the-here-and-now*. In addition to theoretical conjectures, self-expansiveness is operationalized by the Self-Expansiveness Level Form (SELF; Friedman, 1981; 1983). Its cartographic representation locates the expanding self-concept at the temporal dimension, positioned on the ordinate, and the spatial dimension, positioned on the abscissa. The ordinate includes the *past* temporal dimension followed by the *present* temporal dimension and then by the *future* temporal dimension. The abscissa consists of the *contracted* spatial dimension followed by the *here-and-now* and then by the *enlarged* spatial dimension (see Figure 1). The area within these two axes comprises the *personal level, middle level,* and *transpersonal level* as follows.

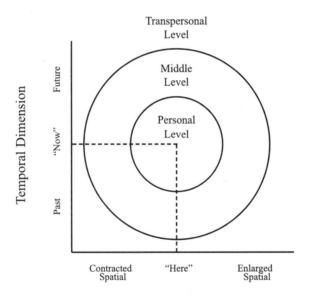

Spatial Dimension

Figure 1. The original cartography of self-expansivesness. *Note*: Adopted from Friedman (1981, 1983).

The *personal level* situates the self-concept in the present and is represented by the intercept point between the here-and-now, which is neither contracted spatially nor enlarged spatially and does not exist in the past or future. Whereas the spatial dimension is limited to the boundaries of the body or physical dimension, which contain the phenomenological functioning of the individual, the temporal dimension indicates the present experience of time within the physical confines of the body. The *middle level* is an extension of the personal level to the extent that the self-concept temporally and spatially expands within the physical as well as in the present. At the *transpersonal level*, the self-concept expands beyond the middle level to an identity that goes beyond phenomenological boundaries of time-space reality: Temporally, identity expands beyond linear time to encompass ancestral past experiences as well as distant future experiences; spatially, identity expands to from atomistic conceptions to ultimate unifications with aspects of reality. Friedman (1981) writes that the "transpersonal level is also viewed as including possible transcendence of both dimensions through an incorporation of all of reality, beyond any notion of time or space" (p. 13). Most importantly, at the transpersonal self-expansiveness level, the self is not bounded and can continually expand to encompass a larger sense of reality similar to that of a universe expanding towards infinity.

This cartography, however, only allows for an expansion beyond materialistic space-time reality without accounting for the inverse vector (Friedman & Pappas, 2006). To reconcile these, Friedman introduced the construct of self-contraction, which inverts the original cartography by placing the transpersonal level, where transcendence is primary, within materialistic boundaries (see Figure 2). The inverted cartography represents self-contraction

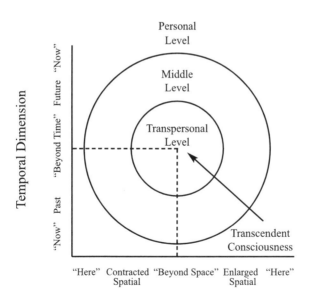

Spatial Dimension

Figure 2. A cartography of Self-contract with transcendent consciousness as primary. *Note*: Adopted from Friedman (1981, 1983).

according to a top-down approach, the transpersonal to the personal; the original cartography, in contrast, is a bottom-up approach, the personal to the transpersonal. This dialectical process allows for both immanence and possible transcendence to be understood as antithetical, yet complementary, processes.

SELF-EXPANSIVENESS USED TO CLARIFY THE CONSTRUCTS OF RELIGIOUS, SPIRITUAL, AND TRANSPERSONAL

Friedman's (1981, 1983) model of self-expansiveness provides an alternative understanding of the terms religious, spiritual, and transpersonal. Insofar as religion prescribes only the externals of religious beliefs and practices, the concept of religion loses its utility and accuracy when describing the individual's internal relationship to the sacred. In fact, religion, seen in this way – devoid of spirituality – is reduced to just a psychosocial variable. For example, many studies clearly link religion with positive health outcomes, but these results can be explained by fact that those who are already healthier are more likely to physically be able to attend religious services, likely take better care of themselves because they see their body as a "temple," generally limit or abstain from tobacco and alcohol for moral reasons, and have more social support networks because of church groups (Elmer, MacDonald, & Friedman, 2003). Likewise, the term spirituality also lacks scientific precision, for it entails idiosyncratic ways of knowing or experiencing that are simply not amenable to empirical research. Unfortunately, research in this area often relies on self-reports that are framed in supernatural or other ambiguous language. Both spirituality and religion are understood typically through a grid of faith-based, internal or external assumptions that inherently rest on metaphysics that are often inconsistent with scientific premises (Slife, Hope, Nebeker, & Scott, 1999). Thus, the salient question becomes, how can we bridge the divide between the consensual, but mundane, world of religiosity and the uniquely private world of spirituality?

Coinciding with its prefix *trans,* the concept of the transpersonal might provide such a bridge. However, the transpersonal has also not been consensually defined (Friedman, 2002). For example, Lajoie and Shapirio (1992) reviewed thirty-seven definitions of transpersonal over the past thirty years, concluding that transpersonal psychology is "concerned with the study of humanity's highest potential, and with the recognition, understanding, and realization of unitive, spiritual, and transcendent states of consciousness" (p. 91), but they are quite varied in their approaches. A recent review of forty-one viewpoints based on descriptions of transpersonal psychology by transpersonalists emphasized this multitudinal nature of transpersonal psychology (Caplan, Hartelius, & Rardin, 2003). Nevertheless, many strands of the transpersonal literature suggest that notions similar to self-expansiveness have a central role as a core theme. For example, Maslow (1968) called for a psychology that was "transpersonal, transhuman, centered in the cosmos rather than in human needs and interest, going beyond humanness, identity, self-actualization and the like" (p. iii-iv). For Grof (1985), the transpersonal emerges when "consciousness has expanded beyond the usual ego boundaries and has transcended the limitations of time and space" (p. 129), or, defined concisely, transpersonal implies "transcending the personal" (Grof, 2003, p. 67). Walsh and Vaughan (1993) defined transpersonal psychology based on viewing the self as "beyond (trans) the individual or personal to encompass wider aspects of humankind, life psyche, and cosmos" (p. 3) to where there is a "dissolution of ego boundaries" (Walsh & Vaughan, 1996, p. 63). Braud (1998) proposed that transpersonal is suggestive of a "connectedness of oneself with others and with all of Nature" (p. 39). These trends suggest the centrality of an expanded sense of self as a major or core theme in transpersonal psychology.

We believe the concepts of spirituality and religiosity could both be better understood by a transpersonal psychology based on scientific assumptions (Pappas & Friedman, 2004). Adopting transpersonal psychology as an explanatory paradigm avoids the limitations of unscientific assumptions based on a theocentric Judeo-Christian framework that marks the majority of contemporary psychology of religion. When rigidly applied to different cultural settings, using a Judeo-Christian notion of God to understand non-theocentric cultures that employ "God-language" differently inevitably leads to parochial biases. In this regard, transpersonal psychology should not also become encumbered with any one tradition but, instead, seek a different type of knowledge: one based on science, though grounded within the wisdom gained from various religious or spiritual traditions. We believe that science offers a naturalistic arena by which transpersonal phenomena can be studied, because the rigors of science yield relatively – but never completely – value free empirical results. We believe that science is a cultural systemic practice, a belief system in-and-of-itself, which pursues observable universal truths based on a-posteriori knowledge. Transpersonal constructs, such as Friedman's self-expansiveness, that are based on materialistic conceptual assumptions lend an objectivity open to measurement that is consistent with the operational quality found in the standard view of science. As such, transpersonal constructs are relatively freer of value judgements than approaches based on supernatural and/or metaphysical notions that are not amenable to falsification and have limited reproducibility for findings, especially in different cultural contexts.

Given this, Friedman's (1981, 1983) construct of self-expansiveness, a term expressing how the self-concept may vary through an identification process from a narrow personal identity to an expanded transpersonal identity, is based on several key materialistic assumptions consistent with nomological science:

1. There is no way to firmly delineate where the sense of self starts or stops, such that the relationship between the self and the world is radically open and "all absolute distinctions between the two are untenable" (Friedman, 1983, p. 3).
2. The self-concept can be mapped temporally to involve identifying with a past, present, and/or future self-concept.
3. The self-concept can be mapped spatially to involve identifying with a contracted and/or enlarged self-concept, and a here-and-now identity that involves a personal level of self-concept.
4. When self-concept greatly expands, temporally and/or spatially, this involves a transpersonal level of identity.
5. In between the personal and transpersonal are middle levels of identities.

These assumptions fit well into the consensual scientific frameworks of other approaches to the self-concept. First, by restricting focus on the notion of self-concept, a cognitive construct, rather than on the self per se, a self-expansive construct becomes amenable to research in conventional scientific ways. Similarly, Frager and Fadiman (2005) concluded that the overall "concept of the self veers more defiantly away from the world of pure science, refusing to submit to objective measurement" (p. 12).

Since a naturalistic framework grounds the self-expansiveness model, it avoids many metaphysical dilemmas inherent in discussing supernatural notions that commonly adhere to the terms of religiosity and spirituality. Moreover, the model provides a view of the self-concept that links transpersonal with mainstream psychology and, perhaps, can be integrated into conventional perspectives. Even so, the self-concept literature itself suffers from a proliferation of terms, such as self-construal (e.g., Marx, Stapel, & Muller, 2005), self-definition (e.g., Robbins, Pis, & Pender, 2004), self-esteem (e.g., Esposito, Kobak, & Little, 2005), self-knowledge (Lieberman, Jarcho, & Satpute, 2004), self-identity (e.g., Webb, 2004), self-perception (e.g., Weiss, & Amorose, 2005), self-representation (e.g., Reinert, 2005), and more. This disjointed body of literature needs unifying (Byrne, 2002; Wylie, 1979), but no one conceptual model has been accepted. Chen, Chen, and Shaw (2004) call for a comprehensive framework. Additionally, there are many views of an expanded self in conventional psychology, such as ecological views (e.g., Besthorn, 2002; Bragg, 1996), temporal views (e.g., Moore & Lemmon, 2001; Newby-Clark, & Ross 2003), biological views (e.g., Damasio, Grabowski, Bechara, Damasio, Ponto, Parvizi, & Hichwa, 2000; Lieberman, Jarcho, & Satpute, 2004), as well as spiritual views (e.g., Pedersen, 1999), including James' (1890) classic view of the extended self. We believe that the transpersonal perspective, when coupled with the construct of self-expansiveness, may be the most comprehensive scientific framework from which to analyze the self-concept.

To this end, Friedman's operational model of self-expansiveness , SELF, demonstrates both psychometric reliability and validity in a number of studies (Friedman, 1983; Pappas, 2003), including in cross-cultural contexts that would challenge most conventional religious and spiritual approaches (Friedman, MacDonald, & Kumar, 2004). For discussions and compilations of other relevant religious, spiritual, and transpersonal measures, see Hill and Hood (1999), Tsang and McCullough (2003), MacDonald, LeClair, Holland, Alter, and Friedman (1995), MacDonald, Friedman, and Kuentzel (1999), MacDonald, Kuentzel, and Friedman (1999), and MacDonald and Friedman (2002). However, most such religious, spiritual, and even transpersonal measures suffer from several major drawbacks that impede their usefulness in research. For example, George, Larson, Koeing, and McCullough (2000) describe how most measures of spirituality confuse religiosity with spirituality through measuring variables such as church attendance and conflating theological beliefs, such as in God, with spirituality. Although almost all extant spirituality scales suffer from such problems, there are a few exceptions that keep spirituality separate from clearly religious material, such as the Spiritual Orientation Inventory (Elkins, Hedstrom, Huges, Leaf, & Saunders, 1988) and the Psychomatrix Spirituality Inventory (Wolman, 2001). These scales, however, still involve using supernatural constructs that pose inherent difficulties from a scientific perspective, as do most of the avowedly transpersonal measures. For a more in-depth discussion of these methodological problems, see Friedman and MacDonald (1997), MacDonald and Friedman (2001), Slater, Hall, and Edwards (2001), and MacDonald and Friedman (2002). That being said, all measures have their limitations, as pointed out by Friedman and MacDonald (2002):

> Although we are of the opinion that such approaches [measures] are fruitful avenues to gain reliable and useful knowledge, we do not believe that measurement can ever capture the inherent complexity or 'suchness' of many important transpersonal constructs that may, by their very nature, defy language, conceptualization, and exact measurement. (p. ix.)

Transpersonal and spiritual instruments themselves also may suffer from what MacDonald, LeClair, Holland, Alter, and Friedman (1995) refer to as the "illusion of spirituality problem" (p. 174). Individuals may falsely portray themselves as highly spiritual and/or transpersonal for egoic or social reasons revealing, what we term, a "transpersonal-spiritual materialism problem." Specifically, individuals might respond in a socially favorable manner to gratify a need for approval by projecting a positive self-image or have some other similar motivation in terms of transpersonal or spiritual posturing. In other words, socially desirable responses indicate the need to control the self-image of negative affect and egoistic impulse by presenting oneself in a socially desirable manner. This tendency occurs commonly among the general population (Weinberger, 1990). These response biases show that transpersonality or spirituality is not dependent on extrinsic morality or socially desirable behavior; to the contrary, such obedience will inhibit rather than promote transpersonality or spirituality. Note that measures of social desirability have been shown not to correlate highly with self-expansiveness (Friedman, 1981, 1983; MacDonald, Tsagarakis, & Holland, 1994). The lack of correlation suggests that social desirability does not affect scores on this particular instrument, but no extant measure of spiritual desirability exists to validate against these types of measurements.

Finally, transpersonal or spiritual desirability is based on the notion that responding favorably in test situations is possibly predicated on the capacity for self-enhanced ego development and the practice of transformation methods or techniques (Porter, 1995). Spiritual addiction and guilt occurs when spirituality is used to deny, escape, and avoid the difficulties of coping with everyday life as well as when spirituality is used as wishful or magical thinking to work through problems (Vaughan, 1991). Vaughan believes that spiritual guilt or fear is seen consistently in individuals low on self-esteem who deem natural impulses such as anger and sexual desire as inappropriate feelings and thus fear punishment by a supernatural power or by spiritual authorities. These individuals may engage in ritualized behaviors for purposes of purification such as superficial confessions. These rituals may, however, exacerbate fear or guilt by instilling feelings of subordination to the specialness of others in the group. Moreover, such behavior may inadvertently espouse suffering without spiritual refinement, possibly strengthening self-righteousness. What is more, those transpersonal or spiritual experiences may be brought upon by false mysticism or substitute gratifications, including experiences or states brought on by alcohol and various drugs, psychological factors such as co-dependency, and even fanatical patriotism.

CONCLUSION

This chapter reviewed the conceptual status of religious, spiritual, and transpersonal constructs. We emphasized that religions are a culturally bound systems based on ideological and methodological ascriptions of beliefs, attitudes, and practices. We illustrated how spirituality is idiosyncratically bound and not mutually exclusive of religion, such that a felt connection with nature, the universe, or even a deity may not be vested within culturally sanctioned institutions to be seen as spiritual. In this regard, one may be an atheist and also be spiritual, whereas in most views of religion this is not possible. The transpersonal conceptual dimension discussed by classical and contemporary scholars in the field of transpersonal psychology offers various ways in which religious and spiritual phenomena can be located within transpersonal experiences. We also presented a theoretically consistent and empirically driven model of self-expansiveness that stands at the forefront of conceptualizing and measuring transpersonal experiences. Although this model does not depend upon religious beliefs and affiliations, it does allude to possible transcendent states described in several religious traditions. A self-expansive model supports a conceptual understanding of how cultural practices such as meditation, yoga, and prayer may induce expansive states that go beyond the here-and-now, the central theme of transpersonal psychology.

Notwithstanding the conceptual clarification we have offered of the constructs of religion, spirituality, and the transpersonal, we have not fully arrived at an entirely satisfactory solution. All the same, we hope our conceptual delineations of these terms proves useful in understanding their uniqueness and their relative advantages and disadvantages. We also believe that this solution, albeit only partial, provides some evidence of the advantages of using constructs that align better with empirical science (i.e., are more isomorphic to consensual empirical understandings). Any clarification of constructs must be commensurate with science in order to offer scientific utility. Our point is that using empirically based constructs provides an opportunity for an integrated study of human nature irrespective of the beliefs one holds. It is our view that this model provides an escape from a trap that has long limited discussion of both religion and spirituality and, thus, opens a promising avenue for empirical research and practical application.

NOTES

[1] That said, some Buddhist sects essentially deify Buddha.

[2] Ontological questions pertain to the very nature of existence, being, reality, and the sacred, while epistemological concerns deal with knowing, purpose, meaning, and fulfillment)

[3] A secular epistemology is based on the scientific method, which replaces myth and mysticism with empirical truths derived from positivistic methods (Hill et al., 2000; Pappas, 2003; 2004). As a result of secularism, god as a theological entity now becomes *humanized* into science as god.

[4] For example, there are sects that subscribe to totemism where animals, plants, and the earth are regarded as sacred.

[5] For more discussion concerning this point, see Friedman (2002).

[6] The terms are defined as follows: materialistic implies physical or tangible essences; mechanistic assets that the operating nature of the universe is much like a machine, since it is divided into orchestrating parts; reductionistic suggests that everything is reducible to its elementary or atomistic elements; deterministic comes from the notion that for every cause there is an effect such that there is no freewill.

References

Allport, G. (1950). *The individual and his religion*: A psychological interpretation. New York: Macmillan.

Allport, G. (1960). *Personality and social encounter*. Boston, MA: Beacon Press.

Allport, G. (1961). *Pattern and growth in personality*. New York: Holt, Rinehart, and Winston.

Allport, G. (1963). Behavioral science, religion, and mental health. *Journal of Religion and Health*, *2*, 187-457.

Allport, G. (1966). The religious context of prejudice. J*ournal for the Scientific Study of Religion*, *5*, 447-457.

Allport, G. & Ross, J. (1967). Personal religious orientation and prejudice. *Journal of Personality and Social Psychology*, *5*, 432-443.

Assagioli, R. (1971). *Psychosynthesis; a manual of principles and techniques*. New York: Viking Press.

Assagioli, R. (1973). *The act of will*. New York: Viking Press.

Besthorn, F. (2002). Radical environmentalism and the ecological self: Rethinking the concept of self-identity for social work practice. *Journal of Progressive Human Services*, *13*, 55-72.

Bohm, D. (1980). *Wholeness and implicate order*. London, UK: Routledge.

Bragg, E. (1996). Towards ecological self: Deep ecology meets constructionist self-theory. *Journal of Environmental Psychology*, *16*, 93-108.

Braud, W. (1998). Integral inquiry: Complementary ways of knowing, being, and expression. In W. Braud & R. Anderson (Eds.), *Transpersonal research methods for the social sciences: Honoring human experience* (pp. 35-67). Thousand Oaks, CA: Sage Publications.

Brown, M. (2001). A psychosynthesis twelve step program for transforming consciousness: Creative explorations of inner peace. *Counseling and Values*, *45*, 103-117.

Byrne, B. (2002). Validating the measurement and structure of self-concept: Snapshots of past, present, and future research. *American Psychologist*, 57, 897-909.

Burris, C. (1994). Curvilinearity and religious types: A second look at intrinsic, extrinsic, and quest relations. *International Journal for the Psychology of Religion*, *4*, 254-260.

Caplan, M., Hartelius, G., & Rardin, M. (2003). Contemporary viewpoints on transpersonal psychology, *The Journal of Transpersonal Psychology*, *35*, 143-162.

Chen, S., Chen, K., & Shaw, L. (2004). Self-verification motives at the collective level of self-definition. *Journal of Personality and Social Psychology*, *86*, 77-94.

Clark, W., & Schellenberg, G., (2006). Who's religious? In Statistics Canada Summer No. 81, *Canadian Social Trends*, (pp. 2-8). Ottawa, ON: Statistics Canada.

Damasio, A., Grabowski, T., Bechara, A., Damasio, H., Ponto, L., Parvizi, J., & Hichwa, R. (2000). Subcortical and cortical brain activity during the feeling of self-generated emotions. *Nature Neuroscience*, *3*, 1049-1056.

Davis, J. (2003). An overview of transpersonal psychology. *Humanistic Psychologist, 31,* 6-21.

Elkins, D., Hedstrom, L., Huges, L., Leaf, J., & Saunders, C. (1988). Toward a humanistic-phenomenological spirituality: Definition, description, and measurement. *Journal of Humanistic Psychology, 28,* 5-18.

Elmer, L., MacDonald, D., & Friedman, H. (2003). Transpersonal psychology, physical health, and mental health: Theory, research, and practice. *The Humanistic Psychologist, 31,* 159- 181.

Esposito, A., Kobak, R., & Little, M. (2005). Aggression and self-esteem: A diary study of children's reactivity to negative interpersonal events. *Journal of Personality, 73,* 887-905.

Frager, R., & Fadiman, J. (2005). *Personality and personal growth* (6th ed.). Upper Saddle River, NJ: Prentice Hall.

Friedman, H. (1981). *The construction and validation of a transpersonal measure of self-concept: The Self-Expansiveness Level Form.* Unpublished doctoral dissertation, Georgia State University.

Friedman, H. (1983). The Self-Expansiveness Level Form: A conceptualization and measurement of a transpersonal construct. *Journal of Transpersonal Psychology, 15,* 1-14.

Friedman, H. (2002). Transpersonal psychology as a scientific field. International *Journal of Transpersonal Studies, 21,* 175-187.

Friedman, H., & MacDonald, D. (1997). Toward a working definition of transpersonal assessment. *Journal of Transpersonal Psychology, 29,* 105-121.

Friedman, H., & MacDonald, D. (2002). Using transpersonal tests in humanistic psychological assessment. *The Humanistic Psychologist, 30,* 223-236.

Friedman, H., MacDonald, D., & Kumar, K. (2004). Cross-cultural validation of the Self-Expansiveness Level Form with an Indian sample. *Journal of Indian Psychology, March,* 44-56.

Friedman, H., & Pappas, J., (2006). Self-Expansiveness and self-contraction: Complementary processes of transcendence and immanence. *Journal of Transpersonal Psychology, 38,* 41-54.

Gall, T., Charbonneau, C., Clarke, N., Grant, K., Joseph, A., & Shouldice, L. (2005). Understanding the nature and role of spirituality in relation to coping and health: A conceptual framework. *Canadian Psychology, 46,* 88-104.

Garrett, M. (2007). Nuwati: Native American medicine, healing, and the sacred way of being. In A. Eisen & G. Laderman (Eds.), *Science, religion, and society: An encyclopedia of history, culture, and controversy, Vol.2* (pp. 654-664). Armonk, NY: M. E. Sharpe.

Genia, V. (1993). A psychometric evaluation of the Allport-Ross I/E scales in a religiously heterogeneous sample. *Journal for the Scientific Study of Religion, 32,* 284-290.

George, L., Larson, D., Koeing, H., & McCullough, M. (2000) Spirituality and health: What we know, what we need to know. Journal of Social and Clinical Psychology, 19, 102-116.

Greer, B., & Roof, W. (1992). "Desperately seeking Sheila:" Locating religious privatism in American society. *Journal for the Scientific Study of Religion, 31*, 346-352.

Grof, S. (1985). *Beyond the brain: Birth, death and transcendence in psychotherapy.* Albany, NY: State University of New York Press.

Grof, S. (1990). *The holotropic mind.* New York: Harper Collins.

Grof, S. (1992). *The holotropic mind: The three levels of human consciousness and how they shape our minds.* New York: HarperSanFrancisco.

Grof, S. (2003). Implications of modern consciousness research for psychology: Holotropic experiences and their healing and heuristic potential. *Humanistic Psychologist, 31*, 50-85.

Grof, C., & Grof, S. (1990). *The stormy search for the self: A guide to personal growth through transformational crisis.* New York: G. P. Putnam's Sons.

Hill, C., & Hood, R. (1999). *Measures of religious behavior.* Birmingham, AL: Religious Education Press.

Hill, P., Pargament, K., Hood, R., McCullough, M., Swyers, J., Larson, D., & Zinnbauer, B. (2000). Conceptualizing religion and spirituality: Points of commonality, points of departure. *Journal for the Theory of Social behavior, 30*, 51-57.

Hill, C., & Pargament, K. (2003). Advances in the conceptualization and measurement of religion and spirituality. *American Psychologist, 58*, 64-74.

Hout, M., & Fischer, C. (2002). Why more Americans have no religious preference:Politics and generations. *American Sociological Review, 67*, 165-190.

James, W. (1890). *The principles of psychology: Vol. 2.* New York: Henry Holt and Co.

James, W. (1892). *The textbook of psychology.* New York: Macmillan and Co.

James, W. (1908). *Varieties of religious experience.* New York: Longmans, Green, and Co.

Jung, C. (1964). Approaching the unconscious. In C. Jung, M-L. von Franz, L. Henderson, J. Jacobi, & A. Jaffe (Eds.), *Man and his symbols* (pp. 1-94). New York: Aldus Books.

Jung, C. (1971). *The portable Jung.* New York: Viking Press.

Jung, C. (1973). *Memories, dreams, reflections.* New York: Pantheon Books.

Jung, C. (1989). *Essays on contemporary events.* Princeton, NJ: Princeton University Press.

Kasprow, M., & Scotton, B. (1999). A review of transpersonal theory and its application to the practice of psychotherapy. *Journal of Psychotherapy Practice and Research, 8*, 12-23.

Koltko-Rivera, M. (2004). The psychology of worldviews. *Review of General Psychology, 8*, 3-58.

Lajoie, D., & Shapiro, S. (1992). Definitions of transpersonal psychology: The first twenty-three years. *Journal of Transpersonal Psychology, 24*, 79-98.

Lieberman, M., Jarcho, J., & Satpute, A. (2004). Evidence-based and intuition-based self-knowledge: An fMRI study. *Journal of Personality and Social Psychology, 87*, 421-435.

MacDonald, D., & Friedman, H. (2001). The scientific study of spirituality: Philosophical and methodological considerations. *Biofeedback, 29*, 19-21.

MacDonald, D., & Friedman, H. (2002). Assessment of humanistic, transpersonal and spiritual constructs: State of the science. *Journal of Humanistic Psychology, 42*, 102-125.

MacDonald, D., Friedman, H., & Kuentzel, J. (1999). A survey of measures of spiritual and transpersonal constructs: Part one-research update. *Journal of Transpersonal Psychology, 31*, 137-153.

MacDonald, D., & Holland D. (2002a). Examination of the psychometric properties of the Temperament and Character Inventory Self-Transcendence dimension. *Personality and Individual Differences, 32*, 1013-1027.

MacDonald, D., & Holland D. (2002b). Spirituality and the MMPI-2. *Journal of Clinical Psychology, 59*, 399-410.

MacDonald, D., Kuentzel, J., & Friedman, H. (1999). A survey of measures of spiritual and transpersonal constructs: Part two-additional instruments. *Journal of Transpersonal Psychology, 31*, 155-177.

MacDonald, D., LeClair, L., Holland, C., Alter, A., & Friedman, H. (1995). A survey of measures of transpersonal constructs. *Journal of Transpersonal Psychology, 27*, 1-66.

MacDonald, D., Tsagarakis, C., & Holland, C. (1994). Validation of a measure of transpersonal self-concept and its relationship to Jungian and five factor model conceptions of personality. *Journal of Transpersonal Psychology, 26*, 175-201.

Marx, D., Stapel, D., & Muller, D. (2005). We can do it: The interplay of construal organization and social comparisons under threat. *Journal of Personality & Social Psychology, 88*, 432-446.

Maslow, A. (1968). *Toward a psychology of being* (2nd ed.). New York: D. Van Nostrand.

Miller, W., & Thorensen, C. (2003). Spirituality, religion, and health: An emerging research field. *American Psychologist, 58*, 24-35.

Moore, C., & Lemmon, K. (2001). The nature and utility of the temporally extended self. In C. Moor & K. Lemmon (Eds.), *The self in time: Developmental perspectives* (preface). Mahwah, NJ: Lawrence Erlbaum Associates.

Moreland, J. (1998). Restoring the substance to the soul of psychology. *Journal of Psychology and Theology, Special Issue: Perspectives on the self/soul, 26*, 29-43.

National Institute for Healthcare Research (1998). *Scientific research on spirituality and health: A consensus report (A report based on the scientific progress in spirituality conferences).* Rockville, MD: John Templeton Foundation.

Newby-Clark, I., & Ross, M. (2003). Conceiving the past and future. *Personality and Social Psychology Bulletin, 29*, 807-818.

Pappas, J. (2003). A construct validity study of the Self-Expansiveness Level Form: A multitrait-multimethod matrix and criterion approach. *Dissertation Abstracts International, 64* (01), 1545B (UMI No. 3085713).

Pappas, J. (2004). The veridicality of nonconventional cognitions: Conceptual and measurement issues in transpersonal psychology. *The Humanistic Psychologist, 32*, 169-197.

Pappas, J., & Friedman, H. (2004). Scientific transpersonal psychology and cultural diversity: Focus on measurement in research and clinical practice. In W. Smythe & A. Baydala (Eds.), *Studies of how the mind publicly enfolds into being* (pp.303-345). Lewiston, NY: Edwin Mellen.

Pargament, K. (1997). *The psychology of religion and coping: Theory, research, practice.* New York: Guilford Press.

Pedersen, D. (1999). Validating a centrality model of self-identity. *Social Behavior and Personality, 27*, 73-85.

Porter, G. (1995). Exploring the meaning of spirituality and its implications for counselors. *Counseling and Values, 40*, 69-79.

Reinert, D. (2005). Spirituality, self-representations, and attachment to parents: A longitudinal study of Roman Catholic college seminarians. *Counseling and Values, 49*, 226-238.

Richards, S., & Bergin, A. (2000). Toward religious and spiritual competency for mental health professionals. In S. Richards & A. Bergin (Eds.), *Handbook of psychotherapy and religious diversity* (pp. 3-26). Washington, DC: American Psychological Association.

Robbins, L., Pis, M., & Pender, N. (2004). Physical activity self-definition among adolescents. *Research & Theory for Nursing Practice: An International Journal, 18*, 317-330.

Saucier, G., & Skrzypinska, K. (2006). Spiritual but not religious? Evidence of two independent dispositions. *Journal of Personality, 75*, 1258-1292.

Sethi, S., & Seligman, M. (1993). Optimism and fundamentalism. *Psychological Science, 4*, 256-259.

Slater, W., Hall, T., & Edwards, K. (2001). Measuring religion and spirituality: Where are we and where are we going? *Journal of Psychology and Theology, 29*, 4-21.

Slife, B., Hope, D., Nebeker, C., & Scott, R. (1999). Examining the relationship between religious spirituality and psychological science. *Journal of Humanistic Psychology, 39*, 51-85.

Smith, H. (2001). *Why religion matters: The fate of the human spirit in an age of disbelief.* New York: HarperSanFrancisco.

Spaeth, D. (2000). Spirituality in history taking. *Journal of the American Osteopathic Association, 100*, 641-644.

Speck, P., Higginson, I., & Addington-Hall, J. (2006). Spiritual needs in health care. *British Medical Journal, 329*, 123-124.

Spiro, M. (1966). Religion: Problems of definition and explanation. In M. Banton (Ed.), *Anthropological approaches to the study of religion* (pp. 85-126). London, UK: Tavistock.

Strohl, J. (1998). Transpersonalism: Ego meets soul. *Journal of Counseling and Development, 76,* 397-403.

Sutich, A. (1969). Some considerations regarding transpersonal psychology. *Journal of Transpersonal Psychology, 1,* 11-20

Talbot, M. (1999). *The holographic universe.* New York: HarperCollins.

Taylor, E. (1996). *William James on consciousness beyond the margin.* Princeton, NJ: Princeton University Press.

Tsang, J., & McCullough, M. (2003). Measuring religious constructs: A hierarchical approach to construct organization and scale selection. In S. Lopez & C. Synder (Eds.), *Positive psychological assessment: A handbook of models and measures* (pp. 345-360). Washington, DC: American Psychological Association.

Vaughan, F. (1991). Spiritual issues in psychotherapy. *Journal of Transpersonal Psychology, 23,* 105-119.

Vich, M. (1988). Some historical sources of the term "transpersonal." *Journal of Transpersonal Psychology, 20,* 107-110.

Walsh, R., & Vaughan, F. (1993). On transpersonal definitions. *Journal of Transpersonal Psychology, 25,* 199-207.

Walsh, R., & Vaughan, F. (1996). The worldview of Ken Wilber. In B. Scotton, A. Chinen, & J. Battista (Eds.), *Textbook of transpersonal psychiatry and psychology* (pp. 62-74). New York: Basic Books.

Washburn, M. (1988). *The ego and the dynamic ground: A transpersonal theory of human development.* Albany, NY: State University of New York Press.

Webb, J. (2004). Organizations, self-identities, and the new economy. *Sociology, 38,* 719-738.

Weiss, M., & Amorose, A. (2005). Children's self-perceptions in the physical domain. *Journal of Sport & Exercise Psychology, 27,* 226-244.

Weinberger, D. (1990). The construct validity of the repressive coping style. In J. Singer (Ed.), *Repression and dissociation: Implication for personality, theory, psychopathology, and health* (pp. 337-386). Chicago, IL: University of Chicago Press.

Whitmore, D. (1991). *Psychosynthesis counselling in action.* London, UK: Sage Publications.

Wilber, K. (1980a). *The atman project: A transpersonal view of human development.* Wheaton, IL: Theosophical Publishing House.

Wilber, K. (1980b). A developmental model of consciousness. In R. Walsh & F. Vaughan (Eds.), *Beyond ego: Transpersonal dimensions in psychology* (pp. 99-114). Los Angeles, CA: J. P. Tarcher.

Wilber, K. (1986). The spectrum of development. In K. Wilber, J. Engler, & D. Brown (Eds.), *Transformations of consciousness: Conventional and contemplative perspective on development* (pp. 65-106). Boston, MA: New Science Library Shambhala.

Wink, P., Dillon., M, & Kristen., K. (2005). Spiritual seeking, narcissism, and psychotherapy: How are they related? *Journal for the Scientific Study of Religion, 44*, 143-158.

Wolman, R. N. (2001). *Thinking with your soul: Spiritual intelligence and why it matters.* New York: Harmony Books.

World Health Organization Quality of Life Spirituality, Religiousness, and Personal Beliefs Group. (2006). A cross-cultural study of spirituality, religion, and personal beliefs as components of quality of life. *Social Science & Medicine, 62*, 1486-1497.

Wulff, D. (2003). The psychology of religion: An overview. In E. Shafranske (Ed.), *Religion and the clinical practice of psychology* (pp. 43-70). Washington, DC: American Psychological Association.

Wylie, R. (1979). *The self-concept: Vol. 2. Theory and research on selected topics.* Lincoln, NE: University of Nebraska Press.

Yogananda, P. (1968). *Sayings of Yogananda.* Los Angeles, CA: Self-Realization Fellowship.

Zinnbauer, B., Pargament, D., & Scott, A. (1999). The emerging meanings of religiousness and spirituality: Problems and prospects. *Journal of Personality, 67*, 889-919.

CHAPTER TWO

THE SHAMANIC MOTIF IN PSYCHOLOGICAL HEALING

William E. Smythe

With the contemporary renewal of interest in the spiritual aspects of psychological health and dysfunction, the techniques and perspectives of shamanism have become especially relevant to an understanding of psychological healing. As the number of references to the topic in the present volume attest, shamanism is currently undergoing a revival among those seeking alternative approaches to mental health and therapy.[1] Shamans are those visionary healers of indigenous cultures, both ancient and contemporary, whose healing powers derive from their uniquely personal and ecstatic mode of access to spiritual reality, that is, to realms of experience beyond the mundane reality of everyday life. Shamanic phenomena, in the form of ecstatic visionary and healing experiences, were first documented extensively in Siberia and Central Asia and the term shaman derives, by way of the Russian language, from the Tungusic word, *saman* (Eliade, 1951/2004). However, the phenomena of shamanism are not confined to any specific geographical or historical setting and have since been documented in diverse cultures all over the world, from North and South America to The Middle and Far East, Australia, Malaysia, and others (Campbell, 1988; Eliade, 1951/2004). The widespread distribution of shamanism might, as Eliade suggests, reflect a general religious propensity among human beings.

However, as Eliade (1951/2004) takes pains to point out, no form of shamanism can be considered *pure* or *primordial* because shamanism readily adapts itself to the cultural contexts in which it is located. Although grounded in practices and modes of experience characterized as archaic, shamanic phenomena are also a reflection of constantly changing cultural conditions among a wide range of indigenous and non-indigenous traditions. Herein lies the value of shamanism for a comprehensive understanding of psychological healing, for we find a remarkably robust pattern of psychological and spiritual healing in shamanism that admits a wide range of cultural variations. Shamanism thereby constitutes a unique opportunity to examine psychological healing in the context of diverse belief systems. In this chapter, I consider the shamanic healing motif as it manifests in traditional, indigenous forms of shamanism in comparison with some implicit parallels in psychoanalysis and its more explicit incorporation into contemporary personal mythology. I identify some significant similarities and differences among these three variations on the shamanic motif, to work towards a conceptualization of shamanic healing as *myth*, that is, in terms of symbolic expressions of perennial themes of human life.

TRADITIONAL SHAMANIC HEALING

Eliade (1951/2004) defined shamanism as a *"technique of ecstasy"* (p. 4). In traditional indigenous cultures, the shaman is an individual with a special propensity and aptitude for ecstatic or transformative experiences that go well beyond the normal range of human experience among his or her contemporaries. By virtue of these magico-religious sensibilities, the shaman becomes a kind of spiritual authority for the local tribe. Although the main vocation of shamans lies in spiritual healing, their authority extends to other spiritual and religious functions as well.[2] In general, the shaman is a psychopomp, a mediator between everyday, mundane reality and the realm of the sacred, someone with unique access to spiritual reality. Yet, the shaman's techniques of ecstasy do not exhaust either the religious or the healing practices of their communities; the traditional cultural settings in which shamanism thrives also make room for other religious authorities and practices, as involved in tribal ritual, ceremony, and public worship. The shaman's unique functions derive from his or her command of techniques of ecstatic transformation (Eliade, 1951/2004). Their spiritual sensibilities notwithstanding, shamans are not wholly benevolent beings, as their special powers can as readily be used to inflict illness and suffering as for healing. The first written account of a Siberian shaman, for example, described him as a "villain of a magician" who called upon demons (Petrovich, 1672/2001, p. 18). As Joseph Campbell (1988) has remarked in this connection:

Our usual association of the spiritual life with "virtue," in the modern sense of the word as referring to "moral excellence and practice," breaks down here . . . . The elementary mythology of shamanism, that is to say, is neither of truth and falsehood nor of good and evil, but of degrees of power: power achieved by breaking through the walls of space and barriers of time to sources unavailable to others. (p. 168)

SHAMANIC INITIATION AND INITIATORY SICKNESS

In its traditional settings, the vocation of shaman is understood as a calling reserved for individuals with special spiritual aptitudes for visionary and ecstatic experiences and healing. Although frequently passed on by virtue of heredity, the call to shamanism can also arise spontaneously through involuntary ecstatic experience such as dreams, visions, and illness, or as a result of a deliberate quest. The spontaneous mode is more common in Asia, where the shamanic vocation is seen as something inflicted by spirits; in contrast, the voluntary quest is more typical of North American shamanism (Eliade, 1951/2004). In both the spontaneous and more voluntary modes, initiation into the profession of the shaman generally has two distinct phases: the *ecstatic phase*, in which the initiate experiences dreams, visions, and symptoms of a revelatory nature; and the traditional or *didactic phase* of receiving instruction from an experienced shaman before receiving the local community's recognition. The characteristics of the ecstatic phase include not only dreams and visions, but also frequently involve sickness exhibiting characteristic psychopathological symptoms resembling epilepsy, hysteria (now termed *somatoform disorder*) and, possibly, schizophrenia (Campbell, 1988; Eliade, 1951/2004). However, it would be ill-advised to attempt to explain shamanism in terms of psychopathology, for traditional indigenous cultures rarely confuse conditions resembling psychopathology with actual shamanism (Campbell, 1959/1958). Instead, certain types of psychopathology might be understood in terms of shamanism as failed or aborted initiatory illnesses: the psychopathological individual being conceived, in Eliade's (1951/2004) terms as an "unsuccessful mystic" (p. 27). I return to this issue later.

The themes that arise during the ecstatic phase of initiation are remarkably universal among differing cultures. These ecstatic experiences occur in the context of a death-and-resurrection crisis and include experiences of bodily dismemberment, removal and replacement of bodily organs, ascent to the heavens or descent to the underworld, and revelatory encounters with divine beings and helping spirits in animal form (Eliade, 1951/2004). For example, among the Aranda of Australia, ecstatic initiations are said to be performed by spirits of the Dreamtime in the following way:

There is a cave near Alice Springs that is supposed to be occupied by such spirits, and when a man feels that he is capable of enduring their transformation, he goes alone to its entrance and lies down there to sleep. At break of day, one of the spirits, coming to the mouth of the cave and finding him there, hurls at him an invisible lance that strikes and penetrates his neck from behind, goes through his tongue, and leaves there an actual hole large enough to admit the little finger. A second lance goes through his head from ear to ear, and, falling dead, he is carried deep into the cave . . . . There the spirit removes his internal organs and implants an entirely new set, along with a supply of magical stones, after which the man returns to life, but in a condition of insanity. (Campbell, 1988, p. 169-170)

Another less common transformational motif is ritual change of sex, as found in Siberian, Indonesian, and some North and South American variants of shamanism (Eliade, 1951/2004). This involves shamans of either sex taking on the characteristics of the opposite sex and can manifest in various ways, from hair arrangement, to transvestitism, to full imitation of behavior. In extreme form, shamanic sex change may even result in marriage to a member of the same sex (Campbell, 1988).

The shaman's initiation does not, however, end with an ecstatic transformative experience. In almost all cases, the ecstatic phase is followed by a period of instruction administered by an experienced shaman and often, but not always, by a public ceremony in recognition of the shaman's new vocation (Eliade, 1951/2004). Newly initiated Aranda shamans, for example, do not practice shamanism for a full year following their initial transformative experiences and, during this time, they consort with more experienced shamans, acquiring their secrets, which consist mostly of techniques of practical magic and sleight of hand (Campbell, 1988). Other kinds of esoteric wisdom passed on during this phase include instruction in a secret language, the language of birds being especially significant as it gives the shaman access to the secrets of nature and the ability to prophesy. During the second or didactic phase, the newly initiated shaman is also indoctrinated into the traditions of the local tribe and its underlying cosmology. Ritual tree climbing, a symbolic ascent to the heavens, is another frequent practice during this phase. Following this period of instruction, the community formally bestows shaman status upon the initiate, often several years after the original experience. Initiation proper is still considered to have occurred during the ecstatic phase; subsequent public recognition of the shaman's status serves only as a kind of confirmation (Eliade, 1951/2004).

THE LOSS AND RECOVERY OF SOULS

Traditional shamanism attributes disease to various causes, including intrusion of a foreign object into a person's body, possession by evil spirits, breach of taboo, sorcery, and loss of soul (Eliade, 1951/2004; Ellenberger, 1970). Among these possible etiologies, arguably the loss of soul constitutes the disease motif aligned closest to psychology. Treatment of loss of soul uniquely concerns the shaman; as Eliade states, "everything that concerns the soul and its adventure, here on earth and in the beyond, is the exclusive province of the shaman" (p. 216). In North American shamanism, for example, other kinds of diseases – particularly, those caused by the intrusion of a foreign object – can often be successfully treated by other medicine men and lay healers, but the recovery of lost souls requires the intervention of a shaman (Eliade, 1951/2004).

In the affliction called loss of soul, the soul is said to depart from the body for any of a number of reasons: It might be frightened away, or abducted by malevolent spirits, or it might simply wander away by itself "just like a dog that runs away from his master overnight" (Jung, 1968, p. 119). According to this disease motif, the soul is seen as something separable from the body, with which it is tightly linked only during normal waking consciousness. As Ellenberger (1970) portrays it, the underlying belief is that "man bears within himself a kind of duplicate, a ghost-soul whose presence in the body is a prerequisite to normal life, but that is able to leave the body temporarily and to wander about, especially during sleep" (p. 7). In its wanderings, the soul encounters various perils that prevent its safe return; at this point, the services of a shaman are called for.

Each archaic disease type has its own unique treatment: The appropriate therapy for intrusion of a foreign object is its ritual extraction by suction; possession is treated by one form or another of exorcism; breach of taboo by confession or propitiation; and sorcery by counter magic. A common, though by no means the only, treatment for loss of soul is for the shaman to undertake an ecstatic journey to recover the lost soul and restore it to its owner. Eliade (1951/2004) describes a shamanic healing séance among the Yenisei Ostyak of Siberia that exemplifies this healing journey motif:

> The séance begins, as usual, with invoking the spirits and putting them in the drum one after the other. During all this time the shaman sings and dances. When the spirits have come he begins to leap; this means that he has left the earth and is rising toward the clouds. At a certain moment he cries: "I am high in the air, I see the Yenisei a hundred versts away." On his way he meets other spirits and tells the audience whatever he sees. Then, addressing the spirit helper who is carrying him through the air, he cries: "O my little fly, rise still higher, I want to see farther!" Soon afterward he returns to the yurt, surrounded by his spirits. It seems that he has not found the patient's soul, or he has seen it at a great distance, in the land of the dead. To

reach it, he begins dancing again, until trance supervenes. Still carried by his spirits, he leaves his body and enters the beyond, from which he finally returns with the patient's soul. (p. 223)

As this account illustrates, the healing séance, like shamanic initiation, has both an ecstatic and a public or ceremonial component: the ecstatic, personal vision experienced only by the shaman and the public ritual of singing, dancing and drumming witnessed by others. This two-fold character of shamanic healing in terms of the ecstatic and the ceremonial or, in the modern psychological idiom, inner and outer, seems to be a general feature of shamanic phenomena.

To be sure, the ecstatic healing journey is an extreme measure, undertaken often at significant peril to the shaman, who has to bargain, appease, or even do battle with spirits of the underworld to retrieve the lost soul. Before undertaking this perilous journey, the shaman attempts other means of recovery, such as calling back the lost soul. If the soul has wandered only a short distance, recovery is relatively straightforward. Only when it has gone a long way off, or left the ordinary world entirely for the spirit world, does the shaman resort to an ecstatic journey (Eliade, 1951/2004; Ellenberger, 1970).

In contemporary shamanism, these healing journeys are understood to be largely figurative and metaphorical. That said, according to legend, there was a time when shamans literally undertook these journeys and had command of magical powers. One shaman of the modern era, for instance, speaks of ancestors who "lived in the time when a shaman could go down to the mother of the sea beasts, fly up to the moon or make excursions out through space" (Eliade, 1951/2004, p. 290). Most modern shamans no longer claim magical powers to this extraordinary degree and, for the most part, resign themselves to imitating the exploits of their ancestors. This exemplifies the widely acknowledged trend toward the *decadence of the shaman*, a theme I will return to (Eliade, 1951/2004).

The cosmology that underlies the shaman's ecstatic journeys consists of a layered conception of reality. Shamanistic belief divides the world into three distinct levels – earth, sky and underworld – that are connected through a central axis. The axis runs through an opening on each of the three levels and it is through these openings that spirits travel between the heavens, the earth, and the underworld and that shamans navigate on their healing journeys. The privilege of navigating these non-terrestrial realms lies exclusively with the shamans; as Eliade (1951/2004) has remarked, "what for the rest of the community remains a cosmological ideogram, for the shamans (and the heroes, etc.) becomes a mystical itinerary . . . . Only for the latter is *real communication* among the three cosmic zones a possibility" (p. 265). In some traditions, a *Cosmic Mountain* or *World Tree* stands as a connecting link among the three cosmic regions; the World Tree in particular represents "the universe in continual regeneration, the inexhaustible spring of cosmic life" (p. 271), hence the widespread motif of tree and pole climbing in shamanic healing and initiation. As an example, the Tungus of Siberia hold the belief that the souls of children perch like birds on the branches of the Cosmic tree prior to birth. Moreover this belief illustrates the substantial role ornithomorphic symbolism – representing the magical powers of flight among the three realms – plays in shamanism generally (Eliade, 1951/2004).

SHAMANISM AND PSYCHOANALYSIS

The phenomena of shamanism, and of soul loss and recovery in particular, may seem rather far removed from the world of psychoanalysis and of modern psychotherapy generally; as Ellenberger (1970) has pointed out:

> Nothing is further from our principles of treatment than the restoration of a lost soul to a patient. And yet, if we ignore the cultural element and seek the roots of facts, we may find a common ground between those primitive concepts and ours. Do we not say that our mental patients are "alienated," "estranged" from themselves, that their ego is impoverished or destroyed? Could not the therapist who gives psychotherapy to a severely deteriorated schizophrenic patient by trying to establish a contact with the remaining healthy parts of the personality and to reconstruct the ego be considered the modern successor of those shamans who set out to follow the tracks of a lost soul, trace it into the world of spirits, and fight against the malignant demons detaining it, and bring it back to the world of the living? (p. 9)

In this section, I recount a classic case study in the psychoanalytic literature that exemplifies a number of shamanic themes and then explore some parallels between psychoanalytic therapy and shamanic healing.

THE SCHREBER CASE

Dr. jur. Daniel Paul Schreber was a court judge who presided in various jurisdictions in Germany during the late nineteenth-century. He suffered three distinct bouts of psychiatric illness, beginning in the autumn of 1884. During the first of these, he was admitted to an asylum, treated for severe hypochondria, and subsequently released. The final episode, which began in 1907, found Schreber "in an extremely disordered and largely inaccessible state" (Strachey, 1958, p. 6) until his death four years later. It was during his second illness, which began in the autumn of 1893, that Schreber exhibited a pattern of symptoms of interest from a shamanic perspective. Inspired by the conviction that his illness had important religious and metaphysical implications, Schreber published an autobiographical account of his experiences in 1903, entitled *Denhwurdigkeiten eins Nervenkranken* (Memoirs of a Nerve Patient). This work came to the attention of Freud in 1910 and his analysis of the Schreber case was published the following year (Freud, 1911/1958). Although Freud never treated or had any personal contact with Schreber, his analysis of this case is considered significant as an account of his views on paranoia and its relationship to repressed homosexuality and also because it represents Freud's first, tentative foray into the field of mythology (Strachey, 1958).

Schreber's second illness was precipitated by a recurring dream that his previous illness had returned and this was accompanied, on at least one occasion, by fantasies upon awakening of being a woman in the act of copulation. Following a period of sleeplessness, he returned to the clinic where he had previously been treated, whereupon his condition rapidly deteriorated. He became fixated on the idea that he was dead and decomposing and that his body was being manipulated in disgusting ways but, nonetheless, for a holy purpose. He came to believe that many of his internal organs had been removed and subsequently restored by divine miracles, what he called *rays*, that rendered him effectively immortal. This was all in service of his gradual transformation into a woman, which was considered necessary for the divine purpose "to redeem the world, and to restore mankind to their lost state of bliss" (Weber's report, as cited in Freud, 1911/1958, p. 16). Schreber believed that from the enormous number of *female nerves* implanted into his body, a new race of humans would one day be produced via direct impregnation by God, a process that could take several decades, or even centuries, to complete. He also believed that "in the meantime not only the sun, but trees and birds, which are in the nature of "bemiracled residues of former human souls," speak to him in human accents, and miraculous things happen everywhere around him" (p. 17). However, these "miracled birds," which are composed of human souls that have entered into a state of bliss, have nonetheless been reduced to repeating meaningless phrases that have been "dinned into them" and, as such, are an endless source of irritation (p. 35).

As his disease progressed, Schreber's ideas and experiences took on an increasingly mystical and religious character. In his complex theological belief system, the heavenly world was composed of anterior and posterior realms and there was both a *lower* and an *upper* God, which were intimately connected, in a kind of solar myth, with the sun and the starry heavens. Human souls were said to be contained in the nerves of the body. Following death all souls undergo a process of purification before being reunited with God; during this purification, souls learn the basic language spoken by God himself. This process was required because God withdrew to an immense distance from the world after creating it and now neither understands living human beings nor learns anything new from experience (Freud, 1911/1958).

Schreber also suffered a number of paranoid delusions, mostly directed at his former physician, Dr. Flechsig, whom he referred to as a "soul-murderer" (Weber's report, as cited in Freud, 1911/1958, p. 14). He believed that there was a conspiracy against him, involving turning over to Flechsig both his soul and body, the latter which "was to be transformed into a female body, and as such surrendered to [Flechsig] with a view to sexual abuse" (Schreber's work, as cited in Freud, 1911/1958, p. 19). God himself was believed to be an accomplice in this conspiracy.

The shamanic elements in this case history are unmistakable – bodily dismemberment, separation of soul from body, removal and replacement of internal organs, change of sex, manifestations of divine beings and the souls of the dead, the symbolism of birds and trees, learning of a special language, and a layered conception of reality consisting of different regions of heaven.

Did Schreber undergo a kind of aborted shamanic initiatory illness? Was he what Eliade (1951/2004) would call an "unsuccessful mystic" (p. 27)? Eliade describes the experiences of the unsuccessful mystic as lacking in religious content, yet Schreber wrote his *Memoir* with a firm conviction of the religious significance of his experiences. But, perhaps because Schreber suffered his ordeal too late in life or because he did so in a cultural setting that did not recognize or value shamanic illness, the eventual outcome was a debilitating and ultimately fatal mental deterioration rather than a shamanic transformation of being. Or perhaps Schreber's experiences were wholly pathological, consistent with Freud's own diagnosis of paranoia. In either case, a substantial similarity between the phenomenology of shamanic initiatory illness and psychoanalytic symptomatology clearly figures in this account. Freud (1911/1958) analyzed the Schreber case in terms of delusions of persecution in the service of "warding off a homosexual wishful phantasy" (p. 59). However, in a concluding statement, he at least acknowledged the possibility of alternative interpretations: "It remains for the future to decide," wrote Freud, "whether there is more delusion in my theory than I should like to admit, or whether there is more truth in Schreber's delusion than other people are as yet prepared to believe" (p. 79).

THE PSYCHOANALYST AS SHAMAN

Over a half century ago, Levi-Strauss (1949/2001) pointed out some ways in which shamans could be likened to psychoanalysts. The psychoanalyst can also be seen as a type of shaman. The initiatory or *creative illness*, in particular, is not an uncommon pattern among practitioners of psychoanalysis and depth psychology and has been experienced by a number of its more significant pioneers, as Ellenberger (1970) among others has documented. It is not unusual for clients in psychotherapy to attribute shamanic powers to their therapists. One client, who knew nothing about shamanism, reported the following dream:

> My therapist appears as a primitive medicine man, dancing and jumping around a fire in a strange squatting position. He drums and utters peculiar cries. I am puzzled but the performance is spooky and powerful. (Larsen, 1996, p. 112, original italics removed)

To elicit apparently forgotten memories, Freud (1910/1992) reported using a technique somewhat reminiscent of shamanism early in his own practice:

> When I had reached a point with them at which they asserted that they knew nothing more, I would assure them that they did know, that they should just continue to speak, and I ventured to assert that the memory which would emerge at the moment when I placed my hand on the patient's forehead would be the correct one. (p. 408-409)

Freud later abandoned this practice because it was "not suited to be a definitive technique" (p. 409). Nonetheless, the technique is not unlike the sympathetic magic of the shaman, whose healing powers of touch can release demons and liberate souls.

While discernable parallels with shamanic healing might appear in various forms of psychotherapy, these parallels figure especially in psychoanalysis given the intense psychological demands on the psychoanalyst in the practice of therapy. Just as shamanic healing involves shamans taking ecstatic journeys beyond the limits of the everyday world to recover lost souls, psychoanalysis requires analysts to navigate the depths of the unconscious – their client's and their own – in an effort to restore their clients' connection with self. The distinction, in shamanic healing, between the ecstatic and the ceremonial aspects of the healing séance finds a parallel in psychoanalysis between the analyst's exploration of subjective consciousness, on the one hand, and the interpersonal circumstances of the transference relationship, on the other. Like that of the shaman, the work of the psychoanalyst involves intuitive and non-rational considerations in order to mediate the symbols, metaphor, and imaginal constructs of the psyche.

Recent scholarship has brought these intuitive, implicit aspects of psychoanalytic practice to the forefront. A volume edited by Canestri (2006), for example, brings together the work of a number of contemporary psychoanalysts who seek to understand the role of implicit, private, preconscious or *lived* theories in psychoanalytic practice, forms of understanding "to which the analyst at work turns very frequently, often without knowing it" (Canestri, 2006, p. 2). These implicit theories bear the stamp of the analyst's own subjective experience and are not governed by discursive logic; they are part of the *context of discovery* rather than the *context of justification* and their language is that of metaphor and symbol rather than of propositional logic (Canestri, Bohleber, Denis, & Fonagy, 2006).

An example of the metaphorical treatment of the psychoanalyst's intuitive knowledge is Reed's (2006) description of "metaphors of transition" in psychoanalytic therapy (p. 105). In terms somewhat evocative of the shaman's healing journey, she writes:

> psychoanalysis, as a treatment method, requires its practitioners to cross the divide within themselves between inner and outer, known

and unknown, with regularity and to encourage patients to become adept in the same way. Analysts imagine not only that part of ourselves that is only vaguely apprehended, but that aspect of the patient's mind that we need help grasping as well. (p. 106)

Just as shamans navigate the passage between mundane reality and the spirit world in their ecstatic journeys, psychoanalysts move between the known reality of conscious experience and the unknown reality of the unconscious. The role of metaphor in enabling these transitions lies in opening up an imaginal space beyond the restrictive cannons of Aristotelian logic, where "categories are neither one nor the other, but both and neither" (p. 106). Metaphors of transition also become useful in understanding aspects of the transference relationship. This requires a conceptualization of transitional analytic space as both intrapsychic and intersubjective. In Reed's description:

the emphasis is less on the boundaries between the analyst and the patient than on the frequency with which those boundaries may be crossed and on the therapeutic need to sort out parts of self and object in order to re-establish boundaries through the containing function of the analyst . . . . Rather than the materially real analyst observing the fate of a fantasy about himself within the patient's transference, we must account for the materially real analyst discovering elements of the patient within himself and possibly losing elements of himself within the patient. (p. 119)

This reference to mobile elements of self that may pass between individuals is, again, very reminiscent of shamanism.

The discourse in this section is not meant to suggest that the psychoanalyst can be identified with the figure of the shaman nor to diminish the substantial cultural differences between modern psychoanalysis and traditional shamanism. Rather, I have sought to view psychoanalysis through a shamanic lens in order to explore some possible connections between an ancient wisdom tradition and a modern form of psychological practice. This perspective may clarify the significant role of imaginative, non-rational and intuitive considerations in psychoanalysis and in psychotherapy more generally.

SHAMANISM AS PERSONAL MYTHOLOGY

Shamanism is deeply rooted in mythology. Traditional shamanism functions within the cultural mythology of the local community, which provides its underlying cosmology and spiritual belief system. In general, *cultural mythologies* provide a common framework for members of a given cultural group to come to terms with fundamental, perennial themes of human life, such as human mortality, stages of life, and our place in the cosmos. In the cultural pluralism of our postmodern age, *personal mythologies* consisting of individuals' idiosyncratic constructions of existential meaning increasingly supplement or even supplant cultural mythologies. Whereas cultural mythologies are singular and monolithic for members of a given society, personal mythologies are informed by multiple cultural sources: They are patched together from various diverse and conflicting strands amongst the multitude of cultural influences to which the contemporary person is exposed. Personal mythologies, nonetheless, fulfill much the same explanatory, pedagogical, social, and spiritual functions for an individual that cultural myths do for an entire society (Feinstein & Krippner, 1997; Krippner, 1990).

Although sometimes employed as a therapeutic treatment modality, personal mythology would seem to find its main application in self-administered programs for personal development, as evidenced by the substantial self-help literature it has spawned (e.g., Feinstein & Krippner, 1997; Houston, 1992; Keen & Valley-Fox, 1989; Pearson, 1989). All the same, personal mythologies also need to be contextualized in the cultural mythologies they depend upon and remain inextricably tied to. As Krippner (1994) points out: "No major writer currently using the term suggests that personal myths exist independently of the cultural context. A person's cultural milieu, as well as his or her physiological predispositions, interpersonal experiences, and transpersonal experiences, form the basis for personal myths" (p. 130). It is thus not surprising that shamanism, a perennial component of cultural mythology, has been incorporated into personal mythology as well. In contrast to psychoanalysis, where the parallels with shamanism were mostly implicit, in the personal mythology tradition, shamanism has been taken up explicitly as a key theme. I consider two examples below.

THE INNER SHAMAN

One approach is to incorporate the figure of the shaman into the "inner cast of characters" that represents the modern person's experience of self (Larsen, 1990). In the modern idiom of the inwardness of mental life, a common metaphor is that of subpersonalities within the person that represent different aspects of one's self (Smythe, 2005): psychological health being conceptualized in terms of the harmonious functioning among these different subpersonalities. As an inner character, the shaman plays a mediating role in this intrapersonal dynamic. Feinstein and Krippner (1997), for example, outline a systematic program for dialectically confronting and resolving the tension between conflicting personal mythologies, in which the figure of the inner shaman plays an essential mediating role. While the traditional shaman mediates between everyday reality and the spirit world, the inner shaman mediates between old and new ways of understanding oneself; as Feinstein and Krippner state, "as myth-making has become more highly personalized, modern individuals are called on to assume these shamanistic responsibilities personally" (p. 33). The inner shaman has three specific functions in the context of these personal mythological transformations: first, to open up and maintain "a conduit between ordinary reality and the hidden realities that may be accessed through nonordinary states of consciousness" (p. 34); second, to function as a guide to creative choices in response to life's demands and opportunities; and third, to guide the evolution of one's personal mythology based on experience.

The main technique employed in Feinstein and Krippner's program is guided imagery, a step-by-step procedure for transforming experience through deliberate visualization of certain contents. Early in the program, for example, there is a highly evocative visualization exercise that introduces the individual to his or her inner shaman for the first time. Beginning with a symbolic journey back through one's past to the "Graveyard of Lost Illusions," the guided imagery instructions continue as follows:

> Leaving the Graveyard of Lost Illusions, you can now enter more fully into the hidden places of your being. The challenges have proven you worthy of the guidance you desire. Soon you can see a light at the end of the tunnel. As you approach the light, you know you are coming closer to the sacred dwelling of your Inner Shaman. You notice that the tunnel opens into a clearing. In the clearing is a path that takes you into an extraordinary ancient forest. You walk onto the path and begin to explore the trees, the sky, the undergrowth. A river runs nearby. Take a breath. You can be fully present. As you begin to walk, you may ease into the beauty and wonder of the lush green foliage.
>
> Ahead of you, the branches of two large trees touch and form an archway. You know that on the other side of that archway is the home of your Inner Shaman. Mustering your determination, you prepare yourself for the important moment when the two of you will meet. Moving forward, you step through the archway. Behold. In front of you is your Inner Shaman. (p. 36)

The inner shaman subsequently appears in other guided imagery exercises, often as a character in internal dialogues with other inner characters and in a ritually enacted dance.

THE NEW SHAMANISM

Another application of the resources of personal mythology lies in the appropriation of shamanic powers directly by individuals themselves. What Samuels and Lane (2003) call the new shamanism aims to make shamanic healing perspectives and techniques accessible to modern people. They write: "For people to understand shamanism today, they need it to make sense in their vocabulary and worldview" (p. 9). Accordingly, the new shamanism accepts what modern medicine has discovered about the physical causes and treatment of illness but aims to supplement this knowledge with the visionary techniques of the shaman. These visionary techniques are, again, to be understood in terms of the modern idiom of the *inner world of consciousness* rather than according to their more traditional otherworldly cosmological framework. Whereas the traditional shaman's healing work lay in departing from his or her body and travel to other realms, contemporary shamanic healers heal through an act of the imagination and an exploration of the visionary world of their own consciousness.

Again, the main technique for these inner explorations is guided imagery. Samuels and Lane's (2003) recent book contains numerous guided imagery exercises, each addressed to a different aspect of the shamanic healing experience. They all have much the same basic format, beginning with abdominal breathing, followed by progressively deepening relaxation, then the guided imagery proper, followed by grounding and closing to return to one's ordinary awareness of the immediate environment. Only the contents of the guided imagery instructions in the penultimate stage vary from one exercise to the next, depending on the focus of the shamanic experience. The instructions for retrieving lost souls, for example, are as follows:

> Ask for a vision of the person's spirit to come to you. See if you can find his or her soul in the world below. Follow a path, tracks; have your spirit animals go with you on this sacred journey. When you see or feel something, let the vision or inner voice come to you. When you see or feel it, let a healing come to you. Do what you feel is healing, what your spirit animals tell you is healing. If you need to take something out of the person in visionary space, you can do it. If you need to put something back into the person, you can do that now. If you think the person's soul has wandered, you can find it and bring it back. (p. 109)

As this example illustrates, guided imagery instructions are only partly directive; considerable leeway is given to the person's own spontaneous powers of imagination (e.g., "When you see or feel something, let the vision or inner voice come to you").

Samuels and Lane (2003) point out an important difference between traditional shamanism and the new shamanism with respect to the role of belief systems. Whereas traditional shamans function within the context of cultural belief systems that acknowledge the sacred, for the modern person, "it is different. We must re-create a belief system that includes the spirit world" (p. 151). That is, anyone undertaking the modern path of the new shamanism bears more personal responsibility for the belief systems they develop in the process; these practices no longer sit firmly rooted in their own culture. At the same time, Samuels and Lane caution against claiming too much personal responsibility for the products of one's shamanic imagination and recommend a receptive approach to this experiential material:

When you see the spirit, it is natural to say, 'I am making this up. This is really a tree root, a branch. There is nothing there.' That is a judgment. Let the spirits come to you. Invite them to come, then accept what you see. (p. 154).

Inner work of this kind is not, however, exhaustive of the new shamanism. Like traditional shamanism and psychoanalysis, it has both a visionary and a public or ceremonial component. Prior to engaging in visionary work, for example, novice shamanic healers establish a sacred space, both within their own bodies and in their physical environments to provide a context for their inner work.

The new shamanism, and the personal mythology approach in general, contrast with traditional shamanism in at least three important ways; first, as already pointed out, reconstruction of shamanic healing space occurs in terms of psychological *inner* space, in contrast to the cosmological, transcendent space of traditional shamanism; second, the highly programmatic character of the new shamanism's visionary exercises which are structured in terms of a step-by-step sequence of instructions contrasts with the wholly spontaneous character of traditional shamanic visions; third, radical inclusiveness defines the new shamanism. Whereas traditional shamanism was practiced by a select minority of individuals with special spiritual aptitudes, the new shamanism is intended for anyone who might be interested in pursuing it. Samuels and Lane (2003) claim, for example, that "it is probably easier for a modern person to become a shaman, because these tools are deep in our culture; we can all learn about them, and they are part of our way of being a healer already" (p. 10).

With its psychological, programmatic and highly inclusive character, the new shamanism might indeed exemplify yet a further stage of the decadence of the shaman remarked upon earlier: a kind of shallow, superficial imitation of traditional, indigenous practices. In the cultural pluralism of contemporary life, individuals almost certainly cannot achieve the same depth of experience as traditional shamans, whose local cultural contexts strongly reinforce a monolithic mythology of spiritual transformation. Lacking this consistent cultural support, the modern individual wanting to undertake the shamanic path is left adrift on a sea of conflicting mythologies and mythological fragments that do not have the same cohesion found in traditional shamanism. However, while the the new shamanism may be lacking in depth, it nonetheless gains both breadth and flexibility. Lacking a singular cultural belief system or mythology, the modern individual is at least in a position to appreciate shamanism *as myth* and to navigate among different interpretations of the shamanic experience, something that would be unimaginable in the cultural contexts of traditional shamanism.

CONCLUSION

By following the shamanic motif from traditional shamanism through to some implicit parallels in psychoanalysis and its more explicit incorporation and emulation in the personal mythology tradition, this discourse brings to light a number of common features of shamanic psychological healing across all three domains. The first commonality emerges in viewing psychological healing in terms of a navigation between two worlds: mundane versus spiritual reality, conscious versus unconscious, or concrete versus imaginary experience. Second, both share a reliance on intuitive, non-rational, symbolic and visionary healing techniques and practices. Finally, a common distinction occurs between the personal, ecstatic component and the more public or ceremonial component of both psychological healing and shamanic practices. Nonetheless, some profound differences demark these variants of shamanic healing, especially with respect to cultural belief systems. Whereas traditional shamanism operates within a cosmological framework of levels of spiritual reality, contemporary Western approaches to shamanism tend to operate within the psychological framework of the inner world of mental life. Yet even in the midst of this substantial difference in cultural belief systems, the shamanic motif is plainly evident all the same. In the cultural pluralism of modern times, shamanism could therefore provide a bridge among diverse belief systems relating to healing. Just as the individual shaman functions as a mediator between different domains of reality, the shamanic motif itself could prove to be especially valuable in mediating among different cultural belief systems. At present, we are uniquely situated to be able to appreciate shamanism *as myth* by exploring its manifestations in a number of different cultural contexts. The implications of this new fluidity of the shamanic motif for psychological healing are just beginning to be explored.

NOTES

1. The chapters by Krippner, Scotton, and Zausner are especially relevant.

2 On the distinction between the spiritual and the religious, see Pappas and Friedman's contribution to this volume. Consistent with contemporary usage, religious generally refers to culturally and institutionally sanctioned modes of access to the sacred, whereas spiritual refers to more personal and idiosyncratic aspects of this access. The distinction is quite marked in shamanism, as will be seen later in this chapter.

References

Campbell, J. (1988). *Historical atlas of world mythology: Volume one. The way of the animal powers: Part two. Mythologies of the great hunt.* New York, NY: Harper & Row.

Campbell, J. (1991). *The masks of God: Primitive mythology.* Harmondsworth, EN: Penguin Arkana. (Original work published 1959).

Canestri, J. (Ed.). (2006). *Psychoanalysis: From practice to theory.* Chichester, England: Wiley & Sons.

Canestri, J., Bohleber, W., Denis, P., & Fonagy, P. (2006). The map of private (implicit, preconscious) theories in clinical practice. In J. Canestri (Ed.), *Psychoanalysis: From practice to theory* (pp. 29-43). Chichester, England: Wiley & Sons.

Eliade, M. (2004). *Shamanism: Archaic techniques of ecstasy* (2nd paperback ed.). Princeton, NJ: Princeton University Press. (Original work published 1951)

Ellenberger, H. F. (1970). *The discovery of the unconscious: The history and evolution of dynamic psychiatry.* New York, NY: Basic Books.

Feinstein, D., & Krippner, S. (1997). *The mythic path: Discovering the guiding stories of your past-creating a vision for your future.* New York, NY: Putnam.

Freud, S. (1958). Psycho-analytic notes on an autobiographical account of a case of paranoia (dementia paranoides). In J. Strachey (Ed. & Trans.), *The standard edition of the complete psychological works of Sigmund Freud* (Vol. 12, pp. 9-82). London, England: The Hogarth Press. (Original work published 1911)

Freud, S. (1992). On psychoanalysis. In S. Rosenzweig (Trans.), *Freud, Jung, and Hall the king-maker: The historic expedition to America* (1909) (pp. 397-406). Seattle, WA: Hogrefe & Huber. (Original work published 1910)

Jung, C. G. (1968). *The collected works of C. J. Jung: Volume nine, part one. The archetypes and the collective unconscious* (2nd ed.) (H. Read, M. Fordham, G. Adler, & W. McGuire, Eds., R. F. C. Hull, Trans.). Princeton, NJ: Princeton University Press.

Houston, J. (1992). *The hero and the goddess: The Odyssey as mystery and initiation.* New York, NY: Ballantine Books.

Keen, S., & Valley-Fox, A. (1989). *Your mythic journey: Finding Meaning in your life through writing and storytelling.* Los Angeles, CA: J. P. Tarcher.

Krippner, S. (1990). Personal mythology: An introduction to the concept. *The Humanistic Psychologist, 18,* 137-142.

Krippner, S. (1994). Introduction: Some perspectives on myth. *The Humanistic Psychologist, 22,* 122-133.

Larsen, S. (1990). Our inner cast of characters. *The Humanistic Psychologist, 18,* 176-187.

Larsen, S. (1996). *The mythic imagination: The quest for meaning through personal mythology.* Rochester, VT: Inner Traditions International.

Levi-Strauss, C. (2001). Shamans as psychoanalysts. In J. Narby & F. Huxley (Eds.), *Shamans through time: 500 years on the path to knowledge* (pp. 108- 111). New York, NY: Tarcher/Putnam. (Original work published 1949)

Petrovich, A. (2001). The shaman: A villain of a magician who calls demons. In J. Narby & F. Huxley (Eds.), *Shamans through time: 500 years on the path to knowledge* (pp. 18-20). New York, NY: Tarcher/Putnam. (Original work published 1672)

Reed, G. S. (2006). Theory as transition: Spatial metaphors of the mind and the analytic space. In J. Canestri (Ed.), *Psychoanalysis: From practice to theory* (pp. 103- 125). Chichester, England: Wiley & Sons.

Pearson, C. S. (1989). *The hero within: Six archetypes we live by* (expanded edition). San Francisco, CA: Harper & Row.

Samuels, M., & Lane, M. R. (2003). *Shaman wisdom, shaman healing: Deepen your ability to heal with visionary and spiritual tools and practices.* Hoboken, NJ: Wiley & Sons.

Smythe, W. E. (2005). On the psychology of 'as if'. *Theory & Psychology, 15,* 283-303.

Strachey, J. (Ed. & Trans.). (1958). *The standard edition of the complete psychological works of Sigmund Freud* (Vol. 12). London, England: The Hogarth Press.

CULTURAL SYSTEMS OF HEALING

CHAPTER THREE

A PROPOSED APPLICATION OF ETHNOMEDICAL MODELS TO TRADITIONAL HEALING SYSTEMS

Stanley Krippner

Ethnomedicine has become a topic of intensive study in recent years due, in part, to the work of the World Health Organization and other groups attempting to facilitate cooperation between indigenous practitioners and those trained in Western allopathic biomedicine. This chapter describes the ethnomedical systems of the North American Navaho tradition and the South American Peruvian Pachakuti *curanderismo* in terms of two different models: one designed by Siegler and Osmond (1974) and the other designed by a task force of the National Institute of Mental Health (NIMH). These two indigenous systems each offer a comprehensive understanding of health and point the way to possible collaboration between allopathic biomedicine and various indigenous systems of healing, a project that has accelerated due to public demand (Iljas, 2006, p. 190).

The term *ethnomedicine* refers to the comparative study of indigenous or traditional medical systems. Typical ethnomedical topics include causes of sickness, medical practitioners and their roles, and specific treatments utilized. The explosion of ethnomedical literature has been stimulated by an increased awareness of the consequences of the forced displacement and/or acculturation of indigenous peoples, the recognition of indigenous health concepts as a means of maintaining ethnic identities, and the search for new medical treatments and technologies. In addition, Kleinman (1995) finds ethnographic studies an "appropriate means of representing pluralism . . . and of drawing upon those aspects of health and suffering to resist the positivism, the reductionism, and the naturalism that biomedicine and, regrettably, the wider society privilege" (p. 195).

In his exhaustive study of cross-cultural practices, Torrey (1986) concluded that effective treatment inevitably contains one or more of four fundamental principles:

1. A shared world view that makes the diagnosis or naming process possible.
2. Certain personal qualities of the practitioner that appear to facilitate the patient's recovery.
3. Positive patient expectations that assist recovery.
4. A sense of mastery that empowers the patient.

If a traditional medical system yields treatment outcomes that its society deems effective, it is worthy of consideration by allopathic biomedical investigators, especially those who are aware of the fact that less than 20% of the world's population is serviced by allopathic biomedicine (Freeman, 2004; Mahler, 1977; O'Connor, 1995).

However, the definition of *effective* varies from society to society (Krippner, 2002). Allopathic biomedicine places its emphasis upon *curing*, removing the symptoms of an ailment and restoring a patient to health, while traditional medicine focuses upon *healing*, attaining wholeness of body, mind, emotions, and spirit. Some patients might be incapable of being *cured* because their sickness is terminal. Yet those same patients could be *healed* mentally, emotionally, and spiritually as a result of the practitioner's encouragement to review their life, to find meaning in it, and to become reconciled to death. Those who have been cured, on the other hand, may be taught by a healing practitioner procedures that will prevent a relapse or recurrence of their symptoms. An emphasis upon prevention is a standard aspect of traditional medicine, and is becoming increasingly important in of biomedicine as well (Freeman, 2004; Krippner & Welch, 1992).

A differentiation can also be made between *disease* and *illness*. From either the biomedical or the ethnomedical point of view, one can conceptualize disease as a mechanical difficulty of the body resulting from injury or infection, or from an organism's imbalance with its environment. Illness, however, comprises a broader range of dysfunctional behavior, mood disorders, or inappropriate thoughts and feelings. These behaviors, moods, thoughts, and feelings can accompany disease or can exist independently. Thus, one may refer to a *diseased* brain rather than an *ill* brain but still prefer the phrase *mental illness* over *mental disease*. Cassell (1979) goes so far as to claim that allopathic biomedicine treats disease but not illness: "physicians are trained to practice a technological medicine in which disease is their sole concern and in which technology is their only weapon" (p. 18).

THE SIEGLER-OSMOND MODELS

Comparisons between biomedicine and ethnomedicine can be made utilizing hypothetical structures such as the twelve-faceted model proposed by Siegler and Osmond (1974). In the social and behavioral sciences, a *model* is an explicit or implicit explanatory structure used to improve our understanding of the processes that underlie a set of organized group behaviors. Models have been constructed to describe human behavior ranging from conflict, competition, and cooperation to mental illness, personality dynamics, and family interactions. I have modified the Siegler-Osmond model, making it applicable to both physical and mental disorders, although traditional practitioners usually do not differentiate between the two. The utility of the Siegler-Osmond model can be demonstrated by comparing a shamanic medical model – an eclectic folk healing model – and the allopathic biomedical model on twelve dimensions:

1. Diagnosis
2. Etiology
3. Patient's behavior
4. Treatment
5. Prognosis
6. Death and suicide
7. Function of the institution
8. Personnel
9. Rights and duties of the patient
10. Rights and duties of the family
11. Rights and duties of the society
12. Goal of the model.

THE NAVAHO INDIAN HEALING MODEL

The Navaho healing system serves as an example of the application of the Siegler and Osmond model. The term *Navaho* (also Navajo) refers to the largest Native American tribe in the United States; the Navaho reservation in the south west part of the country comprises 16 million acres. The word Navaho comes from the Spanish term for "people with big fields," but in their own language, they call themselves the *Dineh* people. They are members of the southern Athapaskan linguistic group and occupy plateau areas of north eastern Arizona, overlapping into New Mexico and Utah.

Geertz (1973) points out that the entire lifestyle of a culture is built upon its mythic view of reality. The Navaho ethic values "calm deliberativeness, untiring persistence, and dignified caution" (p. 130). As such, they view nature as "tremendously powerful, mechanically regular, and highly dangerous" (p.130). While the dominant U.S. culture attempts to control nature, the Navaho worldview seeks to live in respectful harmony with it. Theories of sickness and methods of healing thus largely focus on harmony in the Navaho culture: The stricken patient receives a vocabulary that defines the nature of his or her distress, relates it to the wider world (Geertz, 1973), provides an explanation, and converts energy into a form that can heal. Sandner (1979) has identified the most important values in Navaho mythology as the acquisition of supernatural power (notably for the maintenance of health), the preservation of harmony in family relationships, and the achievement of adult status, defined by the Navaho as working in cooperation with and holding respect for the other members of the family, clan, and community.

The Navaho diviner discerns the diagnosis through consultation with the patient and the patient's family. The medicine man usually plays a limited role in diagnosis as he later carries out instructions given by the diviner (Sandner, 1979). Navahos have constructed three major diagnostic categories of mental illness. *Moth craziness* is attributed to incestuous activities and is characterized by fits of uncontrolled behavior (e.g., jumping into the fire like a moth), rage, violence, and convulsions. *Crazy violence* has some of the same external manifestations as moth craziness but results from alcoholism instead of incest. *Ghost sickness*, ascribed to sorcery, manifests in nightmares, loss of appetite, dizziness, confusion, panic, and extreme anxiety. When someone knowingly or accidentally breaches taboos or offends dangerous powers, the natural order of the universe is ruptured and *contamination* or *infection* occurs that must be redressed.

In Navaho etiology, disease occurs because the intrusion of a harmful agent destroys the natural harmony between individuals and their surroundings. Circumstances that especially disturb this harmony include exposure to lightning or whirlwinds and inappropriately trapping, killing, or eating such animals as bear, deer, coyotes, porcupines, snakes, and eagles. Sometimes these harmful agents appear in frightening, ominous dreams. Contact with spirits of the dead is especially hazardous, as is sorcery. As noted before, the diviner, the medicine man, the patient, and the patient's family work together in determining the cause of sickness (Sander, 1979).

The patient's behavior determines what type of *Chant Way* will be utilized in his or her treatment. A person who is unable to resolve grief, who harbors fears of accidents, and who speaks of chest pains usually will be told to have an Evil Way ceremony. The patient's dreams are important as a diagnostic aid; the most ominous dreams are those of being burned, falling off a cliff, and drowning; dreams of dead relatives are especially portentous.

During treatment, the Navaho *hataalii* (or singing-shaman) utilizes a number of therapeutic procedures, most notably one or more of the ten basic Chant Ways and their accompanying sand paintings.[1] These are complex rituals that center on cultural myths in which heroes or heroines once journeyed to spiritual realms to acquire special knowledge. The prescription for a chant depends upon the connection between the patient's symptoms and the narrative of the chant myth. For example, the Hail Way is prescribed for muscular fatigue and soreness because the hero, Rain Boy, suffered from these symptoms when he was attacked by his enemies; the Big Star Way protects the patient against the powerful influences of the stars and the dangers of the night. The Night Way alleviates blindness, deafness, and mental illness because the hero of the chant confronted each of these dangers. The difficulties faced by the hero of the Beauty Way makes it effective against rheumatism, sore throats, digestive and urinary problems, and skin diseases.

Ritual chanting takes a multimodal approach that contributes to its effectiveness. The repetitive nature and mythic content is easily deciphered and often repeated at appropriate times by those patients well-versed in tribal mythology. According to Sandner (1979), "The visual images of the sand paintings and the body painting, the audible recitation of prayers and songs, the touch of the prayer sticks and the hands of the medicine man, the taste of the ceremonial musk and herbal medicines, and the smell of the chant incense – all combine to convey the power of the chant to the patient" (p. 215). The *hataalii* usually displays a highly developed dramatic sense in carrying out the chant but generally avoids the clever sleight of hand effects used by many other cultural healing practitioners to demonstrate their abilities to the community.

Sandner proposed that the function of the chant lies in creating suggestibility because the chant shifts attention through repetitive singing and elaborate retelling of culturally specific mythic themes. These activities prepare participants for a lengthy healing ceremony that may involve mythic images and narratives enacted in purification rites or executed in sand paintings composed of sand, seeds, charcoal, and flowers.[2] From a psychological perspective, the patients *translate* these symbols and metaphors as they sit on the painting, but from their perspective, they are interacting with some of the basic forces and energies of nature.

Six steps comprise the typical Chant Way ritual: preparation, in which the patient is *purified*; presentation of the patient to the healing spirits; evocation of these spirits to the place of the ceremony; identification of the patients with a positive mythic theme; transformation of the patients into a condition where ordinary and mythic time and space merge; and release from the mythic world to return to the everyday world where past transgressions are confessed, where new lessons are assimilated, and where life changes are brought to fruition. The *hataalii's* performance empowers the patient by creating an alternative domain of consciousness – a mythic reality – through the use of chants, dances, songs accompanied by drums and rattles, masked dancers, ritual purifications, and sand paintings.[3] Through entering this mythic reality, made especially concrete through the *hataalii's* sand painting, the patient is taken into sacred time and is able to bring a total attentiveness to the healing ritual.

The community has an important role in achieving this focus. Large numbers of people attend the chant and many might be asked to participate, providing social reinforcement and increased motivation. This type of participation appears to increase the patient's sense of personal power and magnify his or her imagination as they attend to the chants. To reinforce this sense of personal power further, the patient follows a specific regimen for the next four days after the ritual to protect members of the community from his or her newly acquired powers. Moreover, the mentation of the practitioner, the patient, and the community may all be affected by the ceremony. The *hataalii* is dusted with the decorated sand and his patients claim to feel the power emanating from the painting. This procedure resembles the enhancement of imagination common to several hypnotic procedures, which the repetitive chanting probably augments.

The *hatallii* uses other rituals in addition to the Chant Way. During a prayer session, one example of a different ceremony, sacred corn pollen may be sacrificed while praying in an attempt to please the spirits needed to heal the patient: This ritual must be performed perfectly and behind locked doors, often at the patient's home.

The setting for treatment usually occurs in the Hogan, a specially constructed octagon made of log walls sealed with mud adobe and decorated with a sand painting on the floor. The door opens to the East and a hole in the center of the domed ceiling lets the smoke out. Men sit on the north, women and children on the south, and the patient sits in the center with family and friends nearby. The door to the darkened Hogan is fastened to prevent the prayer from escaping. Sharpened flints are used to expel the evil from both the patient and the Hogan.

These procedures reduce the patient's symptoms at the same time they stabilize the social and emotional condition of the community. For example, the hataalii instructs the family to make elaborate preparations for their forthcoming visitation. Upon arriving, the patients are told that the prognosis is excellent, thus fostering positive expectations (Torrey, 1986). The most important people in the patient's life often join in the prayers, reaffirming the belief that the patient will recover. Prognosis, to a large degree, depends upon the attitude of the patient. A Navaho practitioner told Sandner (1979): "If the patient really has confidence in me, then he gets cured . . . . If a person gets bitten by a snake, for example, certain prayers and songs can be used, but if the patient doesn't have enough confidence, then the cure won't work" (pp. 17-18).[4]

When a sick person's family determines that a practitioner is necessary, they call for a *hataalii*; frequently, a herbalist and a diviner, both of whom are of lower status, accompany the *hataalii*. There are some two hundred plants in the Navaho pharmacopoeia and the herbalists gather these plants and make medicines, some of which are only used in ceremonies by the *hataalii*. The diviners are usually women who diagnose the problem by *listening* to the spirits and report it to the *hataalii*. This procedure may be accompanied by such diagnostic procedures as hand trembling, stargazing, candle-gazing, and crystal-gazing, all of which involve the inward focusing of the practitioner's attention to bring insight as to the nature of the problem.

Every *hataalii* must go through a long and arduous period of training and apprenticeship; they must earn the approval of their teachers and their community by demonstrating that they can perform successfully (Sandner, 1979). The *hataalii* memory must be impeccable; the effort required to learn one major chant has been compared to that of obtaining a university degree (Sandner, 1979). Moreover, a *hataalii* must also learn many other medical techniques beyond memorizing the Chant Ways. Although, a patient with a break or fracture is usually sent to an allopathic practitioner, Sandner observed a Navaho specialist set broken bones "in a true scientific manner" (p.18).

In the Navaho system, the patient's first priority is to accept treatment, and they assume the role of cooperating with the practitioner by taking an active part in their diagnosis and treatment. The major priority of the patient's family lies in seeking diagnosis and treatment from qualified personnel for their indisposed family members. The family also arranges payment for the *hataalii*, an important responsibility because some Chant Way ceremonies last for several days and the fee may exceed several months' salary.

The major priority of the patient's community rests in supporting the sick patient through attending the Chant Way and facilitating his or her treatment. The community plays the role of preserving traditions and training new practitioners. This latter task is difficult because of the high cost of apprenticeships, especially for the hataalii.

The goal of this healing model is integration within the framework of cosmic harmony and the rejection of the effects of sorcery, which are seen as alien to this harmony (Sandner, 1979). According to Kluckhohn and Leighton (1962), the Navahos are generations ahead of U.S. physicians in treating the whole person. The goal of Navaho healing is to restore the patient's harmony with his or her family, clan, and universe.

THE U.S. OFFICE OF ALTERNATIVE MEDICINE MODEL

In April 1995, the Office of Alternative Medicine (OAM) of the United States National Institutes of Health (NIH) held a conference on research methodology (O'Connor et al., 1997). The charge of this conference was to evaluate research needs in the field of complementary and alternative medicine (CAM), and several working groups were created to produce consensus statements on a variety of essential topics. The panel on definition and description accepted a dual charge: first, to establish a definition of the field of complementary and alternative medicine for purposes of identification and research; and second, to identify factors critical to a thorough and unbiased description of CAM systems, one that would be applicable to both quantitative and qualitative research. The panel defined CAM as follows:

> Complementary and alternative medicine (CAM) is a broad domain of healing resources that encompasses all health systems, modalities, and practices and their accompanying theories and beliefs, other than those intrinsic to the politically dominant health system of a particular society or culture in a given historical period. CAM includes all such practices and ideas self-defined by their users as preventing or treating illness or promoting health and well-being. Boundaries within CAM and between the CAM domain and the domain of the dominant system are not always sharp or fixed. (O'Connor et al., 1997)

The second charge of the panel was to establish a list of parameters for obtaining thorough descriptions of CAM systems. The list was constructed on 14 categories first conceptualized by Hufford (1995, pp. 54ff):

1. Lexicon – What are the specialized terms in the system?
2. Taxonomy – What classes of health and sickness does the system recognize and address?
3. Epistemology – How was the body of knowledge derived?
4. Theories – What are the key mechanisms understood to be?
5. Goals for Interventions – What are the primary goals of the system?
6. Outcome Measures – What constitutes a successful intervention?
7. Social Organization – Who uses and who practices the system?
8. Specific Activities – What do the practitioners do? What do they use?
9. Responsibilities – What are the responsibilities of the practitioners, patients, families, and community members?
10. Scope – How extensive are the system's applications?
11. Analysis of Benefits and Barriers – What are the risks and costs of the system?
12. Views of Suffering and Death – How does the system view suffering and death?

13. Comparison and Interaction with Dominant System –
What does this system provide that the dominant system
does not provide? How does this system interact with the
dominant system?

The fourteenth category regards research methods and it not appropriate for this essay, which focuses on descriptions.

PERUVIAN CURANDERISMO

The utility of the OAM categories can be illustrated by applying them to an Andean ethnomedical system called Pachakuti (meaning world reversal or transformation) *Mesa Curanderismo*, a tradition deeply rooted in the Huachuma and Paqokuna traditions and blended with aspects of Paqokuna *Curanderismo*. I have discussed this system with two of its leading English-speaking practitioners, Oscar Miro-Quesada (2002) and his student Matthew Magee (2002). Because of the complexity and sophistication of Pachakuti *Mesa,* Miro-Quesada has adapted this system to make it more accessible to the industrialized world. In addition, I have observed Magee perform two ritualistic *Mesa* ceremonies. Within the OAM categories the system can be described as follows (O'Connor et al., 1997).

1 – LEXICON.

Specialized terms come from Spanish, Aymara (an Andean language), and two forms of assimilated Quechua language: the rural form *Runasimi* and the high form *Khapaqsimi* spoken by royalty or people in positions of power. In describing the ethnomedical and social communitary function of Peruvian *Curanderismo,* however, it is important to note that several terms have changed over time. For example, the contemporary terms used to describe the shaman and the sorcerer are *maestro* and *brujo,* respectively. However, if one traces the lineage of the Pachakuti *Mesa* tradition, one would find the terms *curandero* and *malero* (post-Conquest), *hampiq* and *layqa* (Inca pre-Conquest), and *kamasqa* and *sonqoyog* (pre-Inca) as well. Furthermore, terminological variations exist between charismatic and non-charismatic healers and, most recently, between Pachakuti *Mesa* practitioners and neo-shamanic practitioners.

2 – TAXONOMY.

The Pachakuti *Mesa* tradition recognizes and addresses a wide variety of physical, mental, emotional, and spiritual classes of health and sickness (Magee, 2002). Within this system, Spanish words are used to describe several types of ailments: *enfermedad de daño* (a sickness caused by human intention), *enfermedad de Dios* (a God-given sickness), *contagio* (contagious sickness), and *encantos* (sickness caused by enchantment). Examples of the most common, *enfermedad de daño*, include harmful intention directed toward the ears, through the mouth, through the air, or by loss of one's *sombra* (soul or *etheric body*). The latter is typically brought about by *susto* or *espanto* (magical shock or fright), or the more extreme cause is *shucaque* (fright by trauma). In addition, there are sicknesses caused by envy and the *mal de ojo* (evil eye) and by *mal aire* (evil wind).

The ritual encounter between the patient and the practitioner can be viewed as a dialogue about *daño* in which the *curandero* or *curandera* (male or female shaman respectively) uses a persuasive rhetoric through speech or song in conjunction with ritualized activities to transform the patient's self-understanding, and, hence, his or her well-being.[5]

Most physical ailments fall into the category, *enfermedad de Dios*. In many traditions, practitioners do not deal with these conditions, but Pachakuti *Mesa* shamans are an exception. The visual symptoms of a God-given sickness are similar to the *vista en virtud* (sight in virtue and power) that practitioners manifest after ingesting the San Pedro cactus, a mind-altering substance. As a result, these symptoms rarely manifest when he or she performs a *diagnostic rastero* (divination or *tracking*) in the *campo medio*, the middle field of the practitioner's healing altar discussed in detail later.

3 – EPISTEMOLOGY.

When tracing the origins of the Pachakuti *Mesa* tradition back through its oral lineage within Peruvian shamanism, one must go back to the Sechin culture, as well as the later Chavin, Tiahuanacu, Paracas, Nasca, Moche, Lambayeque, Chimu, Wari, Inca (or Inka), Aymara, Runa (or Quechua), and Mestiso traditions. Although archeological discoveries in the 1980s suggest that Peru's central highlands were inhabited from 8 000 BCE and the origins of Peru's shamanic technology can be traced back to 2 000 BCE at the latest, many practitioners believe that *Mesa*-related healing practices were utilized far earlier.

4 – THEORIES.

The key mechanisms of the practitioner's power lie in his or her ability to control and direct unseen forces and entities by working with a *mesa*, a practitioner's healing altar. This is accomplished through proper utilization of the *campo ganadero* (field of the magician) as well as the *campo justiciero* (field of the mystic). Mastery of these two skills allows the practitioner to surrender his or her personal will or agenda, becoming an open, transparent vessel for Spirit to flow through unhindered. Symbols of a practitioner's mastery of these fields rests on either side of the *mesa*, while the practitioner, as Master Healer or *maestro*, resides in the *campo medio* (middle field).

The healer also works with a supernatural hierarchy through a process of co-creation with Spirit. This hierarchy is believed to be a unified, interdependent system that provides practitioners with limitless sources of guidance and power. These sources include the *Apukuna* (Sacred Mountains); *Huaringas* (Sacred Highland Lagoons); *Pachamama* (Mother Earth); *Mama Killa* (Grandmother Moon); *Inti Tayta* (Father Sun); *Auquis* (Nature Spirits); *Tirakuna* (the Watchers); *Mallquis* (Tree Spirits); *Machukuna* (Ancestors); *Machula Aulanchis* (Benevolent Old Ones); tutelary animal allies; the elements of nature such as *unu, wayra, nina, allpa*; and various Roman Catholic saints including San Cipriano of Antioch, and Brother Martin de Porres. Working with these sources requires a delicate balance, not only through the practitioner's negotiation of control and surrender, but also through living a lifestyle that reflects this balance, known as *ayni* (sacred reciprocity). Training involves a culturally sanctioned *calling* into the tradition. When a maestro passes on his or her knowledge or bequeaths the practice of Pachakuti *Mesa* to an initiate, an initiatory phenomenon called *karpays* occurs and a *pacto magico* (magical contract) is made.

5 – GOALS FOR INTERVENTIONS.

The Pachakuti *Mesa* practitioners believe healing is a spiritual phenomenon; all sickness originates in the Spirit world. The purpose of life itself is to be initiated into the visionary regions of Spirit and to maintain oneself in concert with all creation (Achterberg, 1985). Hence, the goal for intervention in Pachakuti *Mesa Curanderismo* is a successful *florecimiento* (flowering-of-fortune healing ritual) that is used to strengthen a person's physical and spiritual systems. Strengthening a patient's *runa kurku k'anchay* (luminous body), as opposed to suppressing the symptom, empowers the patient to remove the sickness-causing intrusion with his or her own innate healing capacities.

Once the patient's personal power has been augmented, there is often a need to go further. This is especially true if the problem is extreme, as in *soul-loss*, possession, enchantments, and potent acts of *daño* (e.g., curses, certain types of contagion). In these cases, often a need arises to intervene on behalf of a patient with specific techniques for removal of the *daño*. These techniques take the form of *chupa* (extraction) or counteracting the attack through ritual battle – known as *volteando, volteada,* or *botando* – where the curse is thrown back to its sender. Successful interventions of this kind usually completely disperse the patient's negative condition and symptoms, and generate sickness in the person who initiated the curse. Depending on the original severity of the curse, death of the sorcerer has been reputed to occur.

6 – OUTCOME MEASURES.

A successful intervention is gauged primarily by the quality of the *florecimiento*, which brings about the energetic restoration or supplementation of a person's potentials. This *flowering* of dormant potentialities brings forth qualities in the person necessary to maintain a sustainable livelihood.

7 – SOCIAL ORGANIZATION.

Depending on the level of shamanic mastery attained, practitioners will be assigned various civic units of geographical space in which to work, ranging from the *ayllu* (extended family or community), to the *llaqta* (village or town), and finally the *suyu* (region). A *curandero* performs shamanic functions in this system that include: working with sicknesses brought about by sorcery, imbalance, envy, etc.; providing insight into conditions of the harvest; resolving interpersonal conflicts; influencing the weather, finding lost items (as well as lost persons or souls); and attending to a variety of spiritual, mental, emotional, and physical conditions. These healing sessions are primarily conducted on Tuesdays and Fridays.

The *curandero* also performs specific ceremonial services for the community, such as providing ritual feedings – called *offrendas, despachos,* or *haywarikuys* – for *Pachamama* (Mother Earth), the *Apukuna* (Sacred Mountains), and various other supernatural beings noted already. Specifically, A *despacho* or *haywarikuy* is a ritual offering used to promote a reciprocal exchange of thanks between human communities and the natural world.

In the Paqokuna tradition, the *pampa misayoq* (ritual specialist) may learn to create and perform several hundred different types of *despacho* or *haywarikuy* ceremonial rituals. The performances are quite diverse and comprise twenty-four basic elements, called *recados,* in the form of plant, animal, mineral, and human made products. All of these elements are reverently arranged on a square sheet of paper and either burned or buried as a way to promote the lifestyle of *ayna* (sacred reciprocity). There are offerings for births, deaths, marriages, good luck, prosperity, longevity, and harvests, to name a few. It is also common for practitioners to use *despachos* to bless certain spaces, such as living quarters, work places, and sacred sites.

There are various types of *curanderos*, for example, the *alto misayoq* (herbalists), the *pampa misayoq* (ritual specialists), and the *kuraq akulleq* (literally meaning, master chewers of coca). The latter is considered to have attained the highest level of mastery and rank within the shamanic hierarchy.

The services of a *brujo* or sorcerer can be purchased to adversely affect the health of a rival, or to assure success in business, love, and other aspects of personal gain. The client of a *brujo* may reveal this fact to an ally, who will subsequently pass the news along a network that eventually leads to the intended target. Similarly, the *curandero's* analysis of the source of a patient's suffering is often a topic of subsequent conversation between social intimates of the patient; this is also true of the countermeasures (e.g., the *volteada* or ritual in which sorcery is reversed) often used by the shaman.

Potential patients for both the *curandero* and *brujo* include most of the members of the community, but when seeking medical assistance from the *curandero*, patients also commonly see both a *curandero* and an allopathic physician, often not openly discussing their visit to the former. This reluctance to reveal the use of the indigenous healing system applies to any member of the social system, from the wealthy business executive to the poor farmer. Patients of *curanderos* and *brujos* include owners of businesses, political office holders, educators, military officers, and even a few medical professionals. These persons are willing to spend significant amounts of money and subject themselves to physically exhausting ritual treatments because they have shared with *curanderos* the belief that sorcery can be the cause of sickness.

The majority of patients for both the *curandero* and *brujo* are women. This may stem from the inferior role of the female as a subordinate within the public transcript of male privileged society (e.g., the values of machismo which support gender-based hierarchies, and the subsequent psychological and social conflicts that arise as a result). Through the sorcerer, women can gain access to powers that guarantee spousal fidelity (e.g., love magic), thus eliminating the competition (e.g., *daño*). Even the apprehension that a woman might pursue this alternative can act as an effective sanction. The *curandero*, on the other hand, provides women with the means to redress wrongs and to hold men accountable for their actions.

8 – SPECIFIC ACTIVITIES.

Diagnosis: Diagnosis can be carried out through a variety of activities, for example, a *rastreo* (divining and tracking), coca leaf divination, reading the entrails of a guinea pig, or casting shells, etc. However, the source of diagnosis most commonly utilized in healing situations by *Huachuma curanderos* is the San Pedro cactus. The entheogenic San Pedro imbues the healer with *vista en virtud* (virtue, vision, and insight), which enables him or her to diagnose not only the illness, aliment, or disease of a patient, but often the source of said illness, aliment, or disease and specific ways to cure it. The *curandero's mesa* (personal healing altar) also plays a vital role in the divinatory process of diagnosis by speaking to the *curandero* through the *cuenta* (the history, story, or narrative) of a specific piece or pieces. There are also practitioners who will *read* the energy of a person's *poq'po* or *wayrari* (so-called electromagnetic energy field) to detect imbalances or deficiencies within that energy field and as a means for diagnosis. Ultimately, the above forms of diagnosis are highly effective and are commonly referred to by anthropologists because of the mystical flavor of shamanic healing arts. However, one must not overlook the *curandero's* keen ability to observe with the senses (e.g., simply observing how a person looks, smells, feels, interacts with the world). *Curanderos* will also often check a person's tongue, nose, eyes, ears, glands, etc., as a means for diagnosis. The combination of practical and mystical forms of diagnosis has availed the *curandero* with a high degree of accuracy regarding diagnosis.

Treatment: The various modes of treatment employed by the *curandero* are as diverse as the conditions requiring treatment. However, nearly all treatments involve the use of a *mesa*, the sacred healing altar that the *curandero* uses to mediate with spiritual and cosmic forces for ritual healing. It is a microcosmic embodiment of a macrocosmic reality. This shamanic altar contains ritually empowered objects, which are aesthetically arranged on a unkhuñas (sacred textile) to reflect the system of medicine employed by its carrier: that is, his or her lineage, cosmological background, animal allies, spirit guides, personal *apukuna* and *huaringas* (sacred mountains and lagoons).

There are four kinds of objects primarily incorporated into a *curandero's* mesa: khuyas* (sacred stones), *sepkas* (power objects), *estrellas* (gifts from the spirits of the mountains), and *enqas* (totem fetishes). Among these, it is also common to find *batas*, *palos*, and *espadas* (staffs, sticks, and swords used for protection), *florecimientos* (extractions, infusions, ritual battle), *pututus* (conch shells used to invoke spiritual assistance and loosen blocks in an person's body), *seguros* (good luck charms, protection pieces), *rumikuna* or *khuyas* (stones used for healing), condor feathers (used for directing energy and cleansing a person's *poq'po* or energy field), *huacos* (objects and artifacts from Colonial and pre-Columbian times used to anchor specific energies into the medicine ground, often that of the ancestors), *agua de Florida* or *agua de Kananga* (colognes and perfumes, which are sprayed in the mouth for cleansing and purification), and, last, rattles and whistles (to balance or bring in energy, commonly used when singing *tarjos* or medicine songs).

It is also common to find candles, crosses, images of Roman Catholic saints, meteorites, *chunpis* (ceremonially woven belts), crystals, holy water, water from the melting ice of glaciers, San Pedro cactus, tobacco, coca leaves, *singha* (a combination of coca, tobacco, cane alcohol, and such perfumes as *agua de florida*, taboo), *siete poderes* (which is imbibed through the nose), and incenses such as *palo santo* or copal. An herbal pharmacopoeia can occasionally be found as well. These objects – in addition to the items specific to the individual *mesa* carrier – are arranged in a spatial configuration on *unkhuñas* (sacred textiles) and worked with to assist the patient in the healing session in attaining physical, emotional, spiritual, and mental integration and balance.

When a *mesa* is used in ritual healing the distinction between the symbol and that which the symbol represents dissolves. The objects arranged upon the *mesa* become the mountains, the rivers, the puma, or the empowered representation of the *curandero's* own healing. Within this state of non-ordinary consciousness the line that delineates subject and object blurs and the *curandero* is able to work with the *mesa* to heal the patient at the level of his or her energy, that is, at the source of the condition rather than through medicating the symptoms.

Treatment also commonly involves incorporating the family members of the patient in the healing ceremony. This helps ensure that the patient will not only return to his or her community transformed, but he or she will return to a transformed community as well. *Curanderos* often find themselves acting simultaneously as arbiters for and avengers of social injustices.

9 – RESPONSIBILITIES.

Practitioner responsibilities require a competent level of mastery through apprenticeship and experiential training; the aspiring practitioner must complete a series of rites of passage, known as *karpays*, governed by his or her teacher, elders, and peers in the tradition and the spiritual hierarchy. An example of the latter would be a demonstration of using coca leaves for diagnostic purposes. Once an apprentice is deemed qualified by his or her community, he or she may begin seeing patients on a small scale, but must build a solid reputation as a competent healer. Thus, the *curandero* must consistently provide accurate diagnosis and effective treatment for patients in need of healing. The *curandero* is also responsible to recommend alternative means for healing if he or she is not capable or does not specialize in the condition presented by the patient. In addition to being a qualified and capable healer, the *curandero* must also live a lifestyle of *ayni*, which reflects not only the qualities of the tradition, but the living example of balance mirrored by nature and the living cosmos. This lifestyle requires uninterrupted communion with the spiritual hierarchy, a perpetual willingness to learn from life, and a deepening relationship with the phenomenal world, the internal world, and the living universe.

Patient responsibilities include openness to participate in the healing being offered and willingness to implement the advice or prescription suggested by the *curandero*. The patient is also responsible to provide some form of reciprocal exchange for the healing service provided, either monetarily or through some form of barter or trade.

Family members are responsible to be present for the healing ceremony if possible and to ensure the patient is able to recover in an environment that supports this new, transformed paradigm. They have a responsibility to retain the information gained from the healing session and to communicate this information to pertinent community members who can further reinforce the transformed living environment for the patient. The family is often responsible to help compensate the *curandero*, either through monetary means or through trade if the patient is unable to do so. The community also has a responsibility to be a supplemental presence of support for the patient and to reinforce the transformed living environment for the person in transition.

10 – SCOPE.

This type of Peruvian shamanism has been practiced over the millennium in remote, northern areas of Peru. This isolation has helped Pachakuti practitioners preserve their independence and their prerogatives. The apparent success of the Pachakuti system in its place of origin is an additional reason for its longevity. The scope of this healing system comprehensively covers physical, mental, emotional, and spiritual problems. However, there are allopathic treatments and technologies that would bolster traditional medicine, and well-meaning *curanderos* often endeavor to make referrals to a clinic or hospital (typically, at a distance) if that would help their patient.

11 – ANALYSIS OF BENEFITS AND BARRIERS.

What are the risks and costs of the system? Due to the recent advances in allopathic medical technology, competition between biomedical organizations and indigenous systems is becoming more common. The boundaries that delineate these two systems, and the conditions they address, are often blurred. Poor people often turn to indigenous healers because biomedical treatments are too expensive. However, *curanderos* are not part of a recognized profession and therefore operate in legal and social marginality. Many *curanderos* experience harassment from local police, who use rarely enforced legal restrictions on non-licensed medical practitioners to extort protection payments. Church and civic officials have also been party to repressive measures against *curanderos.*

Curanderos certainly recognize the tenuous position that they occupy in the Peruvian medical system. Some prefer to maintain a very low profile to avoid the notice of local officials by performing ritual sessions in remote agricultural fields, as one solution. Other *curanderos* bank on the support of well-connected patients to keep them out of trouble.

12 – VIEWS OF SUFFERING AND DEATH.

This system holds that there is a basic continuity between life and death. Life and death are not seen as separate, for life cannot exist without death. When the physical body dies it goes into the Earth and feeds it, giving life to the plants and trees. The plants feed the animals, who feed the Earth, ad infinitum, in a self-regulating interdependent relationship seen as the great web of life. All things are born from *Pachamama* (Mother Earth) and all things shall return to her. Views of the afterlife vary from practitioner to practitioner but most believe in life after the physical body dies. All in all, death is seen as a natural process, inseparable from life.

Anthropologists have long noted that life's transitions (i.e., birth, death) are commonly marked by elaborate rituals, the purpose of which is to smooth the disruption to the social order that such changes can cause. The body of the person undergoing the transition is often the target of symbolic manipulations: special decorations (e.g., burial costumes) and purification (e.g., cleansing). A particularly frequent symbolic message conveyed by these rituals is death and rebirth: The person is dying from the social status previously held and being born into a new identity.

In fact, a study of these Indigenous rituals draws interesting parallels to hospital patients in allopathic treatments: the standardized garb required by the institution, the strict fasting enforced before surgery, the cleansing processes required by both the patient and the surgical staff, the process of anesthetization that brings the patient's vital signs and consciousness into a death-like state, and the patient's frequently cited post-surgery sense of being reborn. The fact that all these features have medical justifications and explanations does not diminish their potential symbolic impact.

Much of the suffering experienced by Peruvians is attributed to acts of *daño*, or sorcery. The prevalence of this perspective is especially strong in a society like that of Peru where personal relationships are critical to economic survival and where the powers of the sorcerer and the *curandero* are assumed to have empirically verifiable effects. *Daño*, as a threat or as an accepted diagnosis, can have serious social repercussions no matter how outsiders to the tradition might view the forces that the sorcerers claim to control.

Peruvian society's rigid social hierarchies make people increasingly dependent upon personal networks in order to survive. The resulting burden of economic self-interest loaded onto personal relationships has contributed to a social world in which mistrust inevitably accompanies interdependence. It should not be surprising, therefore, that social relations would be the assumed source of misfortune and suffering for rural Peruvians. This stands in contrast with traditional Andean attributions of sickness to natural forces and supernatural transgressions.

13 – COMPARISON AND INTERACTION WITH DOMINANT SYSTEM.

What does this system provide that the dominant system does not provide and how does this system interact with the dominant system? On the one hand, Miro-Quesada (2002) believes that global shamanism is an emerging phenomenon of the twenty-first century. The Pachakuti teachings are intended to empower all interested persons, allowing them to work with unseen forces in order to promote healing and balance through spiritual mediation. But on the other hand, the dominant role being played by allopathic biomedicine often rules out people's interest and participation in an indigenous healing system (see Levi-Strauss, 1955).

CONCLUSION

On July 14, 2003, Matthew Magee performed a ritualistic ceremony on the top of Mount Tamalpais in Marin County, California, in the spirit of Kamasqa *Curanderismo*, one of the components of the Pachakuti *Mesa* tradition. This ceremony wove together several themes that expressed the participants' reverence for the Earth as teacher and mother. Together, the group created a consecrated *despacho* (Earth offering) to foster a lifestyle of *ayni* (sacred reciprocity) and an awareness of life's interdependence, calling upon participants to live harmoniously with themselves, with others, and with the planet as a whole.

There are ecopsychologists who believe that healing the planet is basically a shamanic journey; if so, traditional medical systems can play a vital role in this endeavor. However, while herbal medicines, indigenous treatments, and shamanism become fashionable but diluted healing practices in Western society, indigenous systems in their original contexts are increasingly endangered. It is crucial to support indigenous cultures and learn what shamanism and related systems of healing have to offer the postmodern world before research in library archives becomes the only method for investigating these healing systems. The longevity of these indigenous health systems indicates that they have served many groups of people quite well over the millennia. The question remains as to what they can offer a world where allopathic biomedicine is not only revered but also powerful, a world in which reality is constricted to measurable physical dimensions and alternative perspectives are dismissed as folk psychology (Kelly, Kelly, Crabtree, Gauld, Grosso, & Greyson, 2007, p. 54).

This discussion of Pachakuti and Navaho healing models has demonstrated the adaptability of many traditional healing systems to conditions in the contemporary world. The eclectic nature of the system bodes well not only for its survival, but also its compatibility with collegial practitioners of allopathic medicine. Finally, the ecological emphasis of the two systems examined here provides inspiration for ecologists and their colleagues who agree with indigenous practitioners that the Earth is at risk, and that collaborative efforts are needed to redress the natural balance.

NOTES

[1] Among the Navahos the *hataalii* are exclusively male

[2] For example, the sand paintings used in the Blessing Way are crafted from such ingredients as corn meal, flower petals, and charcoal.

[3] These ritual purifications include sweat baths, emetics, fumigants, lotions, herbal medicines, ritual bathing, and sexual abstinence

[4] Premature death and suicide are attributed to sorcery, the return of the dead, or to the presence of outsiders. Kluckhohn (Kluckhohn & Leighton, 1962) noted that funeral rituals are designed to prevent or discourage dead persons from returning to threaten their relatives. The fear of spirit possession is connected with the fear of ghosts, spirits, and the dead. High suicide rates are associated with Navaho communities marked by loss of tribal identity

[5] Both genders are employed as healing practitioners in this tradition; however, for the sake of simplicity, I will use *curandero* to signify shamans of both genders.

References

Achterberg, J. (1985). *Imagery in healing: Shamanism and modern medicine.* Boston, MA: Shambhala.

Cassell, E. J. (1979). *The healer's art.* Middlesex, England, UK: Penguin.

Freeman, L.W. (2004). *Mosby's complementary & alternative medicine: A research-based approach.* St. Louis, MO: Mosby.

Geertz, C. (1973). *The interpretation of cultures.* New York: Basic Books.

Hufford, D. (1995). Cultural and social perspectives on alternative medicine: Background and assumptions. *Alternative Therapies in Health and Medicine, 1,* 53-61.

Iljas, J. (2006). *Introduction to psychology: Inner reality, outer reality in diversity.* Dubuque, IA: Kendall/Hunt.

Kelly, E. F., Kelly, E.W., Crabtree, A., Gauld, A., Grosso, M., & Greyson, B. (2007). *Irreducible mind: Toward a psychology for the 21st century.* Plymouth, UK: Rowman & Littlefield.

Kleinman, A. (1995). *Writing at the margin: Discourse between anthropology and medicine.* Berkeley, Cal: University of California Press.

Kluckhohn, C., & Leighton, D. (1962). *The Navajo* (rev. ed.). Garden City, NJ: Natural History Library.

Krippner, S. (2002). Spirituality and healing. In D. Moss, A. McGrady, T.C. Davis, & I. Wickramasekera (Eds.), *Handbook of mind-body medicine for primary care* (pp.191-201). London, UK: Sage.

Krippner, S., & Welch, P. (1992). *Spiritual dimensions of healing: From tribal shamanism to contemporary health care.* New York: Irvington.

Levi-Strauss, C. (1955). The structural study of myth. *Journal of American Folklore, 78,* 428-444.

Magee, M. (2002). *Peruvian shamanism: The Pachakuti Mesa.* Chelsford, MA: Middle Field.Mahler, H. (1977, November). The staff of Aesculapius. World Health, p. 3.

Miro-Quesada, O. (2002). Foreword. In M. Magee, Peruvian shamanism: The Pachakuti mesa (pp. vii-viii). Chelsford, MA: Middle Field.

O'Connor, B. B. (1995). *Healing traditions: Alternative medicine and the health professions.* Philadelphia, PA: University of Pennsylvania Press.

O'Connor, B. B., Calabrese, C., Cardeña, E., Eisenberg, D., Fincher, J., Hufford, D. J., Jonas, W. B., Kaptchuck, T., Martin, S. C., Scott, A.W., & Zhang, X. (1997). Defining and describing complementary and alternative medicine. *Alternative Therapies in Health and Medicine, 3,* 49-57.

Sandner, D. (1979). *Navajo symbols of healing.* New York: Harcourt, Brace, Jovanovich.

Siegler, M., & Osmond, H. (1974). *Models of madness, models of medicine.* New York: Macmillan.

Torrey, E. F. (1986). *Witchdoctors and psychiatrists:.* New York: Harper & Row.

CHAPTER FOUR

PERSONAL, SOCIAL, AND CULTURAL DIMENSIONS OF HEALTH IN KUSASI ETHNOMEDICINE

Charles Mather

Personal health is an emergent property of social, biological, ecological, psychological, and cultural relationships. Ideally, an effective healing system deals with or satisfies concerns in all of these dimensions of health. A biomedical creation for addressing the multifaceted nature of illness is, at least, nominally a biopsychosocial model of health.

This chapter examines the ethnomedical tradition of the Kusasi from Northern Ghana in order to illustrate how local healing systems satisfy the social, psychological, and cultural needs of groups and individuals. The beliefs that underlie Kusasi medicine relate health to personal identity, status, and role, casting it as an outcome of relations that are simultaneously social, natural, and supernatural. Sickness can never be equated to any one of these dimensions of life alone but, rather, exists as a consequence of a plurality of events and circumstances, not all of which are limited to the physical world.

Despite the introduction of Western biomedicine, hospitals, and clinics over the last 70 years or so, the Kusasi maintain their traditional medical system to deal with the health problems they face. The focus of this chapter is on Kusasi medicine and how it treats health as a physical, social, psychological, and cultural phenomenon. Although the chapter focuses on the traditional ethnomedical system, the reader should note that the Kusasi practice medical pluralism, drawing diagnostic methods and treatments from the traditional system and alternative systems that include biomedicine.

In addition to drawing upon ethnographic fieldwork in and around the town of Bawku, I discuss health in Kusasi ethnomedicine by focusing upon shrines, diviners, and ritualistic beliefs. Shrines are vehicles for ensuring the health of individuals, households, and the larger community. People make shrines out of a variety of objects including: animal horns, animal tails, stones, ceramic vessels, iron bars, manilas, trees, and calabashes. According to Kusasi cosmology, shrines house spiritual agents and forces that influence and determine how people live their lives: They are the cause of good fortune, including being healthy, and misfortune, including suffering from disease and illness. Shrines also serve a very important social function in that they connect individuals together into groups of various sizes and types (e.g., residential units, lineages, clans, tribes), and connect smaller groups to form large groups (e.g., connect lineages into clans, clans into tribes).The presence and use of shrines thus embodies the fact that health is a matter of biological, psychological, social, and cultural factors.

BACKGROUND

The home territory of the Kusasi covers parts of Bawku Municipal, Bawku West, and Garu-Tempane Districts, in the Upper East Region of Ghana, West Africa. Colonial administrators made the first ethnographic observations of the Kusasi during the late 1920s and early 1930s (Lynn, 1937; Rattray, 1932; Syme, 1932). These studies examined Kusasi culture in hopes of better administering the territory as part of the Gold Coast. Over the next seventy years, a host of ethnographic studies have looked at the Kusasi from a developmental perspective with a decided interest in Kusasi agriculture and environment (Benneh, 1972; Blench, 1998; Chilalah, 1957; Cleveland, 1980, 1986, 1989, 1991; Department of Agriculture, 1955; Devereux, 1993; Institute of Development Studies, 1988; Overseas Development Administration, 1989; Warner, 1995; Webber, 1996a, 1996b). Moreover, select scholars have conducted research on Kusasi language (Institute of African Studies, 1968, 1972) marital presentations (Awedoba, 1989a, 1989b, 1990), architecture (Bourdier & Minh-Ha, 1985), and history (Hilton, 1959, 1962).

Anthropologists have yet to concentrate explicitly on Kusasi ethnomedicine, though they have provided some related information. Rattray (1932), for example, discusses local remedies in the context of traditional belief systems and provides information about the association of medicines with shrines.

Similarly, I deal with ethnomedicine as part of the network of beliefs and practices built around shrines (Mather, 1999, 2003). Anthropologists working among related populations from Northern Ghana have made comparable observations (e.g., Fortes, 1945, 1949 among the Tallensi; Goody, 1962 among the LoDagaba; Mendonsa, 1976, 1977, 1978, 1979, 1989 among the Sisala; Kroger, 1982 among the Bulsa; Tait, 1967 among the Konkomba; and Kirby, 1986, 1993 among the Anufo).

The Kusasi are one of many societies that anthropologists have documented in the Savannah region of Northern Ghana. Traditionally, the Kusasi were horticulturalists – subsistence farmers who relied on the seasonal planting and harvesting of cereal crops such as millet and sorghum. Anthropologists sometimes refer to horticultural societies from Northern Ghana as politically acephalous societies, meaning that prior to British Colonial rule they lacked a central form of government. Historically, Kusasi residential groups were extended families living in multi-courtyard compounds that formed the basic political and economic units of their society. Kin relations between residential groups formed the ties that made up larger groups within society, which anthropologists divide into lineages, clans, and tribes. These northern groups have a patrilineal social organizations that pass the inheritance down the male line, maintain polygynous relationships, and practice patrilocal postmarital residence that keep newly married couples among the compound of the husband's father.

Due to the environment they live in and the mode of subsistence they follow, the Kusasi must contend with a variety of factors that cause disease or negatively impact their health. Reliant on rainfall for their agriculture, Kusasi farmers are faced with the spectre of famine in times of drought, an ever-increasing problem. Malnutrition is a major cause of concern because it leads to compromised immune systems, making individuals more susceptible to infection and other diseases. As such, climate is a major health concern since it sets the limits of agricultural productivity.

Climate is a health concern for other reasons. The Savannah region that the Kusasi live in is semi-tropical. A wet season occurs from May to October and a dry season happens from November to April (Ojo, 1977). In the rainy season, increased rainfall provides breeding locales for mosquitoes and other vectors of disease. Health risks include malaria, dengue fever, onchocerciasis, schistosomiasis, and yellow fever. The dry season offers little health relief due to the common occurrence of epidemics of cerebrospinal meningitis, caused by an airborne bacillus moving in dust and sand in wind storms that blow southwards off the Sahara.

Apart from the health impact of climate, the Kusasi are increasingly facing the spectre of infection from tuberculosis, hepatitis, and AIDS. National and regional governments take measures to contend with these health problems; even so, the country unfortunately adopted a cash and carry system where the client pays at the point of use that had devastating effects on the majority of Kusasi and, more generally, the entire population of Northern Ghana. Recently, the country has adopted a national health insurances scheme that shows promise of alleviating the burden of having to pay out of pocket for medical services (Sulzbach & Garshong, 2005).

This chapter consists of observations from two separate periods of ethnographic research. The first period of research took place from July 1996 to April 1997 and focused upon shrines and rituals, while the second period of research occurred from July 4 to August 14, 2005 and dealt with the place of pharmaceuticals in the cultures of Northern Ghana (See Mather, 1999, 2000, 2003, 2005). Both periods of research involved interviewing people about health, illness, medicine, divination, and disease. The first period of research included over two hundred interviews, involving one hundred fifty-six individuals and seven months of observations of a variety of events and behaviors including seasonal festivals, funerals, divination, sacrifices, and medicine production. The second research included twelve interviews with twelve individuals, and two weeks of observation at a licensed chemical store and pharmacy.

The analysis of these observations falls into two parts: The first describes how Kusasi medicine deals with health as a personal, social, and cultural phenomenon; the second deals with the Kusasi's concept of health as simultaneously natural, supernatural, and social in character. Both parts of the description use shrines and their associated rituals for the sake of illustration.

KUSASI MEDICINE AND HEALTH

THE PERSONAL

In Kusasi ethnomedicine, health is an innate capacity within people. It is perhaps best represented by the concept of *win*, a phrase that my study participants refer to as personal destiny. Every person has a *win*, it is something we inherit from our parents and it represents both our uniqueness and our sameness; the soul in Christian belief is an apt analogy. We are unique because each of us has our own *win*, but we are the same because all persons ultimately get their *win* from *Na-Win*, the high god who is the chief of *win*. Personal character and disposition are ultimately reflections of the *win* that *Na-win* passes down to us through our forebears. Hence, the foundation of our personality and our personal health is a spiritual force that imbues the world with the power of creation.

One could think of *win* as a life force that connects health with conception and fertility. A powerful *win* amounts to good health, as well as wealth, fertility, and long-life. Notwithstanding, a powerful *win* can also be a troublesome thing – just as it has great potential to create (e.g., to have children, do hard work, help others, be a *big man*) it also has great potential for sickness and trouble. Consequently, the Kusasi regard hernia and leprosy as symptoms of a powerful *win* or life-force. Just as health is an innate capacity, disease is an innate capacity within people. Too much fertility can result in disease just as readily as too little fertility.

People seek to balance their innate capacities by making timely, appropriate offerings to their *win* shrines. Typically, individuals do not have a *win* shrine of their own until they have become parents, or have had some experience that demands their *win* receive libations and sacrifices directly (i.e., not as part of the libation or sacrifice that their parents' *win* shrines receive). A *win* shrine commonly consists of an orange sized stone placed within a small, plastered dirt mound. The mound is often associated with a small ceramic vessel that contains certain plant materials and water from which the shrine owner will prepare certain medicines. The majority of shrines have the same sort of medicines that serve as remedies for other sorts of ailments. The *win* shrine is usually built into the floor of the compound, most often near the entrance to the individual's bedroom. The shrine placement varies when the individual in question is the head of the compound or residential group. Thus, compound heads – who are almost always men – locate their *win* shrines in the center of the main courtyard of the compound, or in the front yard of the compound. Justification for this placement is that the *win* of the compound head looks after the entire compound, not just the individual, and so the shrine has to be located in a place where the win can survey and protect all of the compound residents.

Two things related to *win* that also play a part in determining the base constitution and psychological disposition of the individual are the guardian spirit or *segr* and the normative method of naming children. A person acquires a *segr* either before they are born or during infancy. The *segr* is a guardian spirit that lets it be known that it wishes to take the child as its spiritual ward. It often announces its intentions by causing a family some sort of misfortune (e.g., recurrent bad luck, poor health, financial loss, agricultural failure) that compels the family to seek out a diviner to find out the source of the problem. Through his divining spirits, the diviner will discover that the segr wishes to take the child as a ward.

Like the *win*, the *segr* remains with the child for his or her entire life. It provides part of the base substance of the individual's character and comportment, and guides and guards the individual throughout life. In reciprocity for the spiritual guidance and protection the individual receives, he or she *serves* the spirits by pouring libations and making sacrifices at the spirits' associated shrines. The *win* shrine appears far more often than shrines for a *segr*. Indeed, 153 of the 156 compounds in my study sample include at least one *win* shrine, while only three compounds include a shrine that residents identified as a *segr*.

Normative rules for naming children also play a part in forging personal identity, and therefore have a bearing in determining personal health. Roughly 70% of the compound heads in my study sample are named after shrines. Classic examples include such common names as Awine (note how the middle three letters spell *win* and denote someone named after a *win* shrine), Abugri (someone named after a shrine made from a horn called *bugr*), and Abagri (someone named after a shrine that houses paternal grandparents called a *bagr*). Given that each shrine houses at least one spirit that plays some sort of role protecting or enhancing the health of those who serve it, the names that people have help protect them from sources of disease or illness.

THE SOCIAL

Revisiting the sources of disease and illness should help illustrate the social dimensions of health. People carry the potential for sickness within them and it arises whenever there is an imbalance in their lives. Sickness may arise from the breaking of taboos such as by committing adultery or seducing someone's wife. In turn, these acts lead to making enemies whose shrines and sacrifices become a likely source for illness and disease as well. Ancestors and other spirits can be held responsible for illnesses experienced by individuals who act detrimentally toward the residential group or descent group. Illnesses are often explained as a result of grievances on the part of ancestors and spirits towards living members of the community, perhaps relating to conflicts, events and people from the past.

Disease can be caused by a variety of supernatural agents and forces, including ancestors, ghosts, spells cast by witches, magical attacks made by owners of specific shrines, and nature spirits. Generally, illness in a compound is traced to a particular agent that has some sort of kin relationship to the client. For a variety of potential reasons, the spirit causes the illness because a social rift exists: for example, a rift between the spirit and the client, a rift between the spirit's descendents and the client and/or client's family, or a rift between the person sending a magical attack and the person receiving the attack.

The Kusasi etiology of disease is part of a more general causal system. In this system, agents or circumstances in the unobservable world cause events in the observable world. The unobservable world includes the past (history), supernatural forces and beings, ancestors, and *Na-Win*. One way to think of the observable world is as the immanent facet of life or the realm of effects. In contrast, the unobservable world is the transcendent facet of life or the realm of causes. The predominant metaphors the Kusasi use for the observable and unobservable realms are, respectively, the *house* and the *bush*. The house is the known, human, social world to which all people belong, while the bush is a wild place inhabited by capricious spirits and forces that threaten the stability and order of the house or social group. The dichotomy between house and bush helps the

Kusasi explain all sorts of misfortunes including diseases and it aids in interpreting individual disease at a different scale, as a symptom of social distress or a tear in the social fabric.

The social dimension of health is also apparent in the creation and use of two different types of shrines, the *ya na'am* or grandfathers, and the *tengbana* or landgod. The *ya na'am* are shrines for paternal parents, grandparents, and great-grandparents of the head of the compound: Tthe individual stones in the mound are called *bagr*. Similar to the *win*, the shrines are made from orange size stones set into plaster mounds of earth. The *ya na'am* are universally located outside the front gate, to the north of the entrance, on the external wall of the *zong*, a building that serves both as a chicken coop, a shelter at night for sheep and goats, and the place of divination and compound ancestors. The head of the compound serves the paternal grandparents to ensure the health of the patrilineage at the core of the residential group. Failure to serve the *ya na'am*, or breaking established tradition, custom, and convention can lead to these ancestors causing disease and other problems for the residential group. As a result, the *ya na'am* are emblematic of the health and well-being of the residential group.

A second type of shrine that well illustrates both the social and environmental dimensions of health is the *tengbana* (literally meaning, skin of the earth) or landgod. Landgods are large stones roughly the size of a soccer ball set into the earth at geographically prominent or unique spots on the landscape, including historically important places. Examples of locales for landgods include perennial springs, waterfalls, crocodile ponds, large trees, hills, rivers, and caves. These stones (singular *kugr*) house the spirits of the land with which the social groups that dwell upon the land have established some sort of covenant or agreement. The landgods provide spiritual protection and guidance for those who dwell upon the landscape that they mark in return for libations and sacrifices provided by the representative of the social group, the *tengindana* or earth custodian.

The spiritual guidance and protection extends to the health of the larger group. In exchange for libations and sacrifices during the two major calendrical festivals – the early millet or *nara* festival and the late harvest or *saman piid* – the landgods ensure the health of the land and hence the health of the social group. The landgods provide fertile fields, rainfall, enhance the fertility of members of the social group, and the fertility of the animals upon which the social group depends for survival: including farm animals like chickens, guinea fowl, cattle, and wild animals taken in the hunt. Accordingly, the landgods provide at the level of the largest social group the same sort of service that the ya na'am and *win* provide at the scale of the residential group and individual respectively.

THE CULTURAL

The cultural dimension of health includes beliefs, values, specialized medical knowledge and practices, and ideas about the causes, diagnosis, and treatment of disease. Kusasi ethnomedicine conforms to what Foster (1976) refers to as personalistic medical systems. Personalistic medical systems follow a comprehensive etiology: They explain disease in the same way that they explain other sorts of misfortune. Naturalistic medical systems, in contrast to personalistic systems in Foster's model, have restrictive etiologies that resist referring to the causes of general misfortunes to explain disease.[1] In the case of the Kusasi, the causes of misfortune are ancestors, ghosts, witches, sorcery, and a variety of malicious spirits. These causes require intervention through ritualistic ceremonies or magic, thus, evincing the inseparability of medicine and magic within the Kusasi healing system and personalistic systems in general.

The Kusasi's multilayered system of causality also defines their etiology as personalistic. Disease has an efficient cause (the agent responsible for the disease), an instrumental cause (the agent or object that makes the disease come about), and an ultimate cause (the reason that this particular person got sick at this particular time and in this particular place). An example should help illustrate the three levels of causality in the Kusasi system.

A person I know has a shrine that he keeps buried in the ground near the front of his compound. The shrine is called *tobig* and the person obtained the shrine to protect his compound, his family, and himself from a rival who he accused of seducing one of his wives (the man married one of the study participant's former wives). Acquisition of the *tobig* was essential because the former wife would reveal to her new husband the sorts of shrines her ex-husband had. The new husband could easily launch some sort of magical attack at the ex-husband, a scenario that might have once seemed negligible to the ex-husband but is now quite likely in light of his perception that his wife was stolen or seduced. In other words, he was attacked once and, thus, has reason to suspect further attacks. Following this line of reasoning, the ex-husband would indeed be sensible if he was proactive and launched a magical attack of his own. Of course, the new husband will have also considered this tactic and might very well be compelled to quickly launch a magical attack first.

If the ex-husband falls ill in this instance, the instrumental cause is likely a curse, spell, or spirit. The efficient cause of the disease would be the new husband or adversary who placed the curse, cast the spell, or sent the malevolent spirit using ritual libation and sacrifice. Finally, the ultimate cause turns out to be the ancestors of a woman who was wronged by the ex-husband's deceased great grandfather. It turns out this ancestor once treated a wife in a dishonorable and terrible manner that ultimately led to her untimely death. Her natal patriline swore an oath against his descendent and this ancestral curse is the ultimate cause of his lack of marital success. A select group of ancestors are causing strife and disharmony in his compound, and the only way for him to rectify this sort of situation is to make amends by offering libations and sacrifices to the ancestors causing his problems.

The etiology of Kusasi medicine determines diagnostic and therapeutic methods. If the causes of disease are spiritual forces, then people require a means of identifying these forces; this need falls decidedly in the domain of ritual and magic. People rely on divination to determine the cause of illnesses and, in Kusasi society, there are different types of ritual specialists who practice divination. In some cases, these people might also provide therapies for the diseases they diagnose, though in the vast majority of cases people acquire medicines from other sources that include specialists in herbal remedies.

The diagnoses of disease occur by way of divination, and one of the most important persons in this regard is the *bakalogo-sup* (person with the *bakalogo* shrine), what my study participants refer to in English as a soothsayer. Divination may be classified as a form of spirit possession. Each session begins with the diviner invoking the spirit by singing its specific song, shaking a rattle in the right hand, tossing cowries with the left hand and reading messages from the spirit in the resulting patterns. Several spirits may be invoked during a session. These preliminary stages provide the general context for the session; they introduce the client's character and problems to the spirits, while also revealing to the diviner the relative disposition of his spirits towards him, the client, and the community. At this stage the spirit may provide directives to the client, as read in the cowries by the diviner. If he is satisfied with the spirit's prescription the client may step away from the session. In the majority of cases, however, the client continues the session, which progresses to the use of a divining stick or to the direct possession of the diviner by the spirits.

The setting for consultations with the *bakalogo-sup* is the *zong*. The *bakalogo-sup's* divining spirit, or *bakalogo*, dwells within his divining bag or *bakalog* with other magical paraphernalia. To communicate with the spirit, the client and diviner cooperate in using the *bakalog duur* or divining stick, a forked branch with a small metal sheath at the bottom end. Sometimes the stick is fashioned of iron. The diviner holds the stick loosely at the forked end and the client holds the opposite end. The client asks questions of the spirit but does not vocalize them, a practical measure that ensures the veracity of the spirit. By hiding the question from the diviner the client eliminates the chance that the diviner can manipulate or alter the answers that the spirit sends. Movements of the stick are choreographed by the bakalogo, much like ghosts, demons and other spirits are said to be responsible for the messages one gets from using a Ouija board.

The client begins by silently telling the spirit why he has come and detailing what problems he hopes to solve. As he presents his problems to the spirit, the client directs the stick towards different objects from the diviner's bag that symbolize the people, actions, and events related to his problem. After outlining his reasons for seeking consultation the client asks direct questions of the bakalogo, using closed questions to get yes or no answers. The spirit answers the client's questions by pointing the divining stick towards the words or drawings the client made in the dirt. The wand may also answer questions in a more hermetic way by pointing towards different articles from the diviner's bag, typically laid out on a goat skin nearby, or by pointing towards parts of the diviner's body or the client's body[2]. It is a complicated system of symbols that takes significant training to understand and interpret. The divining stick reveals more particular details about the problem at hand and provides a restatement of the original synopsis and course of action suggested by the spirit in the tossing of the cowries.

One way to think of this system of divination is that it has an etiology that stresses a converging sequence of causality: The responsible agent is picked from a variety of potential past causes for a present condition (Mendonsa, 1979). The answers given by the divining spirit are not always right. These errors do not mean the magic does not work but, rather, that for whatever reason the consultation was not done correctly, and so it must be repeated. The process continues in this way until the condition resolves, presumably because the real responsible agent was identified and, then, appeased or thwarted.

Once the client identifies the responsible agent he or she makes offerings at the appropriate shrines – the shrines that house the agents responsible – and makes arrangements to acquire medicines from an appropriate source. Sometimes the shrine in question is also used to prepare and store specific medicines; hence, the supernatural force or agent in the shrine has the power to both cure and cause disease. In other cases, the client requests medicines from those who do possess the appropriate shrines.

One of the ironies of Kusasi divination as a means of dealing with disease is that the source of a soothsayer's healing power – the divining spirits – also causes illness. Indeed, spirits make known their intent to be used by an individual for divining by causing that individual to become ill, and frequently the illness takes the form of madness. In order to cure the ailment the afflicted individuals have to either enshrine the spirits, if they have yet to be enshrined, or make the appropriate ritual preparations to transfer the spirits' shrines to their own homes. They also have to make arrangements to train in divination under three senior soothsayers. In a sense, becoming a soothsayer is one of the first steps in the therapeutic process of those who are afflicted by the divining spirits. These same spirits will ultimately provide the neophyte soothsayer with the knowledge of new medicines for treating the diseases that afflict his clients.

SOCIAL, NATURAL, AND SUPERNATURAL DIMENSIONS OF HEALTH

In the Kusasi system the cause of illness is ultimately centered on the person. A person for the Kusasi differs from the Western concept of a unique individual personality; a person is a social persona founded on formal and informal social relationships. Personal identity comes from social designations such as mother, father, brother, sister, boss, slave, master, enemy, friend, etc. Disease often stems from the person's failure in social relationships. A woman becomes sick because her great grandfather is angry that his descendent failed to maintain the family farm. A recently divorced husband becomes ill because his ex-wife's new husband magically attacks him. A child becomes ill because her guardian spirits are unhappy with the sacrifices they have received. The social failure might not be the fault of the sick person; past social failures by ancestors can also result in disease.

Social dimensions of disease and health include care-giving through the actions that friends, family, and specialists (e.g., clinicians and herbalists) perform to help the person who is sick. Elder males consult with diviners to help determine the cause while other household members tend to matters of comfort (bathing, feeding, etc.). In search of treatments, compound members make contact with extended relations who possess needed medicines and/or shrines. The manifestation of disease spurs the activation of a large social network that surrounds the sick individual: either direct friends or relatives, or people to whom the sick person is indirectly connected through friends or relatives.

Sickness compels social recruitment, enlisting aid from those with whom the client or client's family have close social relations. In this sense, sickness is different from disease. Disease is the outward physical manifestation of external agents affecting the individual: agents could be ancestors, germs, essential elements, etc. Sickness, in contrast, is the socially recognized condition of the person experiencing disease. Across cultures, when someone is categorized as being sick, she or he is expected to take on a specific role – the sickness role – with expected patterns of behavior. In Canada, a sick person becomes a client in hospital, receives medical treatment from medical specialists, and is expected to comply with his doctor's or other health provider's orders. Invocation of the sickness role, the classification of a person as being sick, also demands a set of standard behaviors from those connected to the sick person, as well as from the specialists who deal with sick people. For the Kusasi, the demands of sickness require that elders consult with diviners, family and friends provide shrine medicines, and participate in treatment rituals, and household members attend to the sick person.

The social dimension of health does not stop at the borders between the physical and spiritual worlds. Just as health is an emergent property of harmonious relations between kin and coresidents, health emerges out of the harmonious relations between the living and the supernatural beings that cause disease. Balanced spiritual relations equate to both personal and collective well-being. Serving the *win* shrine will facilitate personal health, while serving the *ya na'am* and landgods will help ensure the well-being of social groups. Social groups are defined by reference to ancestors – founders of lineages and clans who, despite being deceased, continue to exercise social authority. Thus, the social dimension of life in Kusasi society, including health, is inseparable from the supernatural dimension of life.

The natural world is also difficult to disentangle from the social and supernatural. When a person inherits a shrine he or she also inherits the ritual and herbal knowledge necessary for using the shrine. The latter type of knowledge includes information about the ecology in that the plant parts and other *materia medica* associated with the shrine have to be gathered from certain locales in the local and regional environment. A crocodile pond bordering the villages of Zorse and Yarigungu, for example, serves as the only nearby locale for select tree species. Gathering the right materials for medicine requires ethnobotanical knowledge and a general sense of the local environment.

Landgods also serve as a type of ecological reserve in that prohibitions exist against harming or using plants and animals living in and around the shrines. The paramount landgod in Zorse, for example, a shrine called Abangkasong, is made up of a large stone set into the ground at the base of an enormous baobab tree in which is located an enormous hive of bees. Settlement residents avoid the tree throughout the year and make a very quiet, reserved approach to the shrine during the major calendrical festivals.

The prominent landgod in Bawku Municipal District exemplifies clearly the way shrines link together society, nature, and the supernatural. Historically, the Kusasi were divided into two sub-tribes: the Agole and the Toende. The Agole reside in the territory that during my fieldwork in 1996-97 made up Bawku East District (now comprising Bawku Municipal and Garu/Tempane Districts) while the Toende reside in the territory that then made up Bawku West District. The paramount landgod of Bawku East District has the same name as the historical name for the district, Agole. The term *agole* simply means up, which makes an appropriate name for the landgod given that it is the tallest hill in the district. At the same time, the Kusal dialect spoken in Agole territory is also called *agole*.[3] Thus Agole is a supernatural agent – the spirit of the land upon which the Kusasi are the original settlers. It is also a natural object, a large hill in the largest formation of hills in Bawku Municipal District. And it is a social phenomenon in the guise of a tribe. The health of the spirit, the environment, and the tribe are entangled in such a way that imbalance in one amounts to imbalance in the others, and balance in one amounts to balance in the others.

CONCLUSION

Although the traditional Kusasi medical system is personalistic, in the contemporary Kusasi world people possess a range of ideas and practices they use to explain and deal with disease. These ideas and practices include biomedicine, something that more people would take advantage of if they had the resources. Antibiotics are available in pharmacies, clinics, hospitals, and table vendors in the villages and towns. People inject and ingest pharmaceuticals to deal with the blood parasites that cause malaria. Likewise, people understand the perils posed by waterborne parasites and other insects. Similar to Canadian society, Kusasi society is characterized by medical pluralism, with the traditional system serving as one of many alternatives that people can choose to deal with sickness.

Despite the fact that these alternative health systems have different origins, different etiologies, diagnostic methods, and therapies, they are not mutually exclusive. Any particular ailment or affliction can be treated drawing upon practices and knowledge from several alternative systems. One of my study participants informed me that he often interprets biomedical causes of disease (e.g., bacteria, viruses, and parasites) as instrumental causes; he uses biomedicine to treat the instrumental causes of disease and divination to deal with efficient and ultimate causes.

The melding of different medical systems that is occurring in contemporary Northern Ghana was made strikingly clear to me during my second period of fieldwork in the summer of 2005. One of the soothsayers that I know informed me about the spirits that he uses to treat clients. One of these spirits is a white doctor named Dr. Gibira who works out of a hospital in a nearby town. The spirit specializes in treating clients suffering from epilepsy, and conducts his practice in the same way that doctors in the hospital practice medicine; that is, Gibira, a physician, conducts daily rounds and works in shifts. The soothsayer realizes the overlap between his form of clinical expertise and that of medical doctors. The result is a syncretic medico-ritual system that combines elements from both biomedicine and Kusasi medicine.

These observations highlight the fact that culture is a dynamic, fluid entity. Human beings are not static creatures and tradition is not some sort of concretized set of customs that never change. We are continually in the act of creating our traditions and giving meaning to our lives in the here and now. Medical pluralism and changes in local ethnomedical knowledge and practice in Kusasi society are reflections of the ever-changing, flexible, and adaptive nature of human culture and society.

NOTES

[1] In addition, there is only one level of causality in naturalistic medical systems: The instrumental, efficient, and ultimate categories are collapsed into a single category. Finally, naturalistic systems do not involve ritual and magic.

[2] The contents of a bag from a diviner in Zorse included a handful of cowrie shells, a mica bead, a large fruit seed, a small leather pouch with two cowries sewn on its front, the heads of two birds, a goat's hoof, a cow tail, a ram's horn, a bull's horn, a calabash rattle, a woolen hat, three brass bell, and the *bakalog duur* or divining stick.

[3] This dialect belongs to the family of Gur languages that the Kusasi speak

References

Awedoba, A. K. (1989a). Notes on matrimonial goods among the Atoende Kusasi, part one. *Research Review, 5*(1), 37-53.

Awedoba, A. K. (1989b). Matrimonial goods among the Atoende Kusasi Contingent prestations, part two. *Research Review, 5*(2), 1-17.

Awedoba, A. K. (1990). Matrimonial goods among the Atoende Kusasi: Matrimonial prestations and exploitation, part three. *Research Review, 6*(1) 49-56.

Benneh, G. (1972). The response of farmers in Northern Ghana to the introduction of mixed farming: A case study. *Geografiska Annaler*, Series B, *54*(2), 95-103.

Blench, R. (1998). Developing common property resource management: Upper east and northern regions, Ghana. ODI Project Proposal.

Bourdier, J-P. & Minh-Ha, T. (1985). *African spaces: Designs for living in Upper Volta.* New York: Africana Publishing Company.

Chilalah, G. C. (1957). Advances in agriculture in Kusasi, Northern Ghana. *Ghana Farmer, 1*, 198-201.

Cleveland, D. A. (1980). *The population dynamics of subsistence agriculture in the West African savanna: A village in Northeast Ghana.* Unpublished doctoral dissertation. University of Arizona, Tucson.

Cleveland, D. A. (1986). The political economy of fertility regulation: The Kusasi of savanna West Africa (Ghana). In H. Pennewerker (Ed.), *Culture and reproduction: An anthropological critique of demographic transition theory* (pp. 263-293). Boulder: Westview Press.

Cleveland, D. A. (1989). Developmental stage age groups and African populations structure: the Kusasi of the West African savanna. American Anthropologist, 91, 401-413.

Cleveland, D.A. (1991). Migration in West Africa: A savanna village perspective. *Africa, 61*, 222-246.

Department of Agriculture. (1955). Dry season vegetable gardening in Kusasi. *Quarterly Newsletter*, IX, 3-5. Gold Coast: Wiszniewski.

Devereux, S. (1993). "Observers are worried": learning the language and counting the people in northeast Ghana. In S. Devereux and J. Hoddinott (Eds.), *Fieldwork in developing countries* (pp. 43-56). Boulder: Lynne Reiner.

Fortes, M. (1945). *The dynamics of clanship among the Tallensi.* London: Oxford University Press.

Fortes, M. (1949). *The web of kinship among the Tallensi.* London: Oxford University Press.

Foster, G. (1976). Disease etiologies in non-Western medical systems. *American Anthropologist, 78*, 773-782.

Goody, J. (1962). *Death, property and the ancestors. A study of the mortuary customs of the Lodagaa of West Africa.* Stanford: Stanford University Press.

Hilton, T. E. (1959). Land planning and resettlement in Northern Ghana. *Geography, 44,* 227-240.

Hilton, T. E. (1962). Notes on the History of Kusasi. *Transactions of the Historical Society of Ghana, 6,* 79-96.

Institute of African Studies. (1968). *Collected field reports on the phonology of Kusaal: Collected Language Notes, 10.* University of Ghana: D. Spratt and N. Spratt.

Institute of African Studies (1972). *Kusal Syntax: Collected Language Notes, 13.* University of Ghana: D. Spratt, and N. Spratt.

Institute of Development Studies. (1988). Distributional effect of cash crop innovation: The peripherally commercialised farmers of North East Ghana. *IDS Bulletin, 19*(2), Sussex: Whitehead.

Kirby, J. P. (1986). *God, shrines, and problem-solving among the Anuf of Northern Ghana.* Berlin: Dietrich Reimer Verlag.

Kirby, J. P. (1993). *White, red and black: Colour classification and illness-management in Northern Ghana.* Unpublished manuscript.

Kroger, F. (1982). *Ancestor worship among the Bulsa of Northern Ghana: Religious, social and economic aspects.* Munich: Klaus Renner Verlag.

Lynn, C. W. (1937). Agriculture in North Mamprussi. *Accra: Department of Agriculture Bulletin, 34.*

Mather, C. (1999). *An ethnoarchaeology of kusasi shrines.* Unpublished PhD Dissertation. Department of Archaeology, University of Calgary, Calgary.

Mather, C. (2000). Kusasi ancestor shrines as historical and social Maps. In M. Boyd, J. C. Erwin and M. Hendrickson (Eds.), *Proceedings of the Entangled Past: The 1997 Chacmool Conference,* (pp. 136-143). Calgary: University of Calgary.

Mather, C. (2003). Shrines and the domestication of landscape. *Journal of Anthropological Research, 59,* 23-45.

Mather, C. (2005). Accusations of genital theft: A case from Northern Ghana. *Culture, Medicine, and Psychiatry, 29,* 33-52.

Mendonsa, E. L. (1976). Elders, office-holders and ancestors among the Sisala of Northern Ghana. Africa, *46,* 57-65.

Mendonsa, E. L. (1977) The Journey of the soul in Sisala cosmology. *Journal of Religion in Africa, 7,* 62-70.

Mendonsa, E. L. (1978). The soul and sacrifice amongst the Sisala. *Journal of Religion in Africa , 8,* 52-68.

Mendonsa, E. L. (1979). Etiology and divination among the Sisala of Northern Ghana. *Journal of Religion in Africa, 9,* 33-50.

Mendonsa, E. L. (1989). Characteristics of Sisala diviners. In A. C. Lehmann and J. E. Myers (Eds.), *Magic, witchcraft, and religion: An anthropological study of the supernatural* (2nd ed.), (pp. 278-288). Mountain View: Mayfield Publishing Company.

Ojo, O. (1977). *The Climates of West Africa*. London: Heinemann Educational Books

Overseas Development Administration. (1989). *Food Security, Seasonality and Resource Allocation in Northeastern Ghana*. ESCOR R4481, London: Devereux.

Rattray, R. S. (1932). *Tribes of the Ashanti Hinterland: Volumes one and two*. The Clarendon Press, Oxford.

Sulzbach, S. & Garshong, B. (2005). *Evaluating the Effects of the National Health Insurance Act in Ghana: Baseline Report*. Retrieved December 10, 2006, from http://www.phrplus.org/Pubs/Tech090_fin.pdf.

Syme, J. G. G. (1932). *The Kusasis. A short history*. unpublished mimeograph.

Tait, D. (1967). Konkomba sorcery. In J. Middleton (Ed.), *Magic, witchcraft, and curing* (pp. 155-170). American Museum Sourcebooks in Anthropology. Garden City: The Natural History Press.

Warner, M. W. (1995). *The dynamics of smallholder agriculture in the Guinea savannah zone of West Africa, with particular reference to Northern Region, Ghana*. Briefing Paper 1. Dept. of Agricultural Economics, Wye College.

Webber, P. (1996a). Agrarian change in Kusasi, North-East Ghana. *Africa, 66*, 437-457.

Webber, P. (1996b). News from the village: Agrarian change in Ghana. *Geography Review, 9*, 25-30.

CHAPTER FIVE

PRESERVERS OF PRE-COLUMBIAN MESOAMERICAN SHAMANISM:
HUICHOL BELIEF SYSTEMS AND
THEIR INDIVIDUAL AND CULTURAL RESULTS [1]

Bruce Scotton

Shortly before the Spanish conquistadores arrived in the Americas to eradicate shamanism as devil worship, the developed shamanic leaders from several great Mesoamerican traditions agreed to preserve their knowledge by sending wise representatives from each tradition to the safest and most remote location they knew, the Sierra Madre. These chosen shamans and their families came from the Olmec, Toltec, Maya, and Aztec cultures and banded together in the Sierra to start a new tribe, the Wirarika.[2] It was the Spaniards who later named them Huichol after their flat-brimmed hats. This chapter will examine the belief systems of the Huichols concerning the world, humanity's place in it, human nature and functioning, and the basis of healing, before exploring the results of these beliefs on individuals and the culture. Last, I will present some case studies that come from my personal experience with Huichol shamanism.

My knowledge and experience of Huichol shamanism comes from what I have learned from Jaichima and her brother Rutury, traditional *marak'ames* from the Sierra Madre now residing in Arizona. For fifteen years they have kindly but firmly taught me from their ancient tradition and their own experience. I acknowledge my profound debt of gratitude owed to them for the lessons both personal and universal I have received.[3]

THE WORLD AND HUMANITY'S PLACE IN IT

In the Mesoamerican worldview as preserved by the Huichols, the universe consists of many worlds, simultaneously existing in different times and dimensions. The familiar physical world is no more exclusively *real* than any of the other worlds, which are spontaneously visited regularly in their culture through ceremonies, visions, dreams, and rituals involving hallucinogenic substances. Shamans or *marak'ames* learn to visit and explore the various worlds at will bring back healing for their patients.[4] Western academics might be tempted to dismiss the Huichol as idealists, but the Huichol accept completely the reality of our physical world as well as others. Subjectivism would better define the Huichol paradigm, for their culture validates those worlds observed by the subject. This definition does not say that they naively believe all possibilities, including those advanced by psychotic individuals. Instead, *marak'ames* have a sophisticated understanding of psychopathology and successfully distinguish psychotic delusions from the strange-but-real experiences of a healthy individual. Using such criteria as internal coherence and validation by other observers, the Huichol test the subjective experiences of their members.

Time is ever present for the Huichol, not linear; it is we who move through it. In an important way, the site of an event continues to manifest that event indefinitely. This timeless view of place helps one understand the confrontations between indigenous peoples and land developers reported in the news. The proposed construction of a new container store just outside Teotihuacan presents a current example of this issue. The site is not just a place where ceremonies were done in the past, but will always be the site where those ceremonies exist and, thus, will always require proper reverence. In other words, certain places contain and convey certain experiences forever. A materially oriented reader might note that all places would be sacred at that rate: to which the indigenous reader would respond, "Now you're starting to get it." Vine DeLoria (1992) describes this quality of indigenous spirituality as leading to a religion of place rather than of time.

Time is also cyclic in addition to being ever-present. Perhaps derived from their expertise in observing the heavens, which resulted in designing a calendar that remains more accurate than the current Gregorian model, Mesoamerican cultures saw time as moving in great cycles. The exact details may change but certain key trends and relationships persist and manifest over and over through the millennia.

All objects are beings with a consciousness. In other words, the Great Mother, *Nakaway*, makes up the world and takes manifestation in many different forms. All beings, including humans, are thus siblings and equally part of God. This stands in contrast to, and creates a very different mindset from the Judeo-Christian schema in which God gives to Adam and his descendants dominion over "every living thing" in the creation account (Genesis, 1:28). Rather than exploit the rest of creation, the Huichol believe that humanity is bound to promote nature's health and well-being because it is our family and it is divine. Creation is conscious; therefore, if we are sensitive and listen well enough, it can aid us as we aid it.

Because the world is primarily Spirit, it is much more mutable than it first appears. The Huichol define Spirit as the self-aware consciousness of an individual being that can travel outside its physical manifestation and persists after the death of that physical manifestation. The term *physical manifestation* is chosen here rather than body because such things as winds and fire, which do not have bodies but still physically exist, are also seen as spirits. A person can change her relationship to the world and physical reality will change too. Furthermore, lessons learned and changes made in other realities have observable results in this physical reality. For instance, *marak'ames* often do healing work in states of conscious dreaming. Patient and doctor will share the same dream and, as a result, bring about healing in the physical world.

One of the characteristics of all worlds is that manifest reality inheres in pairs of opposites: All beings and events contain both good and bad, strength and weakness, light and dark. A favorite insight exercise is to consider the opposite qualities of an event of seemingly obvious value. A windfall has arrived; what are the problems caused? My neighbor teases me mercilessly; what do I gain from the situation? Gods were frequently seen as having two sides or a twin of opposing nature: for instance, Quetzalcoatl, God of Light and Spiritual Transformation, and Tezcatilipoca, God of Darkness and Treachery. Like the cyclic nature of existence, this view of opposing qualities of experience is seen by the Huichol as fundamentally important. To better understand this worldview, the Western observer might recall Hegel's (1817/1959) dialectical method of inquiry or Jung's (1970) view that the hallmark of a developed psyche lies in the ability to simultaneously hold pairs of opposites within the mind.

THE NATURE OF HUMANITY

Akin to all of creation, humans are first of all consciousness. This consciousness temporarily resides in a body but is not confined to that body, even during life. Instead, it is free to range out of the body to other locations, other dimensions, other times, and other beings. As with most skills, some are gifted with this ability from birth, but practice under expert guidance can greatly strengthen innate abilities.

Consciousness can be developed to function more efficiently for the benefit of the individual, community, and universe. Intention and focus are particularly important. *Marak'ames* learn to enumerate and keep in attendance each part of their awareness; when all parts are present there is a deeply creative and profoundly knowing awareness. To illustrate, Jaichima, the senior practitioner of my two guides, carefully followed and aided a difficult transplantation surgery by traveling consciously to the operating room while still physically sitting in the patient's room. For hours she remained in this state seeing and hearing all the events in the surgery, including the thoughts of the participants. If necessary, she could intervene to calm or even suggest needed solutions to the surgeons. Furthermore, she could make direct adjustments when needed to the *beings* of the doctors and patient on the spirit plane. She returned to her body and arose to announce it had gone well; at that moment, the patient was wheeled out to the recovery room after what was indeed a successful procedure.

The following traits are also valuable in becoming a developed healer:

1. Great sensitivity to inner and outer stimuli. In the shamanic world everything is interrelated and all events are meaningful. The student needs to notice what he actually knows but mistakenly disregards.

2. Delicate control of one's activities, known as *delicado*. As the extremely manoeuvrable hummingbird is feared by the eagle because of its needle-like beak, so too is the most delicate action often the most powerful.

3. Willingness to endure pain. Self-sacrifice is essential to being a *marak'ame*. Not only is personal growth dependent on such willingness, but healing is often accomplished by the *marak'ame's* ability to enter the wounding situation with the patient.

In summary, due to our divine nature as part of *Nakaway's* body and siblings to all the rest of creation, humans both have access to knowledge of the working of the world and bear responsibility to sustain that world.

WOUNDING AND HEALING

Each human when born is given a unique design that is exquisitely beautiful and never to be duplicated. However, due to the dual nature of the world, each human is inevitably wounded both physically and psychically. Just as the body is subjected to an unceasing wearing process of accidents, invasions by other beings, and self-inflicted wounds, so too is the mind. Before this process inevitably ends in aging and death, beautiful design inevitably gets dented. Psychological wounding often results in a part of the psyche fleeing to avoid the pain of the wounding situation, splitting from the rest. The fleeing, once started, often continues in response to less painful situations leaving the individual feeling incomplete and alienated much of the time. In addition to reducing the individual's ability to function, the persistence of the split perpetuates and recreates the original wound, never allowing it to heal. The Huichol schema of psychological fragmentation to avoid a painful situation nearly mirrors the Western psychological defense mechanism of dissociation that Jung (1967) proposed was the basic building block of psychopathology.

Healing this sort of wound involves retrieving the lost part or *niño*, bringing it to awareness, and being willing to experience the previously denied wounding event. Some *marak'ames* are powerful enough to retrieve lost niño and work directly with them. Other shamans, like even our most developed psychotherapists, must gradually entice the lost *niño* to feel safe enough to return and then gradually build up to facing the trauma. Shamanic ceremonies help to evoke the repressed experience and to appropriately grieve over the wound. Although widely held among Western observers – my own students and patients included – that such ceremonies work on the basis of the shaman's power of suggestion over the primitive, undeveloped consciousness of the patient, my observations of such ceremonies suggest quite the opposite. Shamans stress the need for the patient to see their own wounding experience and, as such, may support the patient through years of working with ceremonies and dream interpretation to find the lost memory. It should be noted that the *marak'ame* usually has seen the episode from the first, yet, unlike iatrogenically induced false memories, the *marak'ame* knows that the patient must make the discovery her- or himself. The power and accuracy of such work should not be dismissed. I have participated in numerous such ceremonies in which the *marak'ame*, the patient, and I saw the same visions of the wounding event and of the *marak'ame's* psychic administrations. Several of these ceremonies were performed by the *marak'ame* over a long distance, after arranging the time and date and giving her background information on the problem. Despite the physical distance, the congruence of experience of the three participants was strikingly consistent.

With her ability to travel in space and time, to see clearly, and to hear the patient's thoughts, the *marak'ame* often finds the source of the patient's wound. By being willing to enter the painful experience with the patient to some degree, the *marak'ame* models for the patient the conscious will to experience the already existing suffering and proceed with life. Personal sacrifice is a central aspect of Huichol healing and spirituality, and willingness on the part of the patient to choose such sacrifice is essential to healing. The pain inherent in the ongoing woundings in life must be experienced so that the wounding is not prolonged indefinitely in a state of suspension in dissociation. In the cases where the *marak'ame* knows the origin of the wound before the patient can recover the experience, she will continue to work in the spirit world toward healing the trauma but will nonetheless leave the patient to discover its nature.

Similarly, ceremonies to acknowledge and grieve the wound powerfully evoke experiences never fully encountered at the time of the trauma. The shaman frequently advises the patient to bring mementos or photos of themselves from the time of the wounding. Using these reminders, the neurological entrainment generated by repetitive drumming or rattling, and the shaman's ability to assist in shifts of consciousness, the patient relives the experience without dissociating this time. Given the opportunity to feel the hurt, the patient can then grieve appropriately. I have seen such ceremonies lead to healing of medical illnesses such as recurrent headaches, pneumonia, depression and, perhaps most surprisingly, personality disorders.

In addition to denying the impact of the trauma, the patient often has made a silent commitment to accept the perpetrator's responsibility. This centuries-old Huichol insight is echoed in our psychotherapeutic observation that abused children often blame themselves for their parents' abuse. The patient must return the responsibility to the perpetrator either through a ceremony or, if possible, through confronting the person. The procedure includes detailed descriptions of the immediate and long term effects of the wounding experiences. It concludes with the clear statement that the patient has been carrying the burden of the wrong behavior when it does not belong to him or her, that he or she refuses to carry it any longer, and that he or she is returning that burden to the perpetrator with this interaction. The response of the perpetrator – whether it is denial or heartfelt apology – does not matter. Healing occurs in the patient's act of returning the weight of the action of the other, which he or she has carried through the years.

In general, illness results from invasion by other beings, both physical and psychic, and from unhealthy sequestrations of dissociated energy of the patient. In all cases, the *marak'ame* can assist by using her consciousness to shift energy directly and to recruit the patient to shift energy in order to release the *nidus* of pathology.

Plants may also help cure by bringing their particular energy to the aid of the patient. Often plants communicate their medicinal powers to the *marak'ame*, many times going so far as to refer the shaman to a specific plant: "Not me but my grandfather up the hill can help." The Huichol maintain that they heal better than Western medicine in most cases because plants constitute a more complex consciousness than chemicals and can heal a broader spectrum of the patient's needs. Working with a plant enlists an ally; working with a chemical medicine applies brute force.

THE CULTURE RESULTING FROM THESE BELIEFS

The Huichol tribe evinces a broad and lasting commitment to the healing and sustenance of the world. The very name of the tribe in their own language means "those who heal" (Jaichima, personal communication). Every day certain tribe members perform a ceremony specifically designed to sustain and heal our planet and its beings. When confronted with the possibility that someday the Huichol youth, like those of other tribes, might be lured away by the gleam of

Western civilization's technology, a Huichol elder expressed concern, not for the welfare of the elders left behind, but for the welfare of *Nakaway*, our Mother Earth. The Huichol see Western civilization's fascination with shiny material objects like fancy cars, compact discs, films, and fashionable clothes as being a kind of hypnosis that distracts people from the important issues like the well-being of the planet and its creatures. Our way of living leads to deforestation, poisoning of the environment, and global warming because too many people are distracted and simply not aware. By imbuing their youth with a traditional perspective, the Huichols have been extraordinarily successful in preserving their culture. The culture continues to involve community-wide participation in many religious rituals that are timed to celebrate and sustain the seasonal changes, plants, animals, and objects in the surrounding world.

The most respected members of the community are the *marak'ames*, who commit many years of their lives – often twenty or more – to learning to heal and then spend the remainder of their years healing others. The rigorous preparation is almost unimaginable to an outside observer. My *marak'ame* guide Jaichima related that her brother Rutury was identified as a *marak'ame* at birth and then spent four years of his early childhood in a totally dark cave – albeit carefully cared for – so that he might grow up capable of seeing the other world. Other aspects of preparing to do shamanic work include long periods of fasting, sleep deprivation and, often combined with the first two, rigorous hiking over mountain and desert trails. At times the hiking is done blindfolded to develop the ability to see differently. Given that many fall to their deaths from the same mountain paths, the commitment to walk there blindfolded is, again, almost unimaginable. The shamanic ethic is that of selfless focus on the task at hand until it is finished.

The next most respected members of the community are laymen who accept "cargoes" or the commitment to carry community responsibilities such as organizing and paying for one of the annual ceremonies and its accompanying feast. Such commitments may extend for years and exhaust the carrier both physically and financially. Those who adeptly fulfilled their roles as *marak'ames*, cargo carriers, and other contributors to the community, become members of the council of elders, which functions as the decision-making body in political, social, religious, and legal matters. Huichols display a general respect for others and more respect for those who give of themselves. Huichols are described by external observers as generally quiet, gentle, and acutely observant. They describe themselves as consistently aware of the beauty and power of the universe.

CASE REPORTS

Three case reports will convey some sense of the depth of healing the Huichol bring about and the breadth of their modes of intervention, modes of healing that are simply unknown in the West or are dismissed as magical.

CASE STUDY ONE

Catherine was a college-educated, married, fifty-two-year-old woman with three children who had worked all her life in positions of responsibility. However, throughout her adult life she had had several breakdowns marked by extreme anger, destructive acts directed against objects and sometimes herself, apparent hallucinations of others trying to hurt her, hypervigilance, and loss of sleep. These episodes were treated through hospitalizations, antipsychotic and antidepressant medications and on one occasion, shock treatments. Despite the seeming depth of her disorder, she would reconstitute herself without chronic loss of function and seemed to fare as well off medication as on it.

Although she saw several psychiatrists over the course of many years and had foresworn seeing any more, she began to see me due to an impending sense of doom. She was not sure why but knew something was terribly wrong and that she could not hold it back much longer. Without the more dramatic symptoms that accompanied her breakdowns, other self-destructive acts like cutting herself superficially had resurfaced, as did thoughts of suicide. During sessions, we began to carefully go over her life history and it emerged that she had been sexually abused by several people over the years, including two psychiatrists. Her hopelessness grew.

I had begun to work with two Huichol shamans just a couple of years before this time. At one session, Catherine announced she had experienced the strangest dream: She had been visited by a Mexican medicine woman in an embroidered white dress who had shown extraordinary compassion for her, actually cradling Catherine in her arms and rocking her while singing in an unknown language. She awoke feeling at ease and optimistic for the first time in months. I had been told by my Huichol guides that they consciously enter people's dreams and work with them there. Catherine's description of the medicine woman was so close to that of Jaichima that I decided to take a risk and showed her a photo of the elder shaman. Catherine gasped and exclaimed: "That's her! That's who was in my dream!" I had not previously mentioned the shamans or my work with indigenous healers. I checked with the *marak'ame* and she confirmed that she had learned of Catherine's problem while performing a ceremony for me and had indeed gone to help her that night.

Other dreams ensued, many with shamanic content, and much more therapeutic work followed; yet through this combined effort, Catherine's crisis passed. Twelve years later, Catherine has had no further breakdowns and has become the pillar of her family. She has advanced professionally and attributes her improvement to her shamanic/psychiatric treatment.

CASE STUDY TWO

Mark was a forty-five-year-old professional with a doctoral degree from an Ivy League school, married with two children. Having completed fifteen years of analysis, he was reasonably happy in his life and successful in his profession. He began to work with a Huichol shaman out of interest in learning about the spiritual tradition. Although he felt that he had encountered and was managing all the major issues in his life, the shaman helped him see that there was a pattern, heretofore unnoticed despite the analysis, of undue emphasis on sexuality coupled with a pervasive distrust of others. When faced with this realization, he allowed that it felt like there was a very early wound around sexuality and that, despite not having specific memories, he suspected he had been molested. She told him flatly that he had been, by several perpetrators, and that he needed to heal the resultant wounds.

Immediately he remembered an episode: When he was ten he had discovered a baby picture of himself naked on a blanket in a box of family photos. In a manner highly uncharacteristic of him, he had become enraged, tearing the photo apart and angrily demanded that his parents explain why they had kept such a thing around. His mother had told him that the photo was taken by a babysitter and that they had always thought it was benign. He was furious with that babysitter! The shaman told him that he had become so angry because the photo reminded him of something he had worked hard to forget, an early episode of molestation. She said she could see the act but wanted him to remember it and the others.

Mark was aware of the controversy about the induction of false memories of molestation, but he trusted the shaman and decided to pursue it. Over the course of several years, he performed ceremonies under the *marak'ame's* guidance and recovered memories of molestations by four perpetrators: his father being the first. The *marak'ame* described the Huichol conviction that children frequently make long forgotten contracts to carry the burden of responsibility for a parent or other perpetrator and made clear the necessity to return that burden to the person. She taught him a ceremony to do with his father and had him prepare carefully, being very precise about what needed to be said and in what setting.

Mark flew to his parent's home and performed the ceremony with his father. At first the father feigned not knowing what Mark was talking about, but when Mark persisted, describing how the molestation continued to affect him to that day, the father admitted it and apologized. Mark and his father grew much closer and Mark has experienced a dramatic reduction in his sense of being driven by sexuality.

CASE STUDY THREE

I had been working with my two Huichol guides about two years when I attended a week-long workshop with them. The workshop concluded with a visit to their house, which was so filled with sacred objects that it looked like a museum. Masks, yarn paintings, beadwork, and sculptures were everywhere. I found myself particularly drawn to a larger-than-life wooden carving of a human skull covered in Huichol beadwork. The fascination with one object was unusual for me and went on for several hours. Finally, I asked one of the shamans if the skull had been taken out for someone in particular. He confirmed that it had. I asked if I was that person and the shaman agreed. I found myself saying that I felt more prepared for my own death than I was prepared to deal with the loss of a loved one. The *marak'ame* replied that he knew that and that was part of the reason for the mask's presence. He also said he could not say all he knew. In response, I did work on facing the death of a loved one. It was only five months later that my younger sister, who was in good health, died suddenly and unexpectedly.

CONCLUSION

Huichol shamanism, which exists explicitly to preserve the ancient pre-Columbian Mesoamerican healing traditions, is a powerful healing system with access to types of knowledge and healing as yet unknown to Western science. This brief chapter has sketched some of its basic beliefs and practices and has noted some of its effects on the form and preservation of Huichol culture and on the sometimes amazing healing experienced by individuals. Rather than attempting to mimic medicine people, a futile attempt given the deep and lengthy study involved in becoming a *marak'ame*, the Western psychiatrist or psychologist should use this brief introduction to broaden her or his sense of what is possible for the human psyche, to understand the importance of cross-cultural study and travel, and to stretch concepts of the proper range of study for the healing sciences.

<u>NOTES</u>

[1] The following work is an edit of another text.

[2] Archaeologists who might think that the Olmec and Toltec traditions were gone by the time of the conquistadores would be mistaken.

[3] For more information please see http://www.indioshuichol.com.

[4] Patient is used rather than client because the *marak'ames* share with Western physicians the belief that healing requires the patient's acknowledgment that something inside is sick and in need of healing. Neither they nor the author believe such an admission lessens the intrinsic worth of the patient since it is true of all of us.

References

DeLoria, V. (1992). *God is red*. Golden, CO: Fulcrum Publishing.

Hegel, G. (1959). *Encyclopedia of philosophy* (G. E. Mueller, Trans.). New York: Philosophical Library. (Original work published 1817)

Jung, C. G. (1967). *The collected works of C. J. Jung: Volume five. Symbols of transformation* (2nd ed.) (H. Read, M. Fordham, G. Adler, & W. McGuire, Eds., R. F. C. Hull, Trans.). Princeton, NJ: Princeton University Press.

Jung, C. G. (1970). *The collected works of C. J. Jung: Volume fourteen. Mysterium coniunctionis* (2nd ed.) (H. Read, M. Fordham, G. Adler, & W. McGuire, Eds., R. F. C. Hull, Trans.). Princeton, NJ: Princeton University Press.

CHAPTER SIX

HEALING AND THE VISUAL ARTS: A MULTICULTURAL STUDY

Tobi Zausner

Since the beginning of time, cultures throughout the world have used the visual arts as a form of healing. Visual art heals in two ways: through creating it and through viewing it. Making art is so beneficial that artists historically and in the present day will turn to creative activity when they are ill (Zausner, 2007c, 1998). Creativity can relieve stress, reduce the perception of pain, enhance physical well-being, and give great enjoyment. Creating art can also help the recovery process and act as an aid to continuing good health. As an accepted healing practice, making art is now an integral part of creative therapies in industrialized nations.

Looking at art can also heal because we relate to what we see in its beauty, imagery, and symbolism. Not only are healing images found in paintings and sculpture, but they also decorate secular objects such as clothing, furniture, and utensils. As a fundamental part of human culture since prehistoric times, healing images appear prominently in religious rituals and civic occasions. Displayed in this manner, such images can become a source for group identification and social cohesion. Recognizing the symbols of our culture produces a sense of solidarity and the healing experience of being part of a greater whole.

Some symbols of healing are local to a particular society (Eberhard, 1986; Joly, 1967; Williams, 1974), while others such as the mother, the sun, and vegetation are found across cultures and throughout time (Biedermann, 1992; De Vries, 1984; Moon, 1991). Carl Jung (1959/1973) calls these universal symbols *archetypes* and says they are part of our collective unconscious, a stratum of mind that all humanity shares beneath the personal unconscious that is shared by all of humanity. The universality of archetypal symbols gives them great power and, according to Jung (1966), "whoever speaks in primordial images speaks with a thousand voices" (p. 81-82).

HEALING THROUGH VIEWING ART

HEALING THROUGH EMPATHY WITH THE ARTIST'S PERSONAL HISTORY

In addition to archetypal symbols, we can also experience healing by seeing paintings that convey the personal history of an artist. Benefits can occur whether the artist makes pleasant images or those that portray distress. Cheerful images can help the person who creates them and delight the people who view them (Zausner, 2007c). The work of the self-taught painter Aaron Birnbaum (American, 1895-1998) exemplifies the ability for cheerful art to heal. Despite experiencing poverty as a child, facing the difficulties of being an immigrant in America, and sadness over the death of his wife, Birnbaum focused only on happy memories in his art (Mai, 1995). His optimistic portrayals of both country scenes and city life were healing to him and a pleasure to his audience. "The painting is a thing that keeps me alive," said Birnbaum. "It keeps me going and people like it" (cited in Mai, 1995, p. 54).

Images that convey distress can also heal (Zausner, 2007c). Artists find release by expressing their anguish through art and others may identify with this experience. Even if artists articulate their feelings unconsciously, other people who view the work may relate to its subject matter, finding strength and healing through the images. I have had this experience in my own life.

In addition to teaching psychology of art, I am also a professional artist. During a difficult time in my life when an unscrupulous landlord forced me out of my loft, I was creating a large oil painting of a woman pulling a cart filled with sacks through a snowy landscape. Although I did not consciously realize it at the time, the painting was a portrait of my experience. I was symbolically depicting my resolution to continue despite the adversity I faced by painting a figure going forward regardless of the load and the weather. While the painting conveyed my personal distress and determination, other people have also felt a strong affinity with the image because it shows them that they too can go forward despite facing obstacles and carrying a heavy load.

HEALING THROUGH VIEWING RELIGIOUS ART

In addition to secular works, healing symbolism is found throughout religious art because religious imagery often represents feeling nurtured and attaining of a higher level of functioning. Artworks of the Madonna and Child can promote a sense of comfort and nurturance, while other images can become vehicles for inspiration and self-evolution. Jesus and Buddha have long been seen as role models for personal potential. Both were born into human lives, yet through effort they progressed to a state of transcendence. In Jungian psychology, they function as symbols of the self, the highest level of personality maturation. According to Jung (1956/1976), Jesus "from the point of view of psychology and comparative religion, is a typical manifestation of the self" (p. 392). By seeing depictions of these divinities and knowing how they surmounted obstacles to achieve transcendence, devotees may be inspired to face their own lives with greater courage and determination. In doing so they may put themselves on a path of self-evolution where their highest aspects can emerge.

HEALING THROUGH VIEWING CULTURAL SYMBOLS

Because it brings us together into the security of a functioning group, art can also be socially healing. Secular symbols like flags promote feelings of national identity and promote healing by bringing individuals into a unified whole, giving them civic pride, a sense of belonging, and social cohesion. Flags function symbolically, both through the individual elements in their design and as unified images symbolizing their countries. The flag of the United States of America, for example, combines the thirteen stripes referring to its original colonies and stars representing its states into a visual whole. The combined image is instantly recognizable within its society and its presence is nearly ubiquitous, appearing on government buildings and postage stamps to voluntary display outside homes and on clothing.

Like flags, clothing and body decoration can also be emotionally healing as signs of belonging and acceptance. These unifying symbols not only bring the feelings of safety that come with membership in a group, but such art also heals by creating the joy of beauty in people's lives. Even in warm climates, like sub-Saharan Africa where clothes are not necessary for protection against the weather, tribal people such as the Nuba of the Sudan decorate their bodies with jewelry, ash, and pigment (Riefenstahl, 1974). These decorations are not only striking but also serve to immediately identify them as Nuba and grant them the full acceptance within their society that is not accorded to people outside the tribe.

In the very cold regions of Northern Canada, Alaska, and Siberia, where clothes are primarily elements of self-preservation, they are also decorated to enhance their attractiveness (Fitzhugh & Crowell, 1988). These decorations beautify the garments and also carry a symbolic message. On the far north Canadian coast the Tlingit tribe uses images of ravens as design motifs for their clothing. In their mythology the raven placed the sun, moon, and stars in the sky, populated the earth, and gave fire to humans (Stewart, 1979). As their most important animal, the raven is considered to be symbol of power, bestowing strength upon the wearer.

The symbolic freight of clothing becomes most obvious in structured subgroups that closely regulate their members' dress, as is the case in the military where standardized uniforms and symbols of rank and achievement signify the individual's specific place in an established hierarchy. By wearing clothing and decoration, individuals promote the stability of their cultural traditions and, in return for this allegiance, they receive membership in and protection from their group.

HEALING IN PREHISTORIC AND ANTIQUE ART: THE GREAT MOTHER

Using visual symbols for healing is so integral to human culture that its origins fade into the mists of prehistory. Some of the earliest examples are the fertility goddesses of paleolithic Europe: the *Goddess of Laussel* found in France (a stone bas relief from c. 22,000-18,000 BCE), the *Goddess* from Dolni Vestonice, Czech Republic (a fired clay statue from c. 20,000 BCE), and the *Venus of Willendorf* unearthed in Austria (a limestone statue from c. 20,000-18,000 BCE) comprise only three examples of this widespread tradition (Baring & Cashford, 1993). All three sculpted figures are very round with full hips, pendulous breasts, and large stomachs suggesting pregnancy. During the difficult life of the paleolithic period, when food could be scarce and the lifespan short, with many dying at birth or in childhood, these voluptuous sculptures were symbols of healing because they denote a time of plenty, successful fertility, and the ongoing existence of the group through new births. Also, as religious objects most likely used in ritual and private devotion, they were probably seen as healing sources of beneficence and prayed to as Mary is in the Christian religion and Kwan Yin is in the traditions of the East.

Like Mary and Kwan Yin, the paleolithic goddess figures are symbolic expressions of the archetype of the Great Mother, which is part of the archetype of the Feminine (Neumann, 1974). As part of the Feminine archetype, the *Goddess of Laussel* and the *Venus of Willendorf* also display associations with the Moon Goddess and the twenty-eight day lunar cycle. The *Venus of Willendorf* has seven rows of carved forms circling horizontally around the top of her head (Baring & Cashford, 1993). Seven is one quarter of the lunar cycle. In her right hand, the *Goddess of Laussel* holds up a bison horn, which is crescent-shaped like the moon. The horn is incised with thirteen notches that Baring and Cashford (1993) believe refer to the thirteen months in a lunar year and the thirteen days of the waxing moon. Since the statue has her left hand on her protruding stomach, it is also possible that the thirteen notches may refer to the thirteenth day of the menstrual cycle, which is during the time of ovulation and heightened fertility.

Women have long been associated with the moon because the lunar cycle approximates the time of the female menstrual cycle; moreover, both cycles are periodic events of renewal (Harding, 1970). The lining of the uterus is shed each cycle so that a new one can take its place and the moon goes through phases of waxing, waning, and disappearing only to reappear after three days of darkness. This periodic renewal implies a healing quality within the Great Mother archetype beyond fertility alone. Lunar symbolism indicates rebirth by showing the renewal of light after darkness. As such, it would give the Paleolithic viewer hope and courage to keep going in spite of difficulties, knowing a time of darkness can lead to rebirth and that, in the cycles of life, light will come again.

Another manifestation of the archetype of the Great Mother is Gula, the Mesopotamian Goddess of Healing. Gula is symbolically associated with the dog: It was unearthing statues of dogs that helped convince McGuire Gibson (1990) of the University of Chicago that the Kassite era temple from 1250 BCE he was excavating belonged to her. Digging in Nippur, an ancient city buried in the Iraqi desert south of Baghdad, Gibson's team found five clay sculptures of dogs and a bronze pendant of a dog to be worn as jewelry. The archaeologists also found small baked clay sculptures of people with their hands on the parts of the body they desired to be cured: One figure was holding its head, another touched its neck, a third placed one hand on its stomach, and the other held its chin. These small votive pieces were undoubtedly used in some form of ritual where seeing images was an integral part of a healing ceremony.

ARCHETYPAL AND LOCAL SYMBOLS OF HEALING

Some archetypal images are associated with healing across cultures. Denoting strength and constancy, the sun is used as a symbol of royalty and national unity. The sun, which supports all life on earth, rises each day undiminished following a night of darkness. King Louis XIV of France called himself the Roi du Soleil (the Sun King), the Japanese flag shows the red rising sun, and lines of solar radiance surround the headdress of the Statue of Liberty to connect the nation symbolically to the sun's power.

Vegetation, which regenerates after being cut down, is a healing symbol of hope and life. One of the most common images worldwide, it is seen in the European-originated style of Art Nouveau (Schmutzler, 1962), the arts of Native America (Penney & Longfish, 1994), and the Japanese decorative arts (Joly, 1967; Kubota, 1984). Prominently featured on the many items we use in daily life – such as clothing, jewelry, rugs, and pottery – vegetation may be the most popular design motif in the world.

While archetypes are found to have similar meanings in many cultures, local symbols exist that only people in a specific society find significant. A local symbol of health in Asian art is the god of longevity called Shou-xing in China and Jurojin in Japan (Eberhard, 1986; Joly, 1967; Williams, 1974). A smiling scholarly old man with a high bald head, he is often shown holding a peach. Because the peach symbolizes immortality, longevity, and springtime, it remains one of the most popular symbols in Chinese art where it often decorates ceramic vases and plates. Another local symbol is the preserved fish found in Japan (Joly, 1967). Objects bearing this motif, such as the small sculptures called *netsuke* and the sword ornaments called *kodzukas*, are given as gifts to people who intend to travel, thereby expressing a wish that their health will be well preserved on the upcoming journey.

Some images have negative connotations in one tradition yet in another place they can carry a positive message of healing. In Europe bats are seen as sinister, while in the Navaho tradition they are the protective guardians of Mother Earth (Moon, 1991). In China, where the word for *bat* and the word for *happiness* (also translated as good fortune) are both pronounced *Fu*, bats are healing symbols of good health, longevity, and joy (Eberhard, 1986; Williams, 1974). The design motif of five bats common throughout Chinese art stands for the Five Blessings: long life, riches, health, love of virtue, and a natural death.

THE ASSIMILATION OF IMAGES AND SYMBOLS

Whether an image is an archetype across cultures or a symbol with local significance, if it is meaningful to the viewer, it has power. One of the reasons symbols are so powerful is that we take them in as we do all other objects in our visual field (Zausner, 2007a). When we view images, they physically enter our body: Looking at an object excites the optic nerve, which then sends impulses into our brain where it is identified. We only realize what we are seeing when its neurologically coded impulses are decoded by the brain into a recognizable object by comparing it with previously stored information. We experience the images in a work of art in the same neurophysiological way we experience the *real* world. We identify images and then respond emotionally by associating them with information from our previous experience.

In a sense, the brain *cross-references* everything we see with everything we have seen and known. This extended line of neural associations also give symbols power because it connects them to everything that they refer to and symbolize. Whether the images are archetypes inherent in collective human consciousness, as Jung theorizes, or symbols with only local significance that are culturally learned, they are powerful because they produce strong associations within us. In viewing these images, we have the feeling that we know what they mean and we respond emotionally to that deep recognition. Recognition is one of our earliest and most powerful experiences. It binds a child to its mother and the mother to her child. Recognition brings the deep immediate comfort of the known, the remembered revisited. Through our profound experience of recognition, symbols become what they symbolize.

HEALING IMAGES AND SYMBOLS IN SHAMANISM AND RELIGIOUS TRADITIONS

The enormous potency of symbols has made them part of religious traditions throughout the world and central to shamanic rituals. Shamans are the healers, the medicine men and women of their tribes (Eliade, 1951/1974). Shamans use a variety of methods to heal people, such as herbal remedies, altered states of consciousness, and rituals to invoke the presence of divinities. These rituals may include only the shaman and the person to be healed or they can be large ceremonies that involve the entire community. To achieve healing in a shamanic tradition, individuals not only view and recognize the images and symbols that are part of the ritual, but, in certain traditions, they may attempt to merge with them through physical contact as a way to absorb their power.

Viewing and physically merging with symbols is central to Navaho sand paintings. These works of art, which are created by using sands of different colors, are meant to heal through their mythological images and through the accompanying prayers that are sung, called a chant or a sing (Moon, 1991; Newcomb, & Reichard, 1975; Reichard, 1977). The Navaho, a Native American tribe living in the southwestern United States, create rituals that can go on for five or nine days. These rites contain songs and a sand painting that are meant to cure a specific illness and to restore physical, emotional, and spiritual well-being. It is through the chants and their images in the sand painting that the deities are invited to participate in the ritual.

Reichard and Newcomb observed that, on the last day of the ceremony, the Chanter paints the body of the individual to be healed with mythological symbols and invites the person to sit down on the painting. Then sand from the feet of the deities symbolized in the painting is pressed onto the individual's feet, sand from their arms onto the person's arms, and sand from their heads onto the person's head. This physical connection between the visual symbols and the individual is made in the hopes of establishing a healing transfer, a spiritual osmosis that passes on the qualities of the divine into the body of the individual desiring a cure.

The Aboriginal people of Australia also pigment themselves with spiritual symbols and create paintings as a form of healing. One of the mythological symbols in their work is the rainbow serpent (Caruana, 1993; Scanlon & Lee, 2001). Signifying water and regeneration, the snake is an icon of hope for a desert land. Because the snake sheds its skin, it forms a cross-cultural image of renewal and an archetypal symbol of healing (Moon, 1991). In Navaho sand paintings, snakes are helpers in the shamanic ritual, and in India, the energies released up the spine during yoga, called *Kundalini*, are represented by entwining snakes (Mookerjee, 1989; Moon, 1991). Even in the West, where snakes have a negative aspect, they still form part of the symbol of the caduceus, which originated in classical Greece (De Vries, 1984).

In Africa, symbolism is central to healing in both Christianity and shamanism. In Christian Ethiopia, works of art showing angels, saints, and biblical figures are often combined with abstract religious designs and used as talismans for protection and healing (Mercier, 1979, 1997). These symbolic images are believed to act on the spiritual causes of illness by exorcising demons and restoring the viewer to good health.

The Kongo peoples of Congo, Zaire, Cabinda, and Angola, create statues called *minkisi* that they used in shamanic rituals to inflict harm or cure illness (Hersak, 2001; MacGaffey, 1993). These statues contain medicine bundles composed of plants, animal products, and earth, which are also adorned with symbols of their power. When an nkisi (the singular form of minkisi) was decorated with shells, which symbolize water, it was considered to have the power to cure diseases of the urinary and reproductive tracts. The shells on the statue were also believed to have an additional benefit as symbols of long life – the shells outlast the animals that inhabited them.

HEALING THROUGH CREATING ART

PSYCHOLOGICAL AND PHYSICAL THERAPY IN CREATING ART

In industrialized societies, the psychological healing power of creativity is central to art therapy because making images facilitates the expression of feelings that may not be available to verbal communication. When these feelings are articulated in art, they are out in the open and can be addressed.

Creating art can also be therapeutic, but art therapy can uncover hidden gifts. The British art therapist Edward Adamson (1990) discusses the case of a woman in-patient who, through creating art, not only resolved emotional difficulties but also acquired such skill that she became an exhibiting artist after leaving the psychiatric hospital. Her creative activity began when she started decorating both the smooth pebbles she collected on visits to the beach and the jagged flint stones that she found in the fields around the hospital. With all of these objects, the woman would let their irregular natural shape suggest the subject matter to depict. A rock with a long projection became the head of an elephant with its trunk, while an approximately oval shaped stone inspired her to paint a Madonna and Child on its surface. "They all demonstrated the release of astounding creative talent which had lain dormant," says Adamson (p. 46), who believed this to be very healing. "She had finally let the outside world in," he explained, (p. 46) "which I felt resonated with the progress in her inner state." The woman's art became so accomplished that a gallery in Ashton, England carried her work.

In addition to its psychological benefits, creating art can also aid physical health. In her work with HIV-positive individuals, the American art therapist Gail Edwards (1993) cites evidence that making art improves immune system functionality. She discusses a thirty-two year old man, whose T-cell count, which is an indication of the body's immune system strength, increased from two hundred to more than five hundred after he started art school. As he continued to make art, the person became even more creative and, although the disease progressed, its course was much slower than expected.

Creativity also heals when it is used as physical exercise in occupational therapy. Making art can provide motivation to restore the use of an arm or hand or to train an alternate hand if the dominant one is no longer available. When a stroke paralyzed the artist Katherine Sherwood's (American, b. 1952) right side, she learned to paint and function with her left hand. "I never appreciated how therapeutic art could be," she said, "until I went through this experience" (Maclay, 1999). At Harlem Hospital's Harlem Horizon Art Studio, Abraham Daniel, who became partially paralyzed after a fall in childhood, uses art as a way to recover both physically and emotionally. "After my accident, I had to learn everything all over again," he said. "It was a slow process, but through painting I was able to use my arm again and, at the same time, express how I was feeling at that moment" (as cited in Vu, 2001).

ARTISTS TURN TO ART FOR HEALING

Most artists are not in occupational therapy or art therapy, yet they have used creativity to heal themselves both physically and emotionally for centuries. When the painter Bartholomeus Spranger (Flemish, 1546-1611) lost his wife and children and felt his health deteriorate as he aged, the artist and art historian Carel van Mander (Dutch, 1548-1606) said, "Art will remain his faithful companion and he will be rejuvenated daily with time-absorbing and pleasure-giving practice" (1604/1936, p. 328).

The following examples only hint at the great number of artists who turn to their creativity to heal. Elizabeth "Grandma" Layton (American, 1910-1993), who used imagery in her recovery from clinical depression, acknowledged the power of creativity by calling one of her works *I'm into Art Therapy* (Lambert, 1995). Even when an illness is incurable, creativity can lessen the experience of pain. Severe rheumatoid arthritis forced Maud Lewis (Canadian, 1903-1970) to support her very crippled right hand with her slightly less crippled left one in order to paint (Woolaver, 1995, 1997). Nevertheless, in spite of ongoing pain, Lewis revealed: "As long as I've got a brush in front of me, I'm all right" (Woolaver, 1997, p. 12). The fabric artist Phyllis Teiko (American, b. 1948) has joint pain and stiffness due to Sjogren's syndrome, an autoimmune disease, but her symptoms seem less severe while she works. "I have Fibromyalgia," she says "but I'm not conscious of it while making art. The pain feels further away and doesn't bother me as much" (Teiko, personal communication, May 15, 2006).

FINDING HEALING WITHIN A CREATIVE TRANCE

Concentrating on the task before them, the artists appear to be in what I call a *creative trance*. This is a dissociative state that gives them pleasure and lessens their experience of pain. Both Hilgard (1977) and Erickson (1967) have found that hypnotic or trance states diminish the perception of pain. In addition, Hilgard believes that hypnotic conditions may enhance creative activity and Gruzelier (2002) found they can also help healing. Csikszentmihalyi (1990, 1996) calls this relaxed and focused state *flow*. He describes flow as an experience of being completely and happily absorbed in an activity. Individuals experiencing a state of flow do not notice distractions from the outside world; they are deeply involved in what they are doing and feel motivated to continue. When challenges are balanced by skills and the goals are clear, the self-consciousness disappears. This state, which is a common occurrence during creativity, is relaxing and can provide needed relief during a time of stress. Francisco Goya (Spanish, 1746-1828) realized this when he said the paintings he made after becoming deaf were not only for income but also "to occupy my imagination, which has been depressed by dwelling on my misfortune" (as cited in Hughes, 2004, p. 130). Creativity provides this relief because it is so consuming. In creating a work of art, the artist loses self-awareness by transferring that awareness onto the work of art.

Cognizance of self becomes cognizance of creativity. The artist dissolves into artwork; the ego becomes submerged in the creative process, and the unconscious comes forward (Zausner, 2007a). This is similar to Hilgard's (1977) connection of a trance state with creativity. When the trance state happens, a person goes beyond their conscious intention to paint the subject matter of their unconscious mind. I have experienced this state during the creative process. While intending to depict a specific person on canvas, there were instances when the face I was painting turned out to look like someone else. Sometimes I did not realize the difference until the face was complete or until another person made me aware of it.

This diminished awareness of self and loss of conscious control during creativity is one of the reasons that artists refer to themselves as channels for creative energy. As Marcel Duchamp (French, 1887-1968) said, "the artist acts like a mediumistic being" (1973, p. 138). The consuming aspect of creativity is so satisfying and centering that artists will fight to stay creative to the point of even making art that only they can see. When Li Kung-lin (Chinese, 1040-1106, also known as Li Lung-mien) was very old and ill, arthritis prevented him from holding a brush (Binyon, 1969). Yet he continued to draw by making lines on the bed sheets with his stiffened fingers. Creating art can restore a feeling of wholeness that physical or emotional illness may have taken away.

MIRRORING, CATHARSIS, CONTROL

Three other healing dynamics in the creative process are mirroring, catharsis, and control (Zausner, 1998). Through mirroring artists see themselves and their world in a work of art, while the experience of catharsis is the deep release of tension that artistic accomplishment provides. Control makes the difficulties in life appear to be more manageable when they are represented in art

HEALING THROUGH MIRRORING IN CREATING ART

Mirroring in a work of art is a reflection of the state of the artist. This act can either be an effort to portray the self and the world as realistically as possible or to alter it to suit our needs. The psychologist and physician Ruth Richards (personal conversation, April, 1998) says that mirroring the self in art can bring forth unexpected material in the form of images and ideas from the unconscious mind. It can make the unconscious conscious. The painted image can inspire a dialogue with the artist who responds to it as an actual person or situation. Although working on cheerful imagery can change the mood of the artist and the viewer, it does not mean that the artist led an easy life. Sometimes a person experiences the exact opposite but chooses to concentrate on subject matter that is positive and pleasurable.

The work of Grandma Moses (Anna Mary Robertson Moses, American, 1860-1961) exemplifies this focus on positive events in creating art. She was born into a poor family in upstate New York and outlived her husband and eight of her ten children. Yet, her paintings show only happy memories, such as the 1951 canvas *Country Wedding* and the 1960 work *Making Horseshoes* (Kallir, 1948; Moses, 1952). Like Aaron Birnbaum, who also focused on optimistic events, Grandma Moses was a memory painter, whose art depicts incidents from her life. Speaking of memory's central role in her work she said, "Memory is history recorded in our brain, memory is a painter; it paints pictures of the past and of the day" (Moses, 1952, p. 3).

Memory paintings, which mirror past experiences, are narratives of an artist's life. Written narratives are associated with improved health (Lepore and Smyth, 2002) and visual narratives also have salutary effects (McNiff, 2004). These positive effects may contribute to the longevity of certain artists. Creativity's positive association with an extended lifespan (Lindauer, 2003;

Richards 2006) is evident in both Moses, who died at 101, and Birnbaum, who died at 103.

Mirroring is intrinsic to self-portraits, where artists define themselves as they are and as they would like to be. We see this mixture of reality and desire in Rembrandt's 1658 (Rembrandt Harmenszoon van Rijn, Dutch, 1606-1669) life-sized self-portrait. His face realistically shows the ravages of time but his gaze is steadfast. Holding his mahl stick (a wooden rod used as an aid in painting) like a scepter, Rembrandt is dressed in a shining gold garment, whose solar symbolism is associated with royalty. Besieged in life, he had already gone bankrupt and lost his great house (Marx, 1960). Nonetheless, in his mirrored self-representation, in creating art he is a king.

Viewing this self-portrait would be very healing for Rembrandt since it provided both hope that his circumstances would change and tangible evidence that he remained powerful in spite of difficulties. By strengthening his optimism for the future and self-confidence in the present, the painting would be emotionally healing through its qualities of empowerment. Because artists often feel divorced from what they create after they finish it, the portrait image would likely inspire Rembrandt's confidence as it appears to be an objective stimulus in the outside world. After completing one of his paintings, Charles Burchfield (American, 1893-1967) said, "It seemed as if it had materialized under its own power" (as cited in Eliot, 1957, p. 236).

All creativity is empowering since observing what has been accomplished can impart a feeling of satisfaction and competence. However, certain pieces of art, like those made by Renée Stout (American, b. 1958), are meant specifically to empower (Harris 1993; Stott, 1998). Fusing the tradition of Kongo *minkisi* with her African-American heritage, Stout created a life-size sculpture showing herself as an *nkisi* in a wish for strength, protection, and healing. Stout also makes art in the hope of healing social violence as seen in her *nkisi* sculpture of the African god Ogun entitled *An Inkisi to Protect Young Black Males 20th Century and Beyond; Ogun-Why Do They Accept Bullets Easier Than They Accept Love?* (Ackland Fund, 1995).

HEALING THROUGH CATHARSIS IN CREATING ART

Through expressing pent up emotions, creativity becomes an ongoing catharsis, a continuing feeling of relief. When it communicates what artists intend to say, it is a conscious catharsis, and when it reveals what they did not realize they had to express, it is an unconscious catharsis. Both serve to release tension during the creative process. As Susan Rothenberg (American, b. 1945) says about finishing a painting, "I'm never satisfied . . . but I stop when the itch is gone . . . when I'm not driven crazy any more" (as cited in Kimmelman, 1997, p. C26). Sometimes artists will create a crisis to start them working because when the tension builds up, they seek catharsis through painting. "Weeks go by and I don't paint until finally I can't stand it any longer," admits Gerhard Richter (German, b. 1932). "Perhaps I create these little crises as a kind of secret strategy to push myself" (cited in Kimmelman, 2002, p. 22).

The physical movements of creating art can also relieve tension. Ch'ên Jung (Chinese, also known as Ch'ên So-Wêng, 13th century), the Taoist painter of dragons, was a tempestuous man who sometimes worked in a wild and furious way, splashing his ink and spitting in his water (Sickman & Soper, 1956, p. 268). In addition, catharsis is part of the feeling of accomplishment that comes when the work is over. Painting is not an action that needs repeating, like housecleaning, where the results are temporary. When a work of art is finished, it gives a sense of completion that brings with it relief and closure.

HEALING THROUGH CONTROL IN CREATING ART

Another healing aspect of art is that artists control what they create. This control becomes especially important when a serious illness has made life seem unmanageable. Since sickness may be perceived as a loss of control over one's body, recreating the illness and its treatment in images can impart a feeling of mastery, a relief from fear, and a changed an attitude of helplessness into one of strength. Through its representation as an image in art, the problem ceases to be an amorphous spectre. Instead, it becomes concrete and less threatening.

Recreating an illness in art is similar to the shamanic technique of displaying the sickness as a tangible object outside the afflicted individual, thus separating the person from the disease. When shamans, such as the Native American Essie Parrish, ritually suck illness out of a person, the affliction may be manifested as an object in the mouth of the healer that is then disposed of ceremonially (Harner, 1982). Creating images of their illness in art also gives artists a feeling of distance from their disease. Like a shamanic extraction, it seems to become an object that is separated from them.

CREATING ART DURING CANCER TREATMENT

Making imagery also helps when aggressive medical treatments alter the body with shunts and scars. In this case, the artist's drive toward perfection can be transferred to the art, not his or her appearance. Both Dan Savage (English, b. 1982), who had testicular cancer, and Darcy Lynn (American, b. 1956), who had immunoblastic lymphoma, made art about their treatment for cancer (Lynn, 1994; Savage, 2004). Their work shows baldness from chemotherapy, radiation markers, bone marrow harvest sites, and vomiting.

Creating images of cancer protocols and their side effects gave the artists a feeling of control in extremely difficult circumstances. Savage and Lynn, who remain well today, say their work strengthened them in a difficult time. Through chronicling the course of their illness and treatment, the art produced became a healing narrative of their experiences. After recovering, they both became public figures who spoke to both medical professionals and general audiences about their sickness and their work. People responded so strongly to these images of cancer, its treatments, and their side effects that one of Savage's paintings was stolen from an auction and Darcy Lynn's work was made in to a book, Myself Resolved: An Artist's Experience with Lymphoma. As Lynn said (1994), "I fought illness with the best weapon I had – my art" (p. ix).

THE NECESSITY OF CREATING ART

Making art is so beneficial that artists have not only recovered their health through creativity but they have also failed to thrive without it (Zausner, 2007c). When Oscar Bluemner's (American born in Germany, 1867-1938) health declined after being badly injured in an auto accident, his doctor forbade him to paint (Barbara Mathes Gallery, 1997; Zilczer, 1979). Sick and denied his creative outlet, Bluemner committed suicide.

In contrast, Lawrence Alma-Tadema (English born in Holland, 1836-1912) and George Tooker (American, b.1920) were fortunately allowed to continue their art after languishing without it. As a young boy Alma-Tadema wanted to be an artist but his family insisted he become a lawyer (Treuherz, 1996). After Alma-Tadema contracted tuberculosis, his doctors, believing the illness was fatal, advised that the boy should be able to do what he wished for the short time remaining to him. In response, the family allowed Alma-Tadema to study art and his health returned. Tooker, who had a chronically inflamed appendix and ulcerative colitis since childhood, also wanted to be an artist but his mother and father directed him toward a career in finance (Garver, 1992; G. Tooker, personal communication, May, 1999). When Tooker was in his twenties, the illness became so severe that his parents relented and let him study art. Tooker's symptoms vanished and he is now eighty-seven and still painting.

CONCLUSION

In conclusion, we see that both viewing and creating visual art have beneficial aspects. As the psychiatrist Silvano Arieti (1976) said, "Although creativity is by no means the only way in which the human being can grow, it is one of the most important. The growth occurs not only in the creative person but in all those who are affected by the innovation" (p. 413).

Evidence for the healing capacity of visual art exists from prehistoric times to the present day in the secular and religious life of cultures around the world. This holds true for non-industrialized societies as well as those that are technologically advanced. Viewing art can heal us through its archetypal images and through symbols local to a specific culture. We can also benefit by seeing narrative paintings of an artist's life, whether the subject matter is pleasant like the imagery in the paintings of Birnbaum and Moses or depictions of serious illness as seen in the art of Savage and Lynn.

Works of art are also beneficial to the people who create them. By expressing themselves visually, artists reduce their stress and enter a state of flow. Here relaxation and concentration combine to produce a condition of trance-like awareness that may reduce the perception of pain and help the healing process. Creating visual art is widely acknowledged as beneficial. It has been incorporated into the creative arts therapy programs of industrialized societies as a way to relieve both physical and emotional difficulties. A multicultural phenomenon since the beginning of human history, visual art continues to beautify our world while also activating the capacities for healing that we all possess.

References

Ackland Fund. Renée Stout. (1995). *Ogun*. Ackland Art Museum, The University of North Carolina at Chapel Hill, 97.6.1. Retrieved September 03, 2006, from http://www.ackland.org/tours/classes/stout.html.

Adamson, E. (1990). *Art as healing*. Boston, MA: Coventure.

Arieti, S. (1976). *Creativity: The magic synthesis*. New York, NY: Basic Books.

Barbara Mathes Gallery. (1977). *Oscar Bluemner: American modernist*. April 12-June 6, 1997. Gallery information accompanying the exhibition.

Baring, A., & Cashford, J. (1993). *The myth of the goddess: Evolution of an image*. London, ENG: Penguin.

Biedermann, H. (1992). *Dictionary of symbolism: Cultural icons and the meaning behind them*. (J. Hulbert, Trans.). New York, NY: Facts on File. (original work published in 1989).

Binyon, L. (1969). *Painting in the Far East*. New York, NY: Dover Publications.

Caruana, W. (1993). *Aboriginal art*. New York, NY: Thames and Hudson.

Csikszentmihalyi, M. (1990). *Flow: The psychology of optimal experience*. New York, NY: Harper & Row.

Csikszentmihalyi, M. (1996). *Creativity: Flow and the psychology of discovery and invention*. New York, NY: HarperCollins.

De Vries, A. (1984). *Dictionary of symbols and imagery*. Amsterdam, NL: North-Holland Publishing Company.

Duchamp, M. (1973). The creative act. In M. Sanouillet & E. Peterson (Eds.), *Salt seller: The writings of Marcel Duchamp* (pp. 138-140). New York, NY: Oxford University Press.

Eberhard, W. (1986). *A dictionary of Chinese symbols: Hidden symbols in Chinese life and thought*. (G. L. Campbell, Trans.). London, ENG: Routledge.

Edwards, G. M. (1993). Art therapy with HIV-positive patients: Hardiness, creativity, and meaning. *The Arts in Psychotherapy. 20*, 325-333.

Eliade, M. (1974). *Shamanism: Archaic techniques of ecstasy*. (W. R. Trask, Trans.). Princeton, NJ: Princeton University Press. (original work published in 1951).

Eliot, A. (1957). *Three hundred years of American painting*. New York, NY: Time, Inc.

Erickson, M. H. (1967). *Advanced techniques of hypnosis and therapy: Selected papers of Milton. H. Erickson*. New York, NY: Grune & Stratton.

Fitzhugh, W. W., & Crowell, A. (1988). *Crossroads of continents: Cultures of Siberia and Alaska*. Washington, DC: The Smithsonian Institution Press.

Garver, T. H. (1992). *George Tooker*. San Francisco, CA: Pomegranate Artbooks.

Gibson M. (1990, September-October). Nippur, 1990: Gula, goddess of healing, and an Akkadian tomb. The University of Chicago, *The Oriental Institute news and notes, 125*. Retrieved August 3, 2006, from http://oi.uchicago.edu/OI/ PROJ/NIP/NN_SEP90/NN_Sep90.html.

Gruzelier, J. H. (2002). A review of the impact of hypnosis, relaxation, guided imagery and individual differences on aspects of immunity and health. *Stress, 5*, 147-163.

Harding, M. E. (1970). *The way of all women*. New York, NY: Harper and Row.

Harner, M. (1982). *The way of the shaman*. Toronto, ONT: Bantam Books.

Harris, M. D. (1993). Resonance, transformation, and rhyme. In M. Wyatt, M. Harris, S. Williams, & D. Driskell, Astonishment & power: *The eyes of understanding: Kongo minkisi / The art of Renee Stout*. (pp. 104-155). Washington, DC: National Museum of African Art and the Smithsonian Institution Press.

Hilgard, E. R. (1977). *Divided consciousness: Multiple controls in human thought and action*. New York, NY: Wiley.

Hersak, D. (2001). There are many Kongo worlds: Particularities of magico-religious beliefs among the Vili and Yombe of Congo-Brazzaville. *Africa; 71*, 614-640.

Hughes, R. (2004). *Goya*. New York, NY: Alfred A. Knopf.

Joly, H. L. (1967). *Legend in Japanese art*. Rutland, VT: Charles E. Tuttle Company.

Jung, C. G. (1966). The spirit in man, art, and literature. (R. F. C. Hull, Trans.). Princeton, NJ: Princeton University Press, Bollingen Series.

Jung, C. G. (1973). *Four archetypes*. (R. F. C. Hull, Trans.). Princeton, NJ: Princeton University Press, Bollingen Series. (Original work published in 1959)

Jung, C. G. (1976). Symbols of transformation. (R. F. C. Hull, Trans.). Princeton, NJ: Princeton University Press, Bollingen Series. (Original work published in 1956)

Kallir, O. (1948). Grandma Moses: American primitive. New York, NY: Doubleday.

Kimmelman, M. (1997, February 21). Two who define today amble in the past. *The New York Times*, pp. C1, C26.

Kimmelman, M. (2002, February 2). An artist beyond isms. *The New York Times*, pp. 18-25, 44, 50, 55.

Kubota, I. (1984). *Opulence: The kimonos and robes of Itchiku Kubota*, (T. Yamanobe, Ed.). Tokyo: Kodansha International.

Lambert, D. (1995). *The life and art of Elizabeth "Grandma" Layton*. Waco. TX: WRS Publishing.

Lepore, S. J., & Smyth, J. M. (Eds.). (2002). *The writing cure*. Washington, DC: American Psychological Association.

Lynn, D. (1994). *Myself resolved: An artist's experience with lymphoma*. Philadelphia: Meniscus Health Care Communications.

Lindauer, M. S. (2003). *Aging, creativity, and art: A positive perspective on late-life development*. New York, NY: Kluwer Academic/Plenum Publishers.

MacGaffey, W. (1993). The eyes of understanding: Kongo minkisi. In M. Wyatt, M. Harris, S. Williams, & D. Driskell (Eds.), *The eyes of understanding: Kongo minkis /The art of Renee Stout.* (pp. 18-103) Washington, DC: National Museum of African Art and the Smithsonian Institution Press.

Maclay, K. (1999, October 13 - 19). A painter reinvents herself: Art professor Katherine Sherwood's stroke forced her to learn to paint left-handed. *The Berkeleyan, 28* (10). Retrieved January 29, 2006, from http://www.berkeley.edu/news/berkeleyan/1999/1013/painter.html.

Mai, A. (1995). A little pepper, a little salt: Aaron Birnbaum. *Folk Art, 20,* Fall.

Mander, C. van. (1936). *Dutch and Flemish Artists.* (C. van de Wall, Trans.). New York: McFarlane, Warde, McFarlane. (Original work published in 1604).

Marx, C. R. (1960). *Rembrandt.* W. J. (Strachan & P. Simmons, Trans.). Paris, FR: Pierre Tisné Éditeur.

McNiff, S. (2004). *Art heals: how creativity cures the soul.* Boston, MA: Shambhala.

Mercier, J. (1979). *Ethiopian magic scrolls.* New York, NY: George Braziller.

Mercier, J. (1997). *Art that heals: The image as medicine in Ethiopia.* New York, NY: The Museum for African Art.

Mookerjee, A. (1989). *Kundalini: The arousal of the inner energy.* London, ENG: Thames & Hudson, 1982. (Reprinted from Destiny Books, Rochester, Vermont)

Moon, B. (Ed.). (1991). *An encyclopedia of archetypal symbolism.* Boston, MA: Shambhala.

Moses, G. (1952). *My life's history.* London, UK: Andre Deutsch Ltd.

Neumann, E. (1974). *The great mother.* (R. Mannheim, Trans.). Princeton, NJ: Princeton University Press, Bollingen Series.

Newcomb, F. J., & Reichard, G. (1975). Sandpaintings of the Navajo Shooting Chant. New York, NY: Dover.

Penney, D, W., & Longfish, G. C. (1994). *Native American art.* Westport, CT: Hugh Lauter Levin Associates.

Reichard, G. (1977). *Navajo medicine man sandpaintings.* New York, NY: Dover.

Richards, R. (2006). Frank Barron and the study of creativity: A voice that lives on. *Journal of Humanistic Psychology, 46,* 352-370.

Riefenstahl, L. (1974). *The last of the Nuba.* New York, NY: Harper & Row.

Savage, D. (2004). *Alluding to illness in art: The pursuit of catharsis.* Unpublished dissertation for the degree of Art: Practice and Theory, University of Lancaster, Lancaster, UK.

Scanlon, J., & Lee, M. (2001). The serpent dreamtime. *Nature Australia, 27,* 36-45.

Schmutzler, R. (1962). *Art Nouveau.* New York, NY: Harry N. Abrams.

Sickman, L., & Soper, A. (1956). *Art and architecture of China.* New Haven: Yale University Press.

Stewart, H. (1979). *Looking at Indian art of the northwest coast.* Seattle, WA: University of Washington Press.

Stott, A. (1998). Transformative triptychs in multicultural America. *Art Journal*, *57*, 55-63.

Treuherz, J. (1996). Introduction to Alma-Tadema. In E. Becker, E. Morris, E. Prettejohn & J. Treuherz (Eds.), *Sir Lawrence Alma-Tadema*. (pp. 11-20). New York, NY: Rizzoli.

Vu, P. (2001, Feb. 10). The art of healing at Harlem Horizon Art Studio. *Columbia University Record*. *26*(14). Retrieved August 2006, from http://www.columbia.edu/cu/record/archives/vol26/vol26_iss14/2614_Healing_Harlem_Studio.html.

Williams, C. A. S. (1974). *Chinese symbolism and art motifs*. Rutland, VT: Charles E. Tuttle Company.

Woolaver, L. (1995). *The illuminated life of Maud Lewis*. Halifax, NS: Nimbus Publishing Ltd./ The Art Gallery of Nova Scotia.

Woolaver, L. (1997). *Christmas with Maud Lewis*. Fredericton, NB: Goose Lane Editions.

Zausner, T. (1998, August). *Mirroring and catharsis: Healing aspects of visual art*. Paper presented at the 106th Annual Convention of the American Psychological Association, San Francisco, CA.

Zausner, T. (2007a), Process and meaning: nonlinear Dynamics and Psychology in visual art. *Nonlinear dynamics, psychology, and life sciences*, *11*, 151-167.

Zausner, T. (2007b). Strength and potential: Everyday creativity and visual art. In R. Richards (Ed.), *Everyday creativity and new views of human nature*. Washington, DC: American Psychological Association.

Zausner, T. (2007c). *When walls become doorways: Creativity and the transforming illness*. New York: Harmony Books / Random House.

Zilczer, J. (1979). *Oscar Bluemner*. Washington, DC: The Smithsonian Institution Press.

CHAPTER SEVEN

KONG (EMPTINESS):
A CHINESE BUDDHIST EMOTION
AND ITS THERAPEUTIC IMPLICATIONS[1]

Louise Sundararajan

According to Frankfurt (1971), while all non-human animals exhibit
desires, only humans exhibit the desire to have certain kinds of desires and not
others. This self-reflexive dimension of desires is referred to by Taylor (1985) as
"second order desires," defined as "the power to evaluate our desires, to regard
some as desirable and others as undesirable" (p. 16, emphasis in original). Thus
we may distinguish between two orders of desires: First order desires are
emotional responses to external stimuli, such as being happy or upset about a
rewarding or frustrating event, respectively; second order desires refer to emotion
in response to one's own experience, for instance pleasure derived from the
experience of pleasure, which constitutes savoring (Sundararajan, in press).
Second order desires have so far been neglected in mainstream psychology
(Sundararajan, 2005): one example being hope theory, examined later (Snyder,
Cheavens, & Michael, 2005). Chinese traditions, in contrast, put a premium on the
self-reflexive dimension of emotions (Averill & Sundararajan, 2006).

This chapter analyzes a second order desire in the Chinese Buddhist tradition known as *kong* (emptiness) and explores its implications for healing. My investigation consists of three parts. First, I situate *kong* in the cultural and historical context of *savoring* and examine the cognitive processes involved in the realization of *kong*, with special focus on cognitive recoding that results in profound transformation of emotional intent. Moreover, the second order desires of savoring and *kong* will be compared and contrasted with the Western contemporary approach to hope as a first order desire.

The main textual sources for this comparative investigation are, on mainstream psychology, the theory of hope by Snyder et al. (2005), and, on savoring and *kong*, a book of aphorisms written by Hung Ying-ming of the sixteenth-century entitled, *Cai-gen Tan,* which translates as discourse on vegetable roots.[2] Although several centuries separate the two books, *Cai-gen Tan* remains an influential book to this day as part of the popular psychology or philosophy of China (something of a Chinese counterpart of the *Chicken Soup for the Soul*). Moreover, to show its relevance to the modern Chinese audience, I consult Wang's (2004) contemporary Chinese commentary of *Cai-gen Tan*. Second, I present selected poems from Chinese classical poetry to illustrate emotions associated with *kong* and savoring. Finally, I explore the therapeutic implications of *kong* with the help of Gendlin's (1981) formulations of *focusing*, a therapeutic approach that approximates the Chinese tradition of savoring.

THE CHINESE NOTION OF SAVORING

An investigation of *kong* needs to start with a review of the Chinese notion of savoring for two reasons: First, phenomenologically, *kong* entails the savoring of loss and grief; second, as a well articulated second order desire, the notion of savoring renders accessible to analysis the cognitive structure and information processing involved in second order desires. Like savoring a taste, a person can also savor an experience. Savoring may be broadly defined as the coming together of experience and meaning, which according to Proust is a rare occurrence: "Proust argued that for the most part experience passes us by – it goes too fast and its sensory basis is dissipated, or our attention moves elsewhere before its meaning can be understood. . . . The coming together of a particular experience and its meaning is rare" (Oatley, 2002, p. 65). Infrequent as it may be, savoring seems to be universal.

There are at least three ways of savoring: Chinese, Indian, and Western. The focus of this chapter is on the Chinese way. The Chinese notion of savoring (Sundararajan, 2004; Sundararajan & Averill, in press) differs from the typical Western formulation as well as from the Indian *rasa*. The Western formulation is confined to positive experiences (Bryant & Veroff, 2007), whereas the Chinese savoring includes negative experiences as well. Also, the concept of *kong* comprises a relatively wider scope of temporality that extends from the subtle incipient phase of things (Sundararajan, 2004) to the aftertaste of an experience (Eoyang, 1993). The Chinese savoring differs from *rasa* in three respects: First, whereas rasa concerns discrete emotions of anger, erotic love, etc. (Shweder & Haidt, 2000), the Chinese savoring gathers multiple emotional states to capture an affective brew; second, whereas *rasa* seeks to transcend the self in its mundane existence, the Chinese savoring is an affirmation of the individual self with its taste, values, and memories as the sole measure of what is worth savoring; and third, whereas *rasa* is oriented towards tasting ultimate reality – Brahman – as its highest aspiration, the Chinese aesthetics of savoring is part and parcel of the Confucian program of self cultivation for social harmony and the art of government (Dehejia, 1996).

To clarify this concept further, I will examine the Chinese notion of savoring along two registers: self-reflexivity and cognitive re-coding.

THE CENTRALITY OF SELF-REFLEXIVITY IN SAVORING

Impetus to the development of savoring may have stemmed from the importance given to self-reflexivity in China (see Sundararajan, 2002; Sundararajan & Averill, in press). According to Berry (2003), the Chinese have five communities, four of which involve interpersonal transactions: the transaction among heaven, earth, and humanity; that between government and the people; that among friends; and that within family. The fifth community, in contrast, entails intrapersonal transactions:

> The fifth community is the community of the individual person with oneself, the harmonious indwelling of the phenomenal ego in the deeper interior self. Because the full development of an authentic self is a basic requirement for the development of the other communities, there is constant mention in Confucian thought of the need for turning inward and reflecting on a person's own thoughts, desires, and actions. (p. 107)

We can differentiate between first order experience and second order awareness: The later becomes available to awareness due to the recursive loop of self-reflexivity, which Zelazo (1996) refers to as "an experience plus an additional experience of that experience" (p. 73). This can be graphically represented as follows:

Experience of X ⟶ experience of (Experience of X).

Zelazo (2000) speculated that there needs to be a mental process "whereby the contents of consciousness are fed back into consciousness so that they can become available to consciousness at a higher level" (p. 158). This phenomenon is generally known as higher-order thought (HOT). According to the HOT theory of Rosenthal (1997), consciousness has a hierarchical structure: First-order consciousness is *expressible* through behavior but not *reportable*; the second-order awareness, in contrast, is *reportable* (see also Lambie & Marcel, 2002). For instance, anger at the level of first order consciousness is expressible through the behavior of slamming the door but not necessarily reportable, as the person may not be aware of his or her own anger. Anger at the level of second order awareness, in contrast, is always reportable: "I am angry when I slammed the door." Likewise, savoring is always reportable: "I am savoring wine." As a reportable experience, savoring entails second order awareness in the hierarchy of HOT.

One major difference between the first order experience of taste and the second order awareness of savoring lies in the fact that the latter is a self-initiated action and cannot be imposed from without. Said differently, an adversary can be given a taste of her or his own medicine, but she or he cannot be made to savor it. This agentic aspect of savoring and its corresponding connotative implications loom large in one of the earliest textual references to flavor, the *Chung Yung*, which stated that: "There is no body but eats and drinks. But they are few who can distinguish flavors" (Legge, 1971, p. 387). The term *zhi*, translated here as *distinguish*, is difficult to translate and literally means cognize. In contrast to the first order experience of taste, to be cognizant (*zhi*) of flavors entails knowing that one knows the flavors. Without the second order awareness of knowing – knowing that one knows – it would not be possible to manipulate one's experience in ways characteristic of savoring, such as prolonging the experience, making fine discriminations of flavor, enjoying unique fusions of taste, and so on.

Even before its aesthetic application to savoring, the second order awareness of knowing played an important role in the moral philosophy of Confucianism. This moral imperative may be a consequence of the immanent notion of the Tao, as Confucius allegedly said in the *Chung Yung*: "The path [Tao] is not far from man" (Legge, 1971, p. 393). Since the Tao is the operative principle of life, a principle followed necessarily by all forms of life from plants to and humans, the difference between the uninitiated and the sage lies in development of consciousness: The former follow the Tao unknowingly, whereas the latter do so knowingly. The main thrust of the Confucian pedagogue was, therefore, to raise consciousness to second order awareness so that people will know that they know, or in Fung's words: "to give people an understanding that they are all, more or less, actually following the Way [Tao], so as to cause them to be conscious of what they are doing" (Fung, 1966, p. 175). The principle of savoring is an aesthetic extension of this moral imperative to develop second order desires.

COGNITIVE RECODING IN SECOND ORDER DESIRES

To recapitulate, second order desire refers to the desire to evaluate the first order experiences. In this self-reflexive evaluation there looms large what Charles Taylor (1985) refers to as the "moral map" that consists of "certain essential evaluations which provide the horizon or foundation for the other evaluations one makes" (p. 39), such as happiness or the good life. Articulation of the moral map has two versions, *strong* or *weak* evaluation (Taylor, 1985). Weak evaluation is based on pragmatic considerations such as the utility value of the object. Strong evaluation, in contrast, is based on moral and ontological categories, such as right or wrong, good or bad, being or non-being. Second order desires tend to be strong evaluations, in contrast to weak evaluations that are prevalent in science.

Strong evaluations with explicit articulation of the moral map can result in cognitive recoding of experiences and even transformation of emotional intent. To illustrate, consider coping with situations in which one's goal attainment is impeded, called *goal block*, from two contrasting perspectives, the scientific theory of hope versus the *Cai-gen Tan*.

The hope theory of Snyder et al. (2005) deals primarily with first order experiences, in which one is immersed on action (Frijda, 2005) such that emotional experiences are understood as the consequences of goal pursuits (Snyder et al., 2005, p. 114), rather than as phenomena in and of themselves. Specifically, emotions "reflect the person's perceived success (positive emotions) or lack of success (negative emotions) in goal pursuit activities" (Snyder et al., 2005, p. 114). The *Cai-gen Tan*, in contrast, deals primarily with second order desires that follow a more complex moral map than the simple laws of stimulus and response. The contrast between the two can be stark. For instance, the hope theory predicts that impediments in pursuit of goals decrease well-being. Not so, says *Cai-gen Tan*. Frustration is good for you and gratification of desires rots like opium or, more literally: "Words that grate on one's ears, and things that frustrate one's desires are the foundation stones for self-cultivation in virtue. A life filled with words pleasant to one's ears, and things gratifying to one's desires is a life buried in opium" (Wang, 2004, p. 24).

Another example of the cognitive recoding of experience via the moral map is the Chinese notion of the golden mean, which is a binocular vision that sees two sides of the same coin – thesis and antithesis – at once. When this principle recodes experience, success is not necessarily positive, nor failure negative, because "extreme engenders its opposite" says *Cai-gen Tan*: "In favor the seeds of calamity are sown, thus it is time to stop and turn around when things are going one's way; after failure things may turn in the opposite direction toward success, thus it is important not to give up when frustrated" (Wang, 2004, p. 31). Like the hinge that maintains equilibrium of a swinging door, one who follows the golden mean treats success and failure alike, since both require the modulation of a delicate sense of balance and proportion, elements that have become definitive of the Chinese notion of well-being.

Second order desires are usually accompanied by second order awareness. At the level of second order awareness, one's attention shifts from awareness of the object that evoked an emotion to reflection on the emotion itself. Such shifts in attention approximate *reflective attending*. This contemplative mode of savoring is different in many respects from the goal pursuits model that marks the hope theory of Snyder et al. (2005). Reflective attending tends to foreground the sensations, feelings, and action readiness – conscious and unconscious tendencies and urges prompted by emotion – that are left out in the calibration of goal pursuits. Reflective attending is also more passive than goal pursuits. Due to its disengagement from goal-oriented reasoning and execution of an action plan, reflective attending is referred to by Frijda and Sundararajan (submitted) as "detachment," which is "an over-arching mental attitude of receptive observation, of unfocused attention that lets information come in from the outside and elicited meanings from within, without prior selection by expectancies and, perhaps, subsequent selection by relevance."

Of particular relevance to savoring is one type of action readiness referred to by Frijda (2007) as *acceptance wriggles*, the actions that aim at maximizing sensory and affective contact with the object. A few examples given by Frijda include: gustatory savoring, which entails inhaling smell and having the food circulate around one's tongue, and aesthetic savoring, which involves being still, turning away from distractions, seeking to let imagination flow, relaxing the body so to allow virtual participation in the scene, and so on. This type of action readiness signifies the emotional intent of acceptance or letting be, which is diametrically opposed to the intent of mastery or control behind agency and goal pursuit.

Whereas savoring is usually associated with the aesthetic experience in the West, making it an unlikely aid in coping with goal block in everyday affairs, the thin line between refinement of emotions in aesthetics and in regular l life is blurred in traditional China (Sundararajan, 1998, 2002, 2004). Can savoring with its acceptance wriggles function as an effective response to goal block? To the extent that savoring, as a second order awareness of experience, has the potential for cognitive recoding of experiences, resulting in possible novel appraisals and transformations of the original emotional intent, the answer is likely to be in the affirmative. To explore this possibility, the remainder of this chapter analyzes *kong*, the Chinese Buddhist notion of emptiness.

THE CHINESE BUDDHIST NOTION OF EMPTINESS

KONG AND DETACHMENT

The Chinese notion of *kong* can be traced back to the Buddhist concept of sunyata, meaning nothingness or emptiness, which is the logical conclusion of the Buddhist doctrine of impermanence of all things. Similar to the Western proverb "vanity, vanity, all is vanity," the appraisal of *kong* tends to be global, such as: "All glamour is empty in the end" (Wang, 2004, p. 80). Typically *kong* entails an appraisal of not only the possible attainment of particular goals, but also the very possibility of having goals and concerns at all. Otherwise put, *kong* names the existential shudder that shakes up the very foundation of things, the very basis of all goals and concerns that the Buddhists call *attachment*. Indeed a common expression for the word *kong* is "ten thousand desires/concerns have become ashes." Or in the words of *Cai-gen Tan*: "What's life like before you were born and after you are dead? Upon such reflections all desires are rendered cold ashes" (Wang, 2004, pp. 303-304). However, *kong* does not spell nihilism: with the deconstruction of attachment comes the consolation of detachment.

Detachment entails a very complex emotional state, a phenomenon aptly captured by the following statement of Meister Eckhart: "Therefore, detachment is the very best thing. It purifies the soul, cleanses the conscience, inflames the heart, arouses the spirit, quickens desire, and makes God known" (as cited in O'Neal, 1996, p. 193). Eckhart's words show how detachment is not to be confused with resignation, nor with social withdrawal in sadness. In comparison to these negative manifestations in response to goal block, detachment is much more complex in structure; it is second order awareness – or savoring – of loss and grief. As such, detachment entails cognitive recoding of the experience resulting in transformation of the original emotional intent. In Eckhart's statement above, this emotional transformation takes the form of a creative combination of opposite emotional intents – *purifies* (the soul) and *cleanses* (the conscience), on the one hand, and *inflames* (the heart) and *arouses* (the spirit), on the other.

Another possibility with radical emotional transformation is taste aversion. In the Buddhist tradition, salience of mortality has often been the trigger for *kong* with its characteristic taste aversion: "Fame and material gain are sweet, but upon the thought of death they both taste like chewing wax" (*Cai-gen Tan*, as cited in Wang, 2004). For individuals with sufficient understanding of the Buddhist notion of impermanence, taste aversion can set in on seemingly innocuous occasions such as when the party is over:

> The guests are crowded in the hall and the revelry is at its height. What a happy occasion! All of a sudden, the water in the clepsydra comes to an end, the candles and the incense go out, and the tea grows cold. What a dreary scene! Disgusting and utterly tasteless. This is the way most things are. (*Cai-gen Tan*, adapted from Isobe, 1926, p. 202)

EMOTION REGULATION AND SAVORING

The emotional transformation involved in the realization of *kong* differs radically from the variety of emotional regulation (Bonanno, 2000) known to psychology.[3] In contrast, the radical cognitive reappraisal of things in *kong* is different from the top down kind of inhibition in emotion regulation by reason or cognition. Emotion regulation through savoring comes close to a relatively neglected type of emotional transformation, which is emotion modified by emotion, a phenomenon quite common in aesthetic experiences (Oatley, 2004). This dynamic process of emotion-to-emotion interaction is usually non-conscious. However, the *kong* experience has a high degree of transparency characteristic of the second-order awareness intrinsic to savoring. For instance, consider the clearly delineated sequence of transformation (in italics) in terms of antecedent, cause, and effect in the above quotation from *Cai-gen Tan*:

> The guests are crowded in the hall and the revelry is at its height [*the initial state*]. What a happy occasion [*original emotion*]! All of a sudden, the water in the clepsydra comes to an end, the candles and the incense go out, and the tea grows cold [*change as antecedent*]. What a dreary scene! Disgusting and utterly tasteless [*new emotion*]. This is the way most things are [*new insight*]. (*Cai-gen Tan*, adapted from Isobe, 1926, p. 202)

In this type of emotional regulation known as savoring, affect and experience are acutely felt. Indeed, the phenomenon of savoring suggests that the goal of emotion regulation may not be inhibitory so much as excitatory – to enhance and deepen emotional experience. In the final analysis, the difference between the Western notion of emotion regulation and the Chinese notion of savoring may be akin to that between a vintner and a connoisseur, as suggested by James Averill:

> The vintner may know all about the production of fine wines but have little appreciation for fine nuances in flavor; his aim is simply to control the processes of production. By contrast, the connoisseur may know little about how wine is produced, and yet have great appreciation for differences in flavor among wines. In the Chinese tradition of savoring, the goal is not so much to regulate one's emotions, but to become an emotional connoisseur. (personal communication, September, 2005)

EMPTINESS IN CLASSICAL CHINESE POETRY

To examine the emotions associated with *kong*, detachment, and savoring more closely, I present in the following pages selected poems from classical Chinese poetry. Consider first the three poems by Meng Chiao (751-814), lamenting the premature death of his child.

Apricots Die Young

Apricots die young: their flowers are nipples which the frost cuts and they fall. They lead me to grieve my late child and to write these poems.

A.

Don't let freezing hands play with these pearls–
If they play with these pearls, the pearls will surely fly loose.
Don't let the sudden frost cut off spring time–
If it cuts off spring, no bright flowering.
Scattering, falling, small nipple buds
In colorful patterns like my dead baby's robes.
I gather them – not a full hand's grasp,
At sunset I return home in hopeless [*kong*] sorrow.

B.

In vain [*kong*] I gather up these stars from the ground,
Yet on the branches I see no flowers.
Sad – a solitary old man,
Desolate – a home without children.
Better the duck that sinks in the water,
Better the crow that gathers twigs for nesting.
Duckling in the waves, breaks through them, still flies,
Fledglings in the wind, ruffled, boasting to one another.
But blossoms and baby will live no more,
I sigh in vain [*kong*], facing these creatures.

C.

Nipping chill, the frost killed spring,
From branch to branch it seemed a tiny knife.
Since the flowers have fallen from the tree's trunk,
Like mountain caves the hollows cry out in vain [*kong*].
Spot after spot – the blossoms that fell to earth,
Dot after dot – like oily drops of light.
Now I know that between heaven and earth,
The millions of things are all fragile.
     (Tr. Steven Owen, as cited in Liu and Lo, 1975, p. 160-161)

Emotions depicted in all three poems by Meng Chiao are variants of the sadness theme: bereavement, grief, loss, sadness, etc. Translated as hopeless in line eight of the first poem, "I return home in *hopeless* sorrow," *kong* is not merely the *hopelessness* or *helplessness* of depression. Indeed, there is a structural difference between *kong* and the rest of the terms in the loss and grief cluster: *kong* is the second order awareness of loss and grief. The instances of *kong* are as follows:

> At sunset I return home in hopeless [*kong*] sorrow
> In vain [*kong*] I gather up these stars from the ground
> I sigh in vain [*kong*], facing these creatures
> Like mountain caves the hollows cry out in vain [*kong*]

Kong expresses the futility – emptiness, uselessness, and meaninglessness – of having sorrow, of gathering the fallen blossoms from the ground, of expressing grief by sighing, or of grieving like the mountain hollows howling in the wind. In all these instances, the term *kong* is a feeling about feeling, a higher order representation of emotions made possible by the recursive loop of self-reflexivity.

Another crucial difference between *kong* and the rest of the loss and grief cluster is that the latter is unequivocal in its negative valence with the former. *Kong* is loss with a consolation. The consolation of illumination or enlightenment is expressed in the realization of impermanence in the envoi of poem C: "Now I know that between heaven and earth,/The millions of things are all fragile."

Consider another example. The following lyric is written by the last ruler of Southern T'ang, Li Yü (937-978), who, in addition to personal tragedies – the death of his wife and their young son – lost his throne and was taken as a captive to the new capital of the usurping Sung dynasty, where he stayed for the rest of his life until his forty first birthday, upon which occasion he was forced to drink poisoned wine and died. This lyric was written during Li Yü's captivity away from his palace:

> Tune: "Ripples Sifting Sand"
> The things of the past may only be lamented,
> They appear before me, hard to brush aside:
> An autumn wind blows in the courtyards and moss invades the steps;
> A row of unrolled beaded screens hangs idly down,
> For now no one comes for all the day.
>
> My golden sword now lies buried deep,
> And all my youth is turned to weeds.
> In the cool of evening, when the heavens are still and the moon
>   blossoms forth,
> I think of all those towers of jade and marble palaces reflected,
> Shining emptily [*kong*] in the Ch'in-huai.
> (Tr. Daniel Bryant, in Liu and Lo, 1975, p. 303)

As can be expected, there is much nostalgia, loss and grief in the last emperor's reminiscences, but the sense of *kong* that concludes the poem extends beyond that of grief. The last emperor thought of the gleaming reflection of his palaces in the river Ch'in-huai and felt empty (*kong*). The translator selected *empty* to express *kong*, but *in vain* would do as well here. In vain is the beauty of the former palaces – all their grandeur in reminiscence only mocks the dethroned ruler. Yet, there is more. *Kong* is the feeling that everything is *empty* to the very core. Indeed the imagery of the shimmering reflections of grandeur captures well this Buddhist sense of emptiness: All that gleaming splendor of towers and palaces, of jade and marble, turns out to be sheer reflection on water, a mirage shot through and through with *nothingness*.

In the present context, the poet/emperor's detachment is manifest in a paradoxical combination of antithetical emotions: On the one hand, the *empty* reflections on water suggest the sentiment of disillusionment and emotional withdrawal; on the other, there is a hint of consolation, an appreciation – so characteristic of savoring – for the aesthetic beauty of things. Without this antithetical emotion the most likely would not have captured that enchanted moment when the moonlight shines forth against the coolness and serenity of the evening sky: "In the cool of evening, when the heavens are still and the moon blossoms forth." We may recall an insight from Meister Eckhart that this paradoxical combination of emotions is characteristic of detachment.

To explore further the structure of detachment, consider the following lines of a lyric by Ou-yang Hsiu (1007-1072):

Recollections of West Lake

Flocks of blossoms gone, yet West Lake's *good*,
Shattered scattered residue of red
As willow down comes misting down
The willow hangs across the wind all day long.

Dispersed without a trace are the pipe songs,
Gone are the tourists of the lake,
Not till then do I realize the emptiness [*kong*] of spring.
I let the thin gauze curtain fall
Fine rain, a mated pair of swallows, coming home.
        (adapted from Tr. Jerome P. Seaton, as cited in Liu and Lo,1975, p. 331, emphasis added)

It is quite common, at least in the Chinese tradition, for a sense of *kong* to follow on the heels of the feeling that the party is over; the tourists are gone and the music bands left the famed West Lake. But more than the realization that spring has come to an end, *kong* produces a self-reflexive appraisal of the poet's attachment to spring as well. The concomitant detachment consists of, again, a paradoxical combination of emotions: On the one hand, there are the sentiments of resignation and emotional withdrawal as suggested by the falling curtain; on the other, there is an appreciation of affective ties as suggested by the return (presumably out of attachment to the nest site) of the mated swallows. Detachment also entails the emergence of a psychological space. It is from this psychological space, cordoned off, as it were, by layers of diaphanous screens – the gauze curtain and the fine rain – that the poet welcomes the returning swallows with renewed appreciation but without attachment. Note the profound transformation of the poet's emotional intent from tenacious attachment to spring – giving up the hope for spring only after the merry making of spring ends – to quiet resignation expressed in letting down the curtain, and then from a sense of loss marked by the departure of spring to a sense of gain as suggested by the returning swallows. But things do not necessarily go full circle; the poet has come to approach loss and gain alike with a grain of detachment.

Along with the emergence of psychological space is the transformation of time. The impetuousness of spring with its festivities is transformed, with the realization of *kong*, into a leisurely, contemplative time, as embodied by the willow that sways gently in the wind all day long. Note the absence of *goal-directed energy* characteristic of *agency thinking* (Snyder, et al., 2005) in this picture. What appears instead are acceptance wriggles (Frijda, 2007): The willow hangs in the wind languidly with as little self determination and purposeful pursuit as the contemplative poet behind the gauze curtain.

Finally, in its movement from attachment to disillusionment, *kong* mimics the taste aversion of disgust, except that in the present context the realization of *kong* entails a double reversal of taste from good to bad, and back again. Shweder and Haidt (2000) found in Medieval Hindu texts a subtype of disgust that entails "horror and disillusionment, as well as world-weariness associated with the quest for detachment, transcendence, and salvation" (p. 403).

The possible connection between disillusionment and disgust as "the rejection response to bad-tasting foods [and by extension, experiences]" (Rozin, Haidt, & McCauley, 2000, p. 644) is intimated at the beginning of the poem in reference to the spoliation of spring: "Flocks of blossoms gone . . . Shattered scattered residue of red" (lines 1, 2). But the implicit disillusionment was countered with the opposite evaluation: Contrary to conventional wisdom, the scene of devastation at West Lake is pronounced "good" (1), in a manner reminiscent of what Rozin (1999) refers to as the *hedonic reversals* characterized by liking objects that initially give rise to aversion, such as preference for the fiery chili pepper. Read along this line, this poem concerns a redefinition of pleasure, and draws the distinction between conventional pleasure that does not survive the spring – or, symbolically, youth – and refined pleasure, which does.

Taken together, this selection of classical Chinese poems demonstrates how the Buddhist notion of emptiness can recode experience to allow for a paradoxical combination of opposite emotional intent – savoring of loss or grief – an interdigitation of the positive emotion of contemplatively savoring and the negative emotion of grief and sorrow. Because of its radical recoding of experience, *kong* signifies a creative response to severe goal block and loss, such a response is best understood in terms of acceptance, not resignation; letting be, not giving up; savoring, not merely coping.

CLINICAL IMPLICATIONS

The Buddhist notion of *kong* brings to light the complexity and creativity inherent in detachment-related phenomena. It also offers an alternative treatment approach to the rhetoric of hope that privileges coping, agency, and goal pursuit. As an alternative response to goal block, the Buddhist *kong* advocates letting be and acceptance that facilitates savoring of experiences, even negative ones.

As a specific instance of savoring, *kong* derives its therapeutic potential from self-reflexive consciousness. In the following paragraphs, I examine more closely the connection between self-reflexivity and healing. Starting with the negative side, deficits in self-reflexive consciousness have been linked to alexithymia (Sundararajan, 2001) and autism (Bogdan, 2000). The positive connection between self-reflexivity and healing is less apparent, but palpably present in one type of psychotherapy that coaches techniques of savoring (see Sundararajan, 2001), namely focusing developed by Gendlin (1981). The following instruction in focusing, for example, is a good approximation of savoring:

> clear a space, stack all your troubles to one side, sit quietly and receptively. Then repeat [to yourself] the most feeling-filled words you have, slowly, a dozen times or so: "I'm scared of it. . . scared of it. . . " And all the time, keep some questions hovering around the words: "What is this "scared"? What does it feel like, inside? Where do I feel it? (Gendlin, 1981, p. 90)

According to Gendlin (1981), this intrapersonal repetition, a self-reflexive feedback loop, eventually inserts a space, a gap, into the assumed unity between words and feeling: "At first the words and feeling may be exactly all one, but after a while you will find the feeling growing somewhat longer, sticking out around the edges of the words" (p. 90). This attempt to get beyond the words in order to immerse more deeply in the ineffable substrata of experience seems to be the information processing strategy shared in common by both savoring and focusing. Gendlin's writing on focusing, therefore, shall serve as our guide in this investigation.

The self-reflexive turn of consciousness consists of a shift of attention on two axes: from external to internal and from physical to mental. Both movements are well articulated by Gendlin's notion of *inward sensing*. First, the term suggests an inward turn of attention from the external environment to internal experiences. Thus Gendlin (1997) writes: "experiencing is simply feeling, as it concretely exists for us *inwardly*, and as it accompanies every lived aspect of what we are and mean and perceive" (p. 15, emphasis added). Second, the term stresses the fact that the self-reflexive turn is simultaneously a transition from the physical to the mental. In cognitive terms, this signifies a transition from the *sensory* experience of physical objects to the *non-sensory* experience of meaning (Mangan, 2001). The shift from bodily sensations to felt sense, from the physical to the mental, is a transition generally considered important for emotional development (see Taylor, Bagby, & Parker, 1997). This inward turn is also important for cognitive development. According to Karmiloff-Smith (1995), this inward attention signifies "the specifically human capacity to enrich itself from within by exploiting knowledge it has already stored, not by just exploiting the environment. Intra-domain and inter-domain representational relations are the hallmark of a flexible and creative cognitive system" (p. 192). However, cognitive accounts of reflexivity fail to differentiate between savoring and self-reflection.

Although both involve self-reflexivity, savoring is not to be confused with the garden varieties of self-reflection. If higher order thought (HOT) (Rosenthal, 1997), characteristic of self-reflexivity, can be divided into two subtypes of hot and cold HOT, savoring would fall under the former and self-reflection under the latter. As a hot HOT, savoring entails a reflexive consciousness that, instead of becoming detached from experience, as abstract thoughts tend to do, moves in the opposite direction to serve the purposes of the pre-reflective and the non-propositional strata of experience, a movement referred to by Wiley (1994) as the *reflexive undertow* of mental representations. The proposed distinction between two types of self-reflexivity, cold HOT and hot HOT, corresponds to two forms of self-focus, variously referred to as analytical versus experiential (Watkins & Teasdale, 2001), conceptual-evaluative versus mindfully aware (Teasdale, 1999), or abstract-evaluative versus concrete process focused (Watkins & Moulds, 2005). Experimental manipulation of the abstract-evaluative self-focus consists of encouraging participants to "think about the causes, meanings, and consequences" of feelings, whereas manipulation of the experiential self-focus, to "focus attention on the experience of" feelings (Watkins & Moulds, 2005, p. 320), a procedure more akin to savoring. The experiential self-focus, relative to the abstract-evaluative self-focus, was found to improve social problem solving in depressed patients (Watkins & Moulds, 2005);

experiential self-focus (Teasdale, 1999), and mindfulness-based cognitive therapy were found to decrease depressive relapses (Williams et al., 2000).

The therapeutic potential of the experiential self-focus involved in savoring may be understood in terms of its information processing strategies. Rogers (1959) draws a distinction between two types of information processing strategies: defensiveness versus openness to experience. According to Pribram and McGuinness (1975), defensive information processing is characterized by "a defensive 'effort' to cope with the situation . . . . to shut off further input, and is reflected in an elevated heart rate and other changes indicative of a lack of readiness to respond meaningfully to the input" (p. 123). Savoring, in contrast, is a receptive mode of information processing, a capability to *let it be*. Further characterized by awareness and acceptance of one's own emotional states, this capacity for savoring is generally known as *affect tolerance* (see Krystal, 1988). Affect tolerance is best described by Hartman (1964) when he refers, in the context of Wordsworth's poetry, to a consciousness that "expresses the freedom of a mind aware of itself, aware and not afraid of its moods or potentialities" (p. 12). The importance of affect tolerance (see Taylor, et al., 1997, and Krystal, 1988) is very well recognized in focusing, as a focusing trainer Cornell (1996) puts it: "The inner climate of *letting it inwardly be* is necessary for inner change" (p. 16). And again, invoking the metaphor of "a welcoming presence," Cornell writes: "A welcoming presence means you are interested in everything you become aware of inside. A welcoming presence gives it [each feeling] the space to be and breathe, evolve and transform" (p. 18).

CONCLUSION

This chapter has examined the Chinese Buddhist notion of emptiness (*kong*) and its therapeutic implications. The phenomena of *kong* were situated in the cultural historical context of savoring, identified as a second order desire, and compared and contrasted with a prominent psychological theory of hope which approaches emotions as first order experiences. Using classical Chinese poetry as illustration, the cognitive processes of *kong* were analyzed in terms of self-reflexivity and cognitive recoding, which evinced potentials for profound transformation of emotional intent. The therapeutic properties of *kong* were further examined in the context of focusing, which is a psychotherapeutic technique that has large margins of overlap and affinity with savoring. For emotion researchers, the Chinese notions of *kong* and savoring help to shed some light on the connection between self-reflexivity and healing, a connection found in both empirical studies of experiential self-focus as well as focusing. For clinicians, the Chinese notion of *kong* offers a valuable set of therapy tools by extending the scope and benefits of savoring to negative experiences as well. For the general reader, *kong* makes possible a serenity that transcends the dichotomy – characteristic of the first order experience – between positive and negative emotions, thereby reiterating the insight of Heidegger: "The soul's greatness takes its measure from its capacity to achieve the flaming vision by which the soul becomes at home in pain" (1971, p. 180).

NOTES

[1] A draft of this paper was presented at the Conference on Religious Emotions, Antwerp, Belgium, September 2005.

[2] I am working from Isobe's (1926) English translation if the *Cai-gen Tan*

[3] Experimental psychology has studied extensively the modification of emotion by something external to the affect system, such as pharmacological or cognitive interventions, for instance cognitive reappraisal (Gross & John, 2003).

References

Averill, J. R., & Sundararajan, L. (2006). Passion and Qing: Intellectual Histories of Emotion, West and East. In K. Pawlik & G. d'Ydewalle (Eds.), *Psychological concepts: An international historical perspective*. Hove, UK: Psychology Press.

Berry, T. (2003). Affectivity in classical Confucian tradition. In W. M. T., & M. E.Tucker (Eds.), *Confucian spirituality* (pp. 96-112). New York: Crossroad.

Bogdan, R. J. (2000). Minding minds/Evolving a reflexive mind by interpreting others. Cambridge, MA: MIT Press.

Bonanno, G. A. (2000). Emotion self-regulation. In T. J. Mayne & G. A. Bonanno (Eds.). *Emotions: Current issues and future directions* (pp.251-285). New York: Guilford Press.

Bryant, F. B., & Veroff, J. (2007). *Savoring: A new model of positive experience*. Mahwah, NJ: Lawrence Erlbaum.

Cai-gen Tan (1926). [Musings of a Chinese vegetarian]. (Y Isobe, Trans.) Tokyo: Yuhodo, Kanda. (Original work published in 16th Century)

Cornell, A. W. (1996). *The power of focusing*. Oakland, CA: New Harbinger.

Dehejia, H. V. (1996). *The advaita of art*. Delhi, India: Motilal Banarsidass.

Eoyang, E. C. (1993). *The transparent eye*. Honolulu: University of Hawaii.

Frankfurt, H. (1971). Freedom of the will and the concept of a person. *Journal of Philosophy, 67*, 5-20.

Frijda, N. H. (2005). Emotion experience. *Cognition and Emotion*, 19, 473-498.

Frijda, N. H. (2007). *The laws of emotion*. Mahwah, NJ: Erlbaum.

Frijda, N. H., & Sundararajan, L. *Emotion Refinement*. manuscript submitted for publication.

Fung Yu-lan. (D. Bodde, Ed.) (1966). *A short history of Chinese philosophy*. New York: The Free Press.

Gendlin, E. T. (1997). *Experiencing and the creation of meaning/A philosophical and psychological approach to the subjective*. Evanston, IL: Northwestern University (Original work published 1962).

Gendlin, E. T. (1981). *Focusing*. New York: Bantam.

Gross, J. J., & John, O. P. (2003). Individual differences in two emotion regulation processes: Implications for affect, relationships, and well-being. *Journal of Personality and Social Psychology, 85*, 348-362.

Hartman, G. H. (1964). Wordsworth's poetry. New Haven: Yale University.

Heidegger, M. (1971). *On the way to language* (P. D. Hertz, Trans.). New York: Harper & Row.

Karmiloff-Smith, A. (1995). *Beyond modularity: A developmental perspective on cognitive science*. Cambridge, MA: MIT Press.

Krystal, H. (1988). *Integration & self-healing:Affect, trauma, alexithymia*. Hillsdale, NJ: The Analytic Press.

Lambie, J., & Marcel, A. (2002). Consciousness and emotion experience: A theoretical framework. *Psychological Review, 109*, 219-259.

Legge, J. (1971). The doctrine of the mean. In *The Chinese Classics* (Vol. I). Taipei: Wen Shih Chi. (Original work published1893)

Liu, W. C., & Lo, I. Y. (Eds.). (1975). *Sunflower Splendor: Three thousand years of Chinese poetry*. Garden City, NY: Anchor.

Mangan, B. (2001). Sensation's ghost: The non-sensory "fringe" of consciousness. *Psyche, 7* (18), http://psyche.cs.monash.edu.au/v7/psyche-7-18-mangan.html.

Oatley, K. (2002). Emotions and the story worlds of fiction. In M. C. Green, J. J. Strange, & T. C. Brock, (Eds.), *Narrative impact: Social and cognitive foundations* (pp. 39-69). Mahwah, NJ: Lawrence Erlbaum.

Oatley, K. (2004). Scripts, transformations, and suggestiveness of emotions in Shakespeare and Chekhov. *Review of General Psychology, 8*, 323-340.

O'Neal, D. (1996). *Meister Eckhart from whom God hid nothing: Sermons, writings, and sayings*. Boston, MA: Shambhala.

Pribram, K. H., & McGuinness, D. (1975). Arousal, activation, and effort in the control of attention. *Psychological Review, 82*, 116-149.

Rogers, C. R. (1959). A theory of therapy, personality, and interpersonal relationships as developed in client-centered framework. In S. Koch (Ed.), *Psychology: A study of a science* (Vol. 3, pp. 184-256). New York: McGraw-Hill.

Rosenthal, D. M. (1997). A theory of consciousness. In N. Block, O. Flanagan, & G. Güzeldere (Eds.), *The nature of consciousness*. Cambridge, MA: MIT Press.

Rozin, P. (1999). Preadaptation and the puzzles and properties of pleasure. In D. Kahneman, E. Diener, & N. Schwarz (Eds.), *Well-Being: The foundations of hedonic psychology* (pp. 109-133). New York: Russell Sage Foundation.

Rozin, P., Haidt, J., & McCauley, C. R. (2000). Disgust. In M. Lewis, & J. M. Haviland-Jones, (Eds.), *Handbook of emotions* (2nd ed., ch. 40). New York: Guilford.

Shweder, R. A., & Haidt, J. (2000). The cultural psychology of the emotions: Ancient and new. In M. Lewis, & J. M. Haviland-Jones, (Eds.), *Handboodk of emotions* (2nd ed. ch. 26). New York: Guilford.

Snyder, C. R., Cheavens, J. S., & Michael, S. T. (2005). Hope theory: History and elaborated model. In J. Eliott (Ed.), *Interdisciplinary perspectives on hope* (pp. 101-118). New York: Nova Science.

Sundararajan, L. (1998). Reveries of well-being in the *Shih-p'in*: From psychology to ontology. In A-T. Tymieniecka (Ed.), *Analecta Husserliana* (Vol. 56, pp. 57-70), Netherlands: Kluwer.

Sundararajan, L. (2001). Alexithymia and the reflexive self: Implications of congruence theory for treatment of the emotionally impaired. *The Humanistic Psychologist, 29*, 223-248.

Sundararajan, L. (2002). The veil and veracity of passion in Chinese poetics. *Consciousness & Emotion, 3*,197-228.

Sundararajan, L. (2004). Twenty-four poetic moods: Poetry and personality in Chinese aesthetics. *Creativity Research Journal, 16*, 201-214.

Sundararajan, L. (2005). Happiness donut: A Confucian critique of positive psychology. *Journal of Theoretiocal and Philosophical Psychology, 25*, 35-60.

Sundararajan, L. (in press). Enjoyment. In D. Sander & K. Scherer (Eds.), *Oxford Companion to the Affective Sciences*. Oxford, UK: Oxford University Press.

Sundararajan, L., & Averill, J. R. (in press). Creativity in the everyday: Culture, self, and emotions. In R. Richards (Ed.), *Everyday creativity and new views of human nature*. Washington, DC: American Psychological Association.

Taylor, C. (1985). *Human agency and language*. Cambridge, MA: Cambridge University.

Taylor, G. J., Bagby, R. M., & Parker, J. D. A. (1997). *Disorders of affect Regulation: Alexithymia in medical and psychiatric illness*. Cambridge, MA:Cambridge University Press.

Teasdale, J. D. (1999). Emotional processing, three modes of mind and the prevention of relapse in depression. *behavior Research and Therapy, 37*, 553-557.

Wang, Q. J. (2004). *The Wisdom of Life in Cai-gen Tan* (in Chinese). Taibai: Cong-wen Guan.

Watkins, E., & Teasdale, J. D. (2001). Rumination and overgeneral memory in depression: Effects of self-focus and analytic thinking. *Journal of Abnormal Psychology*, 110, 353-357.

Watkins, E., & Moulds, M. (2005). Distinct modes of ruminative self-focus: Impact of abstract versus concrete rumination on problem solving in depression. *Emotion, 5*, 319-328.

Wiley, N. (1994). *The semiotic self*. Chicago, Il: University of Chicago.

Williams, J. M. G., Teasdale, J. D., Segal, Z. V., & Soulsby, J. (2000). Mindfulness-based cognitive therapy reduces overgeneral autobiographical memory in formerly depressed patients. *Journal of Abnormal Psychology, 109*, 150-155.

Zelazo, P. D. (1996). Towards a characterization of minimal consciousness. *New Ideas in Psychology, 14*, 63-80.

Zelazo, P. D. (2000). Minds in the (re-)making: Imitation and the dialectic of representation. In J. W. Astington (Ed.), *Minds in the Making: Essays in honour of David R. Olson* (pp. 143-164). Oxford, UK: Blackwell Publishers.

RELIGIOUS BELIEF SYSTEMS AND HEALING

CHAPTER EIGHT

THE INTERFACE AMONG SPIRITUALITY, RELIGION, AND PSYCHIATRY

Andrea Grabovac
&
Nancy Clark

In recent decades, religion and spirituality have figured more prominently within the discipline of psychiatry. The impetus for integrating religion and spirituality within psychiatric practice has been influenced by several factors. First, the world's population has become more migratory, as reflected by diverse cultural and religious traditions that exist amidst Western cosmopolitan cities (Boehnlein, 2006; Kirmayer & Minas, 2000). The impact of migration and globalization requires psychiatrists and other mental health professionals to increase their knowledge of the cultural traditions and belief systems among immigrants and refugees seeking mental health services. In addition, many cultures practice traditional healing methods that are derived from spiritual and religious roots indigenous and salient to their understanding of wellness. This factor challenges clinicians to take on new interpretations and explanations of human behavior and raises the issue of cultural competency (Alarcon, Westermeyer, Foulks, & Ruiz, 1999). Second, spiritual and religious beliefs often define the identity of individuals and communities beyond boundaries of ethnicity and even national identity (Kirmayer, Rousseau, Jarvis & Guzder, 2003; Post,

1998). To overlook spiritual aspects of a patient's culture may devalue the patient's perspective, undermine a successful working alliance, and impede successful negotiation of treatment (Clark, 2005; Kirmayer, Corin, & Jarvis, 2004; Koenig & Pritchett, 1998). Understanding the spiritual and religious belief systems of psychiatric patients allows the clinician to develop a better understanding of health-seeking behaviors and provides insight into the patients' explanatory models for mental health issues, which in turn impacts treatment acceptance and adherence. Third, there is a growing interest in complementary and alternative therapies by patients, in order to have the religious or spiritual component addressed as part of healing (Grabovac & Ganeson, 2003; Sirois & Gick, 2000).

In this chapter, we discuss research in biomedicine and cultural psychiatry that supports the integration of spirituality and religious belief systems with psychiatric clinical practice. The positive associations between mental health and religion and spirituality lie in such factors as salutogenic mechanisms and pathways that may contribute to mental health. Several studies are reviewed that have shown a positive association between mental health outcomes and religion and spirituality even when controlling for confounding variables (Koenig, 1998; Larson, Swyers & McCullough, 1998; Levin & Chatters, 1998; Oman & Thoresen, 2002). The current understanding of the neurobiology of spiritual and religious experience is discussed, which highlights biological mechanisms that may be associated with positive health outcomes.

Cultural psychiatry is described by Kirmayer & Minas (2000) as understanding the impact of social and cultural difference on mental illness and its treatment. From this standpoint, religion, spirituality, and psychiatry are concerned with how identity is defined and affected by interpersonal, social, and cultural processes (Boehnlein, 2006).

We therefore conceptualize the constructs of spirituality and religion through a cultural lens, which offers an alternative epistemology for addressing the complex relationships among religion, spirituality, mental health, and illness. We provide clinical examples of ways to bridge the gap between the Western medical model of mental health and illness and beliefs about healing and wellness from other cultures using the current nosology of the Diagnostic and Statistical Manual of Mental Disorders (American Psychiatric Association, 2000). We conclude this chapter with a review of several clinical assessment tools, including the cultural formulation tool, which may assist clinicians to integrate spiritual and religious domains into practice where appropriate.

DEFINITIONS OF TERMS

In Western society, the terms religion and spirituality have historically varied in meaning and continue to be subject to diverse interpretations influenced by cultural and historical events (Chiu, Emblen, Van Hofwegen, Sawatzky &

Meyerhoff, 2004; Hill et al., 2000; Miller & Thoresen, 2003). Although religion and spirituality differ in their root origins, they are considered almost as synonymous within many cultures (Dein, 2005). Prior to the Enlightenment (1800s), early Christian religion was associated with the concept of faith and included both the subjective experience of worshippers as well as hierarchical organization of the church and monastic life (Dien, 2005). Contemporary Western theorists and social science scholars, however, have focused on the association of religion with fundamental faith, bound by systems of social organization and membership (Dien, 2005; Miller & Thoresen, 2003), whereas spirituality is associated with an individual experience and personal search for meaning (Chiu et al., 2004; Dien, 2005; Zinnbauer, Pargament, Cole et al., 1997; Zinnbauer, Pargament & Scott, 1999). Although conceptual distinctions exist between the constructs of religion and spirituality, how one understands these terms is culturally determined (Dien, 2005; Stewart, 2002). Because of these conceptual distinctions, both terms are used throughout this chapter. Where necessary to maintain clarity, we will refer to these combined concepts as *religion/spirituality*. Currently, there is no accepted single definition of either construct in the social science literature; nevertheless, religion and spirituality form an integral part of the way in which culture can be understood.[1]

HISTORICAL BACKGROUND

Psychiatry as a scientific discipline has recently undergone much criticism for neglecting spirituality and religion in its endeavor to understand mental disorders (Cook, 2004). This neglect is in part related to a lack of cultural understanding by, and education of, mental health professionals about the historical and social processes related to spirituality, religion and mental health. Thus, the influence of religious, spiritual, and cultural beliefs on mental health and illness often remains overlooked in clinical practice (Clark, 2005; Grabovac, Clark, & McKenna in press). In order to understand the current challenges associated with integrating religion/spirituality with mental health delivery, it is important to review first the historical origins of the complex relationship between religion/spirituality and psychiatry. For the purpose of this review we draw heavily on the work of Samuel Thielman (1998) and Harold Koenig (2005), who provide detailed historical accounts on the history of mental health care in the West.

Historically, both Eastern and Western cultures considered mental illness to be caused by natural and supernatural forces. In some cultures, these views have prevailed and continue to determine the care and treatment of those living with mental illness. In the time of Plato (fourth-century BCE), biological or natural causes for mental illness were attributed to the imbalance of four humors.

Plato later described the nature of diseases of the soul as humoral excess (yellow bile, black bile, blood and excess phlegm); it was excess of humors that led to mood variability, such as delusions and hallucinations (Koenig, 2005; Thielman, 1998). Hippocrates in the fifth-century BCE and Galen in the second-century BCE classified the four humors into a taxonomy that described personality types, however, therapy and treatment consisted of what Plato called *charm* or use of soothing words that were capable of healing (Thielman, 1998). Although natural or biological explanations co-existed with supernatural views, early treatment for the mentally ill generally took place in a religious context and may have confounded future interpretations, explanations, and care (Koenig & Larson, 2001; Thielman, 1998). For example, this classical period was heavily influenced by demonological ideas supported by the church and religious orders in the West that downplayed biological explanations of mental illness, using terms such as *possession* and *insanity* interchangeably (Thielman, 1998). Thus, the treatment of individuals was based on a complex history of care that included compassion and persecution (Koenig, 2005).

In the early Middle Ages, religious philosophers such as Bartholomaeus, a Franciscan monk, and Thomas Aquinas made an attempt to support biological mechanisms and workings of the unconscious; these views became widely accepted by 1230-1274 CE (Koenig & Larson, 2001). Demonology lost favor again during the Renaissance (CE 1400-1700) leading to the rise of asylums. With the aid of Johann Weyer, the founder of the modern study of psychopathology, the demonological view declined. Compassionate care arose out of religious faith and personal experience with suffering: For example, St. John of God of the sixteenth-century experienced a psychological breakdown after having a vision of baby Jesus and thereafter devoted his life to care of the sick and mentally ill (Koenig, 2005). Similar movements developed through Christian charity, such as in Gheel, Belgium, where the mentally ill have been cared for by entire communities and families devoted to St. Dymphna (Koenig, 2005). In addition, St. John of the Cross (1542-1591) described depression in his writing *Dark Night of the Soul* as two kinds of melancholy; the first type was described as a kind of spiritual distress that could lead to spiritual growth, the second led to further despair and hopelessness. St. John of the Cross instructed priests of the day to distinguish among the two kinds of depression and to treat those afflicted with compassion (Thielman, 1998).

The Enlightenment introduced the moral movement and the development of asylum care promoted by French physician Phillippe Pinel, who viewed religion as a negative force (Thielman, 1998). Although many factors contributed to the rise of asylum care, its shortcomings contributed to reform motivated by religious commitment and moral obligation to care for the sick. For example, a devoted Quaker, William Tuke, established the York retreat centre in England. Compassionate care was based on the premise that "insanity was a disruption of the mind and the spirit, not just the body," thus providing a more holistic framework for mental health care and practice (Koenig, 2005, p. 24). These movements initiated health promotion for the mentally ill by assisting them to build social connections, find meaning through work activities, and develop a sense of self. The central tenets of care revolved around Christian virtues of self-discipline and work (Koenig & Larson, 2001).

The scientific revolution caused a more radical shift in the way the mind, body, and spirit are viewed. This shift, in the West, discounted the role of supernatural forces and explanations for disease by seeking biomedical explanations, supported by the advent of pharmacological therapies for the effective treatment of mental illness (Josephson, Larson & Juthani, 2000; Koenig & Larson, 2001; Thielman, 1998). Despite these breakthroughs, Koenig (2005) suggests that many of the most important breakthroughs in mental healthcare have been made by persons of faith around the world.

Another important influence on the opinion of religion and spirituality in the psychiatric community comes from early psychoanalytic and cognitive-behavioral approaches. In an effort to have psychiatry accepted as a bonafide science, analysts such as Freud and behaviorists such as Ellis discounted supernatural explanations to follow instead the principles of determinism and naturalism. They went as far as to claim that religion and spirituality are detrimental to mental health. Freud's overt antagonism toward religion has been the subject of much analysis in current research related to spirituality and mental health. Freud's influence on how religion and spirituality have been perceived by the psychiatric community factors into the failure to integrate spiritual and religious matters with psychiatric care for decades (Josephson et al., 2000; Koenig &Larson, 2001; Thielman, 1998). Thielman (1998) describes Freud's concept of religion, not as an individual psychopathology but, rather, as a failed social phenomenon, or pathology of culture. It should be noted, however, that early psychoanalytic theories about religious beliefs were not substantiated by research nor did they take into account the cultural and social context of the individual. Despite its negative views towards religion, psychoanalysis became one of the bases for the development of the clinical pastoral education movement in the mid-twentieth-century (Thielman, 1998).

In contrast to Freud's views, Carl Jung believed in the benefits of religious faith for resolving mental conflict. Jung's concepts of spirituality and the collective unconscious are valid for many cultures (Turbott, 1996). Thus, throughout Western history, biological and supernatural explanations for mental illness have been accepted or refuted by Western scholars. The implications of the debate continue to challenge traditional psychiatric frameworks and practices.

PRESENT CONTEXT

Perhaps because of the historical tensions between religion/spirituality and psychiatry there has been a lack of attention to these issues within psychiatric practice, creating what Lukoff, Lu, and Turner (1992) describe as the *religiosity gap*. Our assumption is that the tensions are lessening and the gap is narrowing with the present resurgence of interest by the scientific community in understanding spirituality. Moreover, recent population health studies and surveys that document increasing public interest in spirituality and religion indicate the necessity for narrowing the religiosity gap. Assumptions made by Freud and others are being challenged by results from rigorous studies in multiple disciplines on the relationships among religion/spirituality and mental health. Furthermore, cultural psychiatry contributed greatly to clarifying the relevance of religious/spiritual beliefs and practices in trauma and loss amongst migrant populations (Boehnlein, 2006), in addition to helping us to understand the cultural implications for religious and spiritual belief systems that exist within cultures (Brown, 1998).

In this section, cultural implications for integrating spirituality and religion in current psychiatric practice are discussed. We review studies pertaining to the positive association between religion/spirituality and mental health and discuss some of the challenges that exist to incorporating spirituality and religion with psychiatry.

The belief in God has been found in 89% of Canadians, 94% of Americans, 95% of people in South America, 96% on the African continent, 98% in India, 76% in the European Union, 65% in the Netherlands and north Europe, and 80% in Australia (Gallup Poll: 1976, cited in Oman & Thoresen, 2003). Since the 1970s, there continues to be a growing interest and need for religion among the general public in the West. Currently, it is estimated that at least 90% of medical patients in the US consider themselves both religious and spiritual (Koenig, 2004). Similarly, in Canada at least 79% of mental health patients consider themselves spiritual and/or religious in some way, believe that spirituality and religion play an important role in their recovery process, and have requested to have their spiritual/religious needs addressed in their mental health care (Baetz, Griffin, Bowen & Marcoux, 2004).

Some authors have suggested, however, that mental health consumers often do not discuss their spiritual and/or religious beliefs because they fear that they will be pathologized; that is, they fear that their beliefs will be misunderstood as part of a psychotic or delusional experience (Baetz et al, 2004; Clark, 2005; Corrigan, McCorkle, Schell, & Kidder, 2003; Lindgren & Coursey, 1995). Concurrently, some mental health professionals may find the incorporation of religion and spirituality into clinical practice challenging (Clark, 2005). Some of these challenges include a lack of consensus on conceptual definitions pertaining to religion and spirituality, an emphasis on biomedical approaches to care and treatment, psychiatric bias toward the association of religion and spirituality with psychopathology, ethical implications for addressing religious and spiritual issues with patients, and the lack of education among many health disciplines pertaining to religion/spirituality and health (Baetz et al., 2004; Corrigan et al.,2003; Grabovac et al., in press; Grabovac & Ganesan, 2003; Hill et al., 2000; Josephson, et al, 2000; Longo & Peterson, 2002; Sheridan, Bullis, Adcock, Berlin & Miller, 1992).

We surmise that the lack of formal training may be related to the historical tension between psychiatry and religion beginning with early psychoanalytic perspectives. Although there is evidence in favor of implementing formal education and training in religion and spirituality within psychiatry, the significant lack of formal training in this area makes it unlikely that mental health professionals will soon incorporate these important aspects of individual culture in practice. A recent survey and comparison of Canadian versus US curricula found that not all psychiatric residency programs offer mandatory didactic and clinical components pertaining to religion/spirituality and psychiatry (Grabovac & Ganeson, 2003).

Research on culture and mental health has also shown that traditional cultural belief systems strongly influence symptomatology, attitudes towards seeking mental care, and the course of mental illness. Recent evidence exists to suggest that some cultural groups do not access the conventional mental health system or seek care because of their own cultural values that emphasize traditional healing methods (Chiu, Morrow, Ganesan, & Clark 2005). In their study of spirituality and treatment choices by South and East Asian women with serious mental illness, Chiu et al. (2005) found that both East and South Asian women had scarce resources and limited options in the current mental health systems. The ability of these women to make choices was significantly tied to their culture and spiritual worldview. For example, the explanatory model of mental illness as well as healing practices for the majority of East Asian women was influenced by Confucianism, Taoism, and Buddhism (Chiu et al., 2005). The use of conventional psychiatric treatment occurred concurrently with the use of specific traditional healing methods. Although cultural and linguistic barriers may play a role in decreased use of mental health services, use of traditional healing methods that involve the spiritual and religious forms of healing may also contribute to the underutilization of the conventional mental health care system (Chiu et al., 2005). Social and cultural factors such as these are major determinants of the use of health care services and generally leave psychiatric services underutilized among the cultural majority (Kessler et al., 1994).

Another example can be found in the communities of people of Aboriginal ancestry in Canada, who rarely seek conventional psychiatric aid (Kirmayer, Brass, & Tait, 2000; Smye, 2004). This eschewal of psychiatry may be related to an emphasis on biomedical approaches that fail to take into account traditional healing methods and cultural explanations for mental health and illness. Globalization and colonization has affected Indigenous cultures that define their spirituality by their connection to the land, local wildlife, and their ancestors (Tanner, 1993; Turbott, 1996). Clinicians need to be aware of the social implications of this and of the effect on the mental health of individuals and the community. For many Aboriginal people, spirituality is a key to recovery and healing and is closely linked to a sense of life-purpose, identity, and place in the world. Traditional beliefs are still a major influence on contemporary Aboriginal cultures despite the mostly negative impact of Christianity on their belief systems. However, not all Aboriginal people subscribe to their traditional beliefs only. More commonly a kind of biculturalism, or what Joe Couture (1994) calls *bispiritualism*, exists in which people are exposed to many different traditions and adapt or integrate different faiths as part of their culture

For the Maori, a religious understanding of reality is at the heart of their culture, to the extent that the New Zealand Ministry of Health documents include culturally safe services (Turbott, 1996). Unfortunately, Canada, the US and Australia have yet to include cultural understandings of spirituality and religion in their mental health policies. We conjecture that spiritual and religious beliefs are an important aspect of culture and may play an important role in resilience and healing for many individuals, thus it is important for psychiatrists and other mental health clinicians to understand their patients' spiritual and/or religious beliefs and how this may ameliorate the challenges associated with diagnosis and assessment.

SPIRITUALITY AND RELIGION: RELATIONSHIP TO MENTAL HEALTH

The relationships among spirituality and religion, and both physical and mental health have been studied extensively. In the following section, we briefly summarize recent studies that explore the relationship of spiritual and religious belief systems with mental health. Before the year 2000, more than seven hundred studies had examined the relationship among religion, well-being, and mental health, with nearly five hundred of those studies demonstrating a significant positive association of religion with better mental health, greater well-being and lower substance abuse (Ellison & Levin 1998; Koenig, McCullough & Larson, 2001; Koenig 2004; Larson, Swyers, & McCullough, 1998). Results of this early research were often confounded by lack of clarity and subsequent overlap in the constructs being studied. For example, early measures of religiosity often measured the same or overlapping factors, resulting in inconsistent results. Furthermore, the lack of distinction in early research between positive and negative religious or spiritual coping strategies again muddied the results. In

2000-2002, an additional 1,100 studies and reviews on the relation between religion/spirituality and mental health appeared in the psychological literature suggesting greater interest by the scientific community in these issues (Koenig, 2004).

More recent studies have carefully controlled confounding variables and consistently demonstrate a positive correlation between spiritual/religious variables and positive health outcomes: including greater longevity, coping skills, health-related quality of life (during terminal illness), and less anxiety, depression and suicide (Mueller, Plevak & Rummans, 2001; Koenig & Larson, 2001). Other studies have shown that religiosity/spirituality is linked to improvements in cardiovascular, neuroendocrine and immune function (Seeman, Dubin, & Seeman, 2003; Powell, Shahabi, & Thoresen, 2003).

It should be noted that religious variables may be associated with negative health outcomes when beliefs encourage avoidance or discontinuation of medical treatment, failure to seek timely medical care, avoidance of effective preventative health measures (e.g., immunizations, prenatal care), abuse (e.g., allowing physical abuse of children) or social isolation beyond alienation from others who do not share the same beliefs. Early studies conducted in the 1950s and1960s were focused on the association between religion and worse mental health. These studies, however, failed to control for confounding variables and were generally restricted to samples of young college students and cross-sectional research (Koenig & Larson, 2001). Although some patients may experience greater distress from their religious and spiritual practices, increased anxiety for example, there has been no conclusive empirical evidence to support that greater religious activity causes mental distress. That said, more studies are needed to examine the positive and adverse effects of religious/spiritual beliefs and practices on mental health.

Addressing the above concern, McCullough and Larson (1999) reviewed the mental health literature, examining the relationship between depression and religion and found that people with high levels of *intrinsic religious motivation*, who uphold religious values according to their own inner beliefs, are at reduced risk of developing depressive disorders. On the other hand, people with high levels of *extrinsic religiosity*, namely those who use religion for strictly utilitarian reasons, such as social connectedness or prestige, were at increased risk of developing depressive symptoms. Subsequent research has supported the generally positive impact of intrinsic belief versus the generally negative health impact of extrinsic belief. More recent longitudinal studies have found through examining the relationship between religious involvement, spirituality, and depression that intrinsic religiosity shows significant associations with a more rapid remission from depression (Mueller et al., 2001).

The following studies describe aspects of the relationship between spirituality and mental health in more detail. Nelson, Rosenfeld, Breitbart, and Garlietta (2002) investigated the relationship between spirituality and depression in 84 terminally ill cancer patients and 78 AIDS patients. Higher spirituality scores (meaning/peace subscale) correlated with lower depression scores. Extrinsic religiosity scores had a negligible to small positive association with depression. Pargament, Koenig, Tarakeshwar, & Hahn (2001) found that hospitalized patients with negative religious coping experienced significantly worse mental health and greater mortality, which increased by 28%, in two years following discharge. Koenig, George and Peterson (1998) studied 94 elderly depressed inpatients and found that intrinsic religiosity was associated with faster remission rates of MDE. Every ten-point increase in intrinsic religiosity resulted in a 70% increase in the speed of remission: Twenty-seven potential confounding variables were adjusted for. Other studies have shown that religious involvement and spiritual well-being are associated with higher levels of quality of life even when there is a decline in physical functioning (Mueller et al., 2001). For example, McClain, Rosenfeld, and Breitbart (2003) examined the effect of spiritual well-being on end-of-life despair in 160 palliative care patients and found that spiritual well-being was negatively correlated with desire for hastened death, hopelessness, and suicidal thoughts or intentions.

In another study conducted by Baetz, Larson, Marcoux, Bowen, and Griffin (2002), the association between religious commitment and mental health in 88 Canadian psychiatric inpatients was examined. Frequent worship attendees had significantly less severe depressive symptoms, significantly higher life satisfaction and lower rates of current or lifetime alcohol abuse. Personal spiritual practice was associated with decreased depressive symptoms and decreased current alcohol use. Religious coping was associated with a significantly shorter length of hospital stay (current and past) and accounted for 9.5% of variance in past length of stay (Baetz et al., 2002). This study suggests that religious/spiritual practices could be incorporated with treatment as an alternative resource for coping and have implications for recovery.

Similarly, Tepper, Rogers, Coleman, and Newton Malony (2001) found religious coping to be a salient method of enduring chronic psychiatric symptoms as well as preventing risk behaviors. This study included 406 mental health consumers and assessed the prevalence of religious coping using a 48 item demographic survey, which included total number of years participants had used religious coping and the perceived importance of religion when their symptoms worsened. Religious activity was reported by 92% of participants who engaged in religious coping for an average of 17.65 years. Another 64% reported that their religious practice helped them to cope with symptom severity. These findings suggest that, for many patients, religion and spirituality are important ways of coping with chronic mental illness.

It has been suggested that one of the challenges that clinicians face when incorporating spiritual and/or religious issues with client care is that it may worsen symptoms: For instance, the patient may start to develop a religious delusion about a particular belief system (Baetz et al., 2004; Clark, 2005). To our knowledge, there have been no studies to support this assumption. Phillips, Lankin, and Pargament (2002) explored this concern by investigating the spiritual needs of those with serious mental illness by implementing a seven-week psychoeducational program based on Pargament's theory of religious coping, in which patients discussed religious resources, spiritual struggles, forgiveness, and hope. Spiritual resources such as services and prayer provided socialization and support. Although some participants were burdened by their personal struggles with God and church (i.e., feeling abandoned, spiritual emptiness, stigma by church members), many patients benefited from the connection they experienced in the group. No participants reported that their symptoms had worsened (i.e., delusions, hallucinations). The authors argue that this intervention was highly valued by its participants, as many did not feel that they had a place to discuss their spiritual concerns (Phillips et al., 2002).

Few studies have addressed the influence of spirituality and religion from a cultural point of view other than the Judeo-Christian framework. Yet the value of spirituality extends beyond this framework. In a recent study, Grouzet et al. (2005) explored how spirituality and religion are intrinsic to human psychological development and suggest that spirituality and religion are common goals across cultures. This study examined goals that people typically strive for and the organization of those goals in people's psyches. Eleven different domains of goals were assessed cross-culturally among 1,854 college students from fifteen cultures around the world. The authors hypothesized that people use motivational systems to negotiate through life; these motivational systems include psychological needs, physical survival, desire for pleasure, seeking rewards, and the existential quest to find meaning. The findings of this research suggest that motivational systems include spirituality, regardless of an individual's cultural situation. Spirituality was defined as an intrinsic goal measured through self-transcendence. The self-transcendent dimension included goals of matching society's desires, benefiting society, and seeking out universal meanings that sometimes contradict desires for physical pleasure and material success (Grouzet et al., 2005).

Positive health outcomes such as improved coping, decreased substance and/or alcohol use, decreased hospital stay, and greater subjective states of well-being correlated positively with psychological and social effects that spirituality and religion exert. It has been hypothesized that salutogenic or protective mechanisms play a role in prevention of morbidity and health promotion (George, Larson, Koenig, & McCullough, 2000; Levin & Chatters, 1998; Koenig, 2004).

A number of approaches to understanding the protective mechanisms associated with positive mental health have been offered in the literature and are used to address two key questions: How does the very personal experience of spirituality or religiosity contribute to these positive health outcomes; what are the key elements that are responsible for these positive health effects? Oman and Thoresen (2002) have suggested four causal pathways for the mechanisms leading to positive health outcomes:

1. Social support and improved health behaviors.
2. Enhanced positive psychological states (e.g., inner peace, faith, mystical experience acting through psychoneuro-immunologic or psychoneuroendocrinologic pathways.
3. Support for maintaining health behaviors.
4. Causal influences on health by distant healing or inter-cessory prayer.

These findings challenge researchers and clinicians to develop methods of inquiry that address the multidimensional nature of health that includes religion and spirituality. The neurobiology of spiritual experience must also be examined in consideration with the causal pathways associated with positive health outcomes.

NEUROBIOLOGY OF SPIRITUAL EXPERIENCE

As more evidence accumulates regarding the salutary effects of spirituality and intrinsic religiosity on health, increasing attention is being paid to possible mechanisms for these effects. From the biological perspective, spiritual experience is being researched from a number of different vantage points, including genetics, neurotransmitters, and functional neuroimaging studies. Mental health clinicians need to be aware of the neurophysiological effects of spiritual practice, for research shows that mental states can be altered markedly through spiritual and religious practice.

Genetics. Twin studies have clearly established that there is a strong genetic contribution to the experience of religiosity and spirituality. Over twenty twin studies have been completed and all show that 40 to 50% of the variance in spirituality is due to genetics. One example of the studies documenting this relationship examined over 1,200 twin pairs (Kirk, Eaves, & Martin, 1999). They found the heritability of self-transcendence, as measured by the Temperament and Character Inventory (TCI-ST), to be about 40% and confirmed a marked difference in shared environmental effect for self-transcendence (8%) versus church attendance (58%).

Neurotransmitters. How do we go from the level of the gene to the actual human experience of spirituality? Some research exists that explores the role of specific neurotransmitters in spiritual experience. The role of serotonin in spiritual experience has long been acknowledged through studies of lysergic acid diethylaminde (LSD). Borg, Andree, Soderstrom, and Farde (2003) explored the role of serotonin (5HT) in personality. Using an open exploratory design, they measured 5HT1A receptor densities and correlated this with personality dimensions as measured by the TCI-ST. They found that the people who scored high on the spiritual acceptance scale had low 5HT1A density. This scale measures a person's apprehension of phenomena that cannot be explained by objective demonstration, such as ESP or a belief in God, and contrasts it with material rationalism, described as a belief in a reductionistic and empirical worldview. Interestingly, there was no correlation with any other TCI dimensions (novelty seeking, harm avoidance, reward dependence, persistence, self-direction and cooperativeness) or their subscales. To understand this result, they investigated the role of the 5HT system, which is involved in gating sensory stimuli and arousal. It was hypothesized that low 5HT1A receptor density may represent sparse 5HT innervation and, therefore, subjects with low 5HT1A receptor density might have a weaker filtering function, allowing sensory stimulation to be experienced that would otherwise be filtered out and not registered. A genetic basis for interindividual variability in 5HT1A receptor density has not yet been confirmed in humans and, thus, determining variability in receptor density due to genetics versus possible environmental effects is not possible.

Functional Neuroimaging. It is well established that functional brain changes occur during certain spiritual experiences. For example, increases in limbic blood flow correspond to feelings of ecstasy and bliss. Decreases in parietal lobe blood flow, which processes information about space, time, and the orientation of the body in space, occur during types of meditation that induce feelings of oneness and decreased awareness of physical and other boundaries. When this part of the brain, which weaves sensory data into a feeling of where the self ends, is deprived of sensory input through the meditator's focus on inward concentration, it cannot find the border between the self and the world. Furthermore, subjects who reported a feeling of infinite perspective and self-transcendence during meditation, showed decreased activity in the brain's *object association areas* where perceptions of the boundary between self and other are normally processed (Newberg & D'Aquili, 1998).

Long-term Changes to Brain Function due to Meditation. There is increasing evidence that functional brain changes are related to positive mental health. Initial research shows that changes in baseline brain function can be maintained between periods of spiritual practice, such as meditation. One of the researchers in this area is Richard Davidson, who is the Director of the National Institute for Mental Health (NIMH) funded Laboratory for Affective Neurosciences at the University of Wisconsin-Madison. His research focuses on the functional neuroanatomical substrates of affect. The current understanding of emotion is that the prefrontal cortex (PFC) plays an important role in the balance between positive and negative affect states, including mood. Davidson (2002) found that people who have sunnier dispositions have more left-sided activation, both during an acute positive emotional state, as well as at baseline. Those who suffer more chronic anger, anxiety, and depression have more right-sided frontal activation. A clinical example of this can be found in the stroke and depression literature; people with left-sided strokes have a greater incidence of depressive symptoms because their ability to experience positive emotion is impaired.

The impact of this asymmetrical activation is far reaching. Davidson and his group have found that individual differences in right- versus left-prefrontal activation predict the length of time it takes an infant to cry after separation from its mother. Asymmetrical activation also predicts dispositional mood, behavioral activation and inhibition, reactivity to positive and negative emotion elicitors, baseline immune function, as well as reactivity of the immune system to emotional challenge (Davidson, 2002). Davidson's work, and the work of others in the field, has established the importance of frontal asymmetry in affect regulation. The question now arises whether there are any interventions that can shift those people who have more right-sided activation at baseline – a predisposition to negative affect – to having more left-sided activation.

Davidson et al. (2003) hypothesized that eight weeks of mindfulness meditation practice would increase baseline left-sided anterior activation. They randomly assigned 41 employees of a biotech company to a meditation group that participated in an eight week mindfulness-based stress reduction program, as developed by Kabat-Zinn (1982), or to a waitlist control group. The intervention consisted of two hours of instruction weekly, with the expectation that participants meditate on a daily basis for 45 minutes in between sessions. The meditation group showed significant changes in baseline left-sided activation and significant increases in left-sided activation to both positive and negative affect induction. These results are consistent with the research literature showing that more left-sided activation is associated with more adaptive responding to negative or stressful life events. They also found a reduction in measures of anxiety and negative affect in the intervention group.

This initial research demonstrates that meditation can affect brain function in a sustained manner; more importantly, this work is likely the first to demonstrate a possible neurobiological mechanism to explain the impact of religious/spiritual practices on affect regulation. Further research is needed to relate this neurobiological change to the existing research that shows positive health effects from religious and spiritual activity: for example, the results of McCullough and Larson's (1998) work that relates higher intrinsic religiosity with decreased depressive symptoms or Koenig, George, and Peterson's (1998) results that shows an association between increased religiosity and faster remission of depressive episodes. These studies have just started to understand the possible impact of religious and spiritual practices on neurobiology and, thus far, strongly support the integration of spiritual interventions with selected patient treatment plans.

In summary, the scientific study of religion and spirituality has led to a vast amount of evidence pointing to the therapeutic effects of religious belief. Various theoretical bases for positive mental health outcomes have been put forward ranging from the neurobiology of spiritual experiences to protective mechanisms that are associated with religious/spiritual beliefs and practices. We now turn to a discussion about the challenges of incorporating religion and spirituality within the existing psychiatric framework.

INTEGRATING RELIGION AND SPIRITUALITY INTO THE DSM-IV

The relevance of culture for contemporary psychiatry has been well documented in the research agenda for the Diagnostic and Statistical Manual of Mental Disorders Fourth Edition (DSM-IV, American Psychiatric Association, 2000) and, most recently, on a research agenda for the DSM-V by Alarcon et al. (2002). This research agenda recognizes religion and spirituality as important cultural variables relevant to all steps in the diagnostic and treatment process and focuses on the interpretive and explanatory function of culture in clinical psychiatry (Alarcon et al., 1999; Alarcon et al., 2002). The World Health Organization's (WHO, 2001) research agenda for the DSM-V also includes a focus on mind-body interaction, the stability of classification across cultures, social and political rights, and primary health care intervention protocols, all of which will have an impact on diagnosis of mental disorders (Alarcon et al., 2002). Considerations have also been made to broaden the DSM-V to include a research appendix that includes alternative diagnostic constructs and evolving knowledge (First, 2006).

Culture permeates every facet of human behavior and is closely tied to spiritual and religious beliefs. Post (1998) has asserted that clinicians cannot fully succeed in establishing therapeutic empathy and efficacy without respecting and allowing a place for spirituality and religion. Recently, a need to understand religious and spiritual experiences in the context of culture has lead to terms such as *cultural sensitivity*, *cultural competence*, and *cultural safety* emerging as important markers for efficacious service (Hutchinson & Haasen, 2004). Cultural competence includes attention to religious and spiritual issues in clinical practice (Lukoff & Lu, 1999). We concur with Dein (2005) that, in many cultural traditions, religion and spirituality is an integral part of culture and society

In this section, the DSM-IV approach to spiritual/religious experience is discussed in order to explore the role of culture in mental health. The challenges associated with identifying normative experience versus psychopathology are reviewed. The DSM-IV Text Revision edition or the DSM-IV TR provides a nosology that can assist clinicians to implement and understand the role of spirituality and religion on their patients' mental health in the clinical context. We discuss the current nosology and provide other clinical tools that may support clinicians in incorporating their patients' cultural worldviews to provide comprehensive care.

The diagnostic category of "Religious or Spiritual Problem" was added to the DSM-IV in 1994 in an attempt to encourage the integration of spirituality and religion into clinical assessments and formulations and to decrease iatrogenic harm from misdiagnosis of religious and spiritual issues as major mood or psychotic disorders. A wide variety of experience and phenomena are captured by this diagnostic category. Religious and spiritual problems are recognized as being distinct from psychopathology by being classified with a V code that identifies non-disordered conditions related to contextual or developmentally relevant conditions.

RELIGIOUS PROBLEMS

Clinical examples of religious problems include loss or questioning of faith, problems associated with conversion to a new faith, and intensification of adherence to beliefs and practices. Loss of religious connectedness often results in individuals experiencing feelings commonly associated with other loss situations, including anger, resentment, sadness, and isolation. Sometimes the loss of meaning is so intense that people become suicidal, occasionally committing suicide (Clark, 2005). Though crises of faith are recognized as a normal part of spiritual development, they can trigger adjustment disorders or depressive episodes. Intensification of religious practices may occur as an attempt to deal with feelings of guilt or, conversely, as a means of coping with trauma (Boehnlein, 2006; Connor, Davidson, Lee, 2003; George et al., 2000). It can also serve the purpose of finding meaning in a distressing event in order to avoid a breakdown of identity.

SPIRITUAL PROBLEMS

Types of spiritual problems include questioning spiritual values or loss of connectedness, meditation-related problems, near death experiences (NDEs) and mystical experiences. Psychiatric side-effects of intensive meditation, including anxiety, dissociation, depersonalization, derealization, altered perceptions, and agitation have all been well documented by Western meditation practitioners (Epstein, 1990). The DSM-IV emphasizes the need to distinguish between psychopathology and these meditation-related experiences; for example, "Voluntarily induced experiences of depersonalization or derealization form part of meditative and trance practices that are prevalent in many religions and cultures and should not be confused with Depersonalization Disorder" (Epstein,

1990, p. 488). Engler (1986) and Epstein (1990) both offer useful considerations on this complex topic.

NDEs are characterized by a temporal sequence of stages, beginning with peace and contentment, and followed by detachment from the physical body, entering a transitional region of darkness, seeing a brilliant light, and passing through the light into another realm of existence. Usually, strong positive affect and transcendental or mystical elements accompany NDEs. The person often feels unconditionally accepted and forgiven by a loving source. Life review is also common and the person returns with a mission or vision, believing that there is still more to be done in this life. Intrapsychic problems associated with a NDE include anger or depression related to losing the near-death state, difficulty reconciling the NDE with previous religious beliefs, becoming overly identified with the experience, and fear that the NDE might indicate mental instability (Greyson, 1997). Interpersonal problems associated with NDE include difficulty reconciling attitudinal changes with the expectations of family and friends, a sense of isolation from those who have not had a similar experience, a fear of ridicule or rejection by others, difficulty communicating the meaning and impact of the NDE, difficulty maintaining previous life roles that no longer carry the same significance, and difficulty reconciling limited human relationships with the unconditional relationships experienced during the NDE (Greyson, 1997).

Mystical experiences are often considered an extreme on the spectrum of spiritual and religious experience (Cook, 2004; House, 2001). Mystical experience is a transient, extraordinary experience characterized by feelings of unity, a sense of harmonious relationship to the divine, euphoria, a sense of gnosis (access to the hidden spiritual dimension), loss of ego functioning, alterations in time and space perception, and a sense of lacking control over the event (Cook, 2004). A common feature associated with the construct of mysticism is a relationship with the Ultimate or Absolute Reality; however, this may not be an individual experience as it may also concern members of a community and/or cultural group (Cook, 2004). Few studies have examined the relationship between mysticism and psychosis. However, Chadwick (2001) draws several parallels between mystical and psychotic states. For example, a mystical intuition may include the belief that "there is great harmony and oneness between all things;" similarly, a psychotic intuition being of the belief that "people and the world are all together in communication against me" (p. 86). Lukoff et al. (1992) propose that the concepts of psychosis and mysticism overlap and proposed a diagnostic category, "Mystical Experiences with Psychotic Features" (MEPF) or psychotic disorders with mystical features. Diagnostic criteria for MEPF include two or four experiences, such as "ecstatic moods, senses of newly gained knowledge, perceptual alterations, mythological content of delusions" (p. 157). These criteria are considered positive outcomes of mystical experiences.

The association of mystical experience with positive outcomes has been supported by some studies that found lower scores on psychopathology scales for those reporting mystical experience and higher scores on measures of psychological well-being than controls (Cook, 2004). Mystical experiences can be overwhelming for individuals who do not have a strong sense of self (Clarke, 2001). Cook (2004) reviews the relationship between psychiatry and mysticism and states that mystical experience may easily be misdiagnosed as a psychiatric disorder if clinicians and therapists collude in pathologizing such experiences. Most commonly, though, mental health professionals do not hear about mystical experiences and NDEs, as people tend to avoid discussing these for fear of being misunderstood and misdiagnosed. Detailed reviews of psychiatry and mysticism can be found in Cook (2004) and Clarke (2001).

INTERPRETATION OF CULTURAL NORMATIVE VERSUS PSYCHOPATHOLOGY

Spiritual and religious belief systems are compounded by culture and ethnic identity, which provide a contextual framework for health seeking behaviors and alternative explanations for mental health evaluation (Kirmayer et al., 2003). For example, in Maori culture no distinction exists between physical and spiritual; that is, the spiritual order is the basis for the social and temporal order (Turbott, 1996). Mental illness is based on the belief that individuals are vulnerable to various deities; if one is afflicted with a negative or debilitating illness, traditional healing includes exorcism and rituals performed by elders or specialists (Turbott, 1996). Currently, health practitioners believe that much of Maori ill health is due to cultural damage caused by colonialism.

Waldram (2004) offers another salient example of cultural misinterpretation provided in Devereux's (1969) case study. Two brothers from the Acoma pueblo were on death row, convicted of murder. The prison psychiatrist was, in Devereux's words, "sufficiently sophisticated not to mistake Indianness for psychosis" but being unable to find any "culturally neutral evidence of real mental derangement," declared them legally sane and hence executable (p. 43). Upon interview, Devereux learned that the man they had killed had, in their view, been using witchcraft against them. Witchcraft was a pervasive element of Acoma culture, but the ease with which the brothers began to talk about it struck Devereux as deviant, for such phenomena were only rarely and reluctantly discussed. Further, in killing the witch themselves, rather than using an intermediary and invoking ritual, they had engaged in a second culturally deviant act. They were, in Devereux's opinion, delusional.

Both brothers were spared from execution, however, based on the fact that one was diagnosed with schizophrenia and the other with psychotically tinged psychopathy. Waldram (2004) discusses how the original diagnosis resulted in the delusion being mistaken for "acceptable normative cultural belief by the psychiatrist, and therefore suggestive of sanity" (p. 113). This example illustrates the complexities associated with understanding cultural norms versus psychopathology and underscores the need for a more comprehensive approach to mental health assessment.

To help in making the distinction between pathology and spiritual experience, clinicians should consider how mental illness might be conceptualized in other cultures (i.e., alternative explanatory models).

Similarly, the spiritist tradition in Brazil concerns the survival of the spirit after death and plays an important role in the mental health of people in contemporary Brazil. The belief in spiritism serves as a theoretical framework developed by Kardec in the mid-nineteenth-century and centers on the belief that a spirit world exists and has a direct relationship to the body. In this tradition, mental disturbance is caused by "the persistent action that an evil spirit exerts over an individual" (Moreira-Almeida & Neto, 2005, p. 574). This theory, however, does not discount the social and biological causes of mental disturbances. Spiritism operates on a dualistic interaction model, whereby the aetiology of mental disturbance is organic but may be triggered in individuals who are predisposed to so called obsessions or previous incarnations. This theory offers an alternative cultural explanation, widely adopted in Brazil, for the causes of madness that incorporates spiritual etiology of mental illness (Moreira-Almeida & Neto, 2005).

Another example of how alternative explanations for mental illness may be misunderstood is that of post-traumatic stress disorder (PTSD). Post-traumatic stress disorder is a significant psychological condition suffered by many Indigenous peoples. According to formal diagnostic criteria, there must be exposure to a traumatic stressor that revisits the individual through traumatic memories such as flashbacks or nightmares. Many Indigenous peoples experience intergenerational trauma as the result of residential schooling; this kind of exposure has shaped the personalities, attitudes, and behaviors of survivors, which has in many cases affected younger generations. Waldram (1997) suggests that "if the concept of PTSD is to be useful for Indigenous communities, clinicians must be cognizant of the intergenerational transmission of pathological behaviors, and that trauma becomes the lived experience of a whole culture" (p. 46). Therefore, if the current nosology (DSM-IV TR) is to be relevant it must be integrated with an understanding of social and cultural origins of distress for particular cultural groups.

In order to consider cultural variations and normative cultural behaviors, clinicians must be aware of cultural etiology and the social origins of distress. The expression of mental illness is heavily determined by culture. Symptoms of a disorder that are prominent in one culture may be insignificant or absent in another or may be interpreted within a religious or spiritual view. Clinicians are also challenged by the plethora of alternative healing systems that exist throughout the world. Alternative medicine has become very popular in the West and covers a wide range of services from "New Age Spiritualism to homeopathy, message therapy, and macrobiotic diets" (Finkler, 1998, p.118). Because of these alternatives Finkler stresses that good medical practice involves understanding the patient point of view. To overlook spiritual aspects of a patient's cultural worldview in any clinical encounter may devalue the patient's perspective, undermine a successful working alliance, and impede successful negotiation of treatment.

CLINICAL ASSESSMENT TOOLS

Current guidelines in the DSM-IV TR, such as the ones developed by Lukoff and colleagues in the 1970s, are useful in drawing attention to the challenges of differential diagnosis and inclusion of spiritual and religious experiences. One example of these guidelines proposes that spiritual experience can be distinguished from psychopathology by the following characteristics: doctrinal orthodoxy (content acceptable to a sub-cultural group); sensory elements that are intellectual (experienced as mental contents); predominantly visual hallucinations; beliefs formed with the possibility of doubt; presence of insight; brief duration; volition over the experiences; and other-oriented, self-actualizing, and life-enhancing aspects. These characteristics are contrasted with key elements of psychosis including: bizarre content (particularly claims of divine status or special powers); sensory elements that are corporeal (experienced as veridical perceptions); predominantly auditory hallucinations; incorrigible beliefs; absence of insight; extended duration of psychosis; no control of the experiences; self-orientation and disintegration from groups; and deterioration in functioning (Jackson, 1997).

We discuss three approaches that may be used in the incorporation of spiritual and/or religious factors for psychiatric diagnosis. The first approach, developed by Richards and Bergin (1997), focuses on clinical assessment based on several criteria: metaphysical world views, religious affiliation and orthodoxy, doctrinal knowledge, religious/spiritual health and maturity, ability to solve religious problems, and image of God. In their approach to spiritual assessment, Richards and Bergin (1997) identify how the above factors are addressed through goals. Level one assessment includes the clinician's ability to gain a global understanding of the patient's metaphysical worldview and establish how this view is relevant to the present problems. At level one, clinicians ascertain the patient's beliefs as either theistic (i.e., Christianity, Hinduism, Islam, Judaism) or non-theistic (i.e., Buddhism, Taosim, Zen). Level two assessments include the clinician's ability to determine the health of the patient's religious/spiritual beliefs in regards to the impact of the problem.

Second, the Source of Hope, organized religion, personal practices and effects (HOPE) tool developed by Anandarajah & Hight in 2001 has proven its utility in incorporating patients' religious and spiritual beliefs in clinical practice.

The HOPE uses simple questions broken into four categories to explore how individual faith and belief can be incorporated in care. Questions in the "H" category deal with sources of hope and might include: What are the sources of comfort and peace? "O" questions address the role of organized religion by asking: Are you a part of a religious or spiritual community? "P" stands for questions related to personal beliefs such as: What aspects of spiritual and/or religious practice are most helpful? Last, "E" stands for how individual beliefs influence effects on medical care and end-of-life issues, an example being: How has your situation affected your ability to do things that usually help your spirituality; and also, are there specific issues that may conflict with your spiritual and/or religious beliefs? (Anandarajah & Hight, 2001).

Third, the Faith, Importance, Community and Address/Action in Care (FICA) questionnaire developed by Puchalski in 1996 also uses acronyms to address specific questions related to individual religious and spiritual values. "F" stands for faith and addresses questions regarding the importance of faith; "I" stands for influence of faith, past, and present; "C" stands for addressing questions related to religious and/or spiritual community and; "A" stands for what spiritual needs should to be addressed in patient care (Koenig & Pritchett, 1998; Puchalski, 2000).

Although assessment tools such as the HOPE and FICA forms exist, as well as guidelines established for the DSM-IV TR (diagnostic codes for spiritual and/or religious problems), research remains limited as to the efficacy of assessment tools and their utility across different cultural contexts. Furthermore, some evidence suggests that these guidelines have not been widely adopted by mental health clinicians, most of whom remain uninformed about the phenomenology of spiritual experience due to lack of education, resulting in a tendency to overpathologize (Clark, 2005).

In brief, these assessment tools underscore the need for clinicians to examine the spiritual and religious context of what defines mental health and illness. In order to provide accurate assessment, diagnosis, and treatment of spiritual and religious issues, the clinician must pay attention to the pluralistic health care environment that encompasses alternative healing systems and cultural diversity. As many cultures continue to practice traditional healing methods that are Indigenous and salient to their understanding of wellness, the cultural diversity that clinicians encounter in their practices challenges them to take on new explanations and interpretations of human behavior (Alarcon et al., 1999).

UNDERSTANDING SPIRITUAL AND RELIGIOUS BELIEFS

USING A CULTURAL FORMULATION TOOL

The current DSM-IV TR nosology of culture-bound syndromes has been developed in order to arrive at a diagnosis that reflects cultural understanding of normalcy. As Brown (1998) discusses, the problem of the definition of normality parallels problems of cultural relativity, for boundaries that define health and illness are difficult to set due to the diversity of beliefs that might exist in a particular culture. For example, saintly behavior in one culture may be considered abnormal in another. Therefore, clinicians must take into account cultural belief systems and their implications for the patient's mental health. Although the current DSM-IV TR helps to identify some mental health conditions as culture-bound or culture-specific conditions, clinicians must also consider individual variability and cultural diversity that exists within even small cultural groups (Kirmayer et al., 2003). Although the identification of culture-bound syndromes (CBS) helps the clinician to address spiritual and religious factors through cultural meanings, this nosology has been criticized by medical anthropology and cultural psychiatry for potentially misdiagnosing religious and spiritual states as being psychotic conditions, "such as reporting hearing the voice of a deceased relative in the midst of the grief process" (Alarcon et al., 2002, p. 225). Since different cultures have their own ethnopsychiatric systems for diagnosing and curing mental illness, clinicians need to be aware that not all symptoms of illness are culture-bound as given in the example by Waldram (2004). Similarly, Lopez and Guarnaccia (2000) argue that cultural psychopathology lies not only within a given ethnocultural group but is specific to individual orientation, beliefs and values.

The question of how to integrate spiritual and religious beliefs with mental health practice is an important issue for many clinicians. These domains continue to be sensitive, and often difficult, topics to address in clinical practice. A number of specific factors contribute to the challenge of addressing these areas clinically. Clinicians are challenged by feelings of ambivalence about their professional role and ethical concerns related to imposing one's own spiritual and/or religious beliefs (Foskett, Marriott, & Wilson-Rudd, 2004). Moreover, clinicians who fail to examine their own beliefs and values run the risk of being ineffective or harming the therapeutic relationship. Mental health clinicians may feel uncomfortable using structured interview questionnaires to address spiritual and religious beliefs because of concern regarding the therapeutic relationship with their patients. For example, in Clark's (2005) study on mental health professional's perspectives on incorporating spirituality in their care of clients with serious mental illness, clinicians acknowledged that they do not use the words *religion* or *spirituality* during initial assessments and would prefer to get to know the individual seeking care better. Words such as *connection, purpose, meaning*, and *cultural beliefs* were perceived as neutral substitutes for the constructs of religion and or spirituality. Similarly, Baetz et al. (2004) state that patients often prefer to know the religious/spiritual orientation of the psychiatrist before they feel comfortable in disclosing their beliefs.

We suggest that the cultural formulation (CF) tool can be a useful alternative for incorporating religious and spiritual beliefs within the context of the clinical encounter, which, in and of itself, may be culturally challenging. The contemporary understanding of culture is derived from both sociological and anthropological underpinnings and is broadly conceptualized as non-static, heterogeneous, and constantly in a state of flux (Kirmayer et al., 2000).

The CF is a tool developed by the NIMH Working Group on Culture and Diagnosis in 1991 to assist clinicians to facilitate the "application of a cultural perspective to the process of clinical interviewing and diagnostic formulation in psychiatry" (Lewis-Fernandez, 1996, p.133). A cultural formulation requires "consideration of the patient's religion and spirituality, and covers areas such as religious identity, the role of religion in family of origin, current practice, motivation for religious behavior (i.e., religious orientation) and specific beliefs of individuals and of their family and community" (Kirmayer et al., 2003, p. 66).

CF is an ethnographic narrative that allows clinicians to obtain an emic perspective of the sufferer and to develop an awareness of how individual spiritual and cultural beliefs frame the illness-experience. The cultural formulation is not directly intended to alter the diagnostic process; rather, it provides a comprehensive approach to psychiatric assessment in relation to religion/spirituality and culture. The focus on narrative may help to broaden the clinician's understanding by contextualizing how culture influences presenting symptoms. A narrative can take into account the spiritual dimension of human suffering and enable the clinician to obtain cultural understanding within the following distinct categories of assessment:

1. Cultural identification of an individual (i.e., noting the individual's culture, ethnicity, and reference groups);
2. Cultural explanations of the individual's illness (i.e., possessing spirits, feelings of guilt and shame related to one's religion or spirituality) perceived causes or explanatory models that help the individual to explain illness;
3. Factors related to environment and levels of functioning (i.e., the availability of social supports; meaningful connections with others; the role of religion and kin networks in providing emotional, instrumental, and infor-mational support).
4. The clinician's ability to self-reflect and acknowledge and respect cultural differences (i.e., differences in religious

and spiritual orientation or beliefs, differences in status and perceived power imbalances, differences in language and understanding cultural meanings). Culture defined broadly also includes the context in which the clinical encounter occurs, how the clinician is situated, and acknowledgement of cultural differences. This requires the clinician to take a reflective stance as part of the process of psychiatric evaluation.

These categories serve as a guide to the overall ethnographic narrative which involves the clinician's ability to hear the patient's story and understand the experience of suffering through the individual or family. The CF also allows the clinician to interview using storytelling by others, such as the patient's family or significant social networks, which again provides a deeper cultural context for understanding the social origins of distress. To illustrate how the CF might help to integrate a spiritual, religious, and cultural understanding, we draw on the case of the two Acoma brothers who were wrongly diagnosed due to a failure to incorporate a narrative that might have accounted for cultural norms.

More research is needed to evaluate the use of CF and its unique approach to integrating spirituality and religion within mental health practices. The information clinicians receive through the patient's narrative can help to diminish barriers and accurately define mental health problems. Recent revisions of the CF tool have helped clinicians to understand better the positive and adaptive factors for religion and spirituality; however, the DSM-IV TR categories remain highly biased toward Euro-American constructs (Kirmayer, 2006).

CONCLUSION

While modern perspectives on mental health include dualistic approaches – biological and social components – to treat individuals living with mental illness, there is a call to integrate biomedical approaches with psychosocial aspects such as spirituality and religion. The inclusion of religion and spirituality as important variables for mental health has been supported by scientific research. More studies are needed to explore the relationship between spiritual and religious variables from the cultural perspective in order to inform psychiatric practice. Nevertheless, it is important for clinicians to examine the relationship between mental health and spiritual and religious practices, as it impacts individual care at the level of assessment and therapeutic decisions, and also influences transnational mental health policies and institutions (Bartocci & Dein, 2005).

Our increasing knowledge of the neurobiological mechanisms of spirituality, which show functional changes that support mental health, emphasizes the importance of working with the spiritual concerns of our patients when appropriate. The integration of spirituality and religion in clinical practice remains challenging and not all clinicians feel prepared to address these important issues. We suggest that formal education on the interface between psychiatry and religion/spirituality be a part of mandatory curricula in psychiatry residency programs. Training should include case study as well as didactic approaches in order to help future clinicians incorporate spiritual and religious aspects of the individual into assessment and treatment plans where appropriate.

Taking into account the above factors, it is clinically necessary for mental health professionals to develop a culturally informed knowledge base about the role of spirituality and religion in mental health. Application of the CF may be a useful assessment and treatment planning tool to help clinicians gain awareness of the cultural dimension in the patient's clinical presentation. Using the CF tool may help to lessen some of the challenges associated with addressing religious spiritual beliefs with patients, such as normalizing beliefs and culture-bound or, conversely, pathologizing religious spiritual beliefs that are culturally appropriate. This tool may validate cultural and local explanations for mental illness. While the CF tool provides a comprehensive approach to understanding cultural belief systems, more studies are needed to address its clinical utility. Based on our current understanding and review of spiritual and religious influences in psychiatry, we predict that it is the cultural representations of religious and spiritual experiences that will influence the art of psychiatric practice in the twenty-first century and beyond.

NOTES

[1] See the chapter by Pappas and Friedman for further clarification of the terms *religious* and *spiritual*.

References

Alarcon, R. D., Westermeyer, J., Foulks, F. E., & Ruiz, P. (1999). Clinical relevance of contemporary cultural psychiatry. *The Journal of Nervous and Mental Disease, 187*, 465-471.

Alarcon, R. D., Bell, C. C., Kirmayer, L. J., Lin, K. H., Ustun, T. B., & Winsner, K. L. (2002). Beyond the funhouse mirrors: Research agenda on culture and psychiatric diagnosis. In D. J. Kupfer, M. B. First & D. A. Regier (Eds.), *A research agenda for DSM-V* (pp. 219-281). Washington: American Psychiatric Press.

American Psychiatric Association. (2000). *Diagnostic and statistical manual of mental disorders* (4th Edition-Text Revision). Washington, DC.

Anandarajah, G. & Hight, E. (2001). Spirituality and medical practice: Using the HOPE questions as a practical tool for spiritual assessment. *American Family Physician 63*, 81-89.

Baetz, M., Larson, D. B., Marcoux, G., Bowen, R., & Griffin, R. (2002). Canadian psychiatric inpatient religious commitment: An association with mental health. *Canadian Journal of Psychiatry, 4*, 159-166.

Baetz, M., Griffin, R., Bowen, R., & Marcoux, G. (2004). Spirituality and psychiatry in canada: Psychiatric practice compared with patient expectations. *Canadian Journal of Psychiatry, 49*, 265-271.

Bartocci, G., & Dein, S. (2005). Detachment: Gateway to the world of spirituality. *Transcultural Psychiatry, 42*, 545-569.

Boehnlein, J. K. (2006). Religion and Spirituality in Psychiatric Care: Looking Back, Looking Ahead. *Transcultural Psychiatry, 43*, 634-651.

Borg, J., Andree, B., Soderstrom, H., Farde, L. (2003). The serotonin system and spiritual experiences. *American Journal of Psychiatry, 160*, 1965-1969.

Brown, P. J. (1998). *Understanding and Applying Medical Anthropology*. Mountain View, California: Mayfield Publishing.

Chadwick, P. K. (2001). Sanity to supersanity to insanity: A personal journey In Clarke (Ed.), *Psychosis and spirituality exploring the new frontier.* (pp.75-89). London: Whurr Publishers.

Chiu, L., Emblen, J. D., Van Hofwegen, L., Sawatzky, R., & Meyerhoff, H. (2004). An integrative review of concept of spirituality in the health sciences. *Western Journal of Nursing Research, 26*, 405-428.

Chiu, l., Morrow, M,. Ganesan, S., & Clark, N. (2005). Choice of South East Asian immigrant women with serious mental illness: A socio-spiritual process. *Transcultural Psychiatry, 42*, 630-656.

Clark, N. (2005). *Community mental health professionals' perspectives on incorporating spirituality in their care of clients with serious mental illness: A qualitative inquiry*. Masters Thesis. Vancouver: University of British Columbia.

Clarke, I. (2001). *Psychosis and spirituality: Exploring the new frontier.* London: Whurr Publishers.

Connor, K. M., Davidson, J. R. T., & Lee, L. C. (2003). Spirituality, resilience, and anger in survivors of violent trauma: A community survey. *Journal of Traumatic Stress, 16*, 487-494.

Corrigan, P., McCorkle, B., Schell, B., & Kidder, K. (2003). Religion and spirituality in the lives of people with serious mental illness. *Community Mental Health Journal, 39*, 487-499.

Cook, C. C. H. (2004). Psychiatry and mysticism. *Mental Health, Religion & Culture, 7*, 149-163

Couture, J. E. (1994). Aboriginal behavioral trauma: Towards a taxonomy. Saskatoon: Corrections Canada. In Waldram, B.J., (1997). *The way of the pipe; Aboriginal spirituality and Symbolic Healing in Canadian Prisons.* Peterborough, ON: Broadview Press.

Davidson, R. J. (2002). Anxiety and affective style: Role of prefrontal cortex and amygdala. *Biolological Psychiatry, 51*, 68-80.

Davidson, R. J., Kabat-Zinn, J., Schumacher, J., Rosenkranz, M., Muller, D., Santorelli, S. F., Urbanowski, F., Harrington, A., Bonus, K., and Sheridan, J. K. (2003). Alterations in brain and immune function produced by mindfulness meditation. *Psychosomatic Medicine, 65*, 564-70.

Dein, S. (2005). Spirituality, psychiatry and participation: A cultural analysis. *Transcultural Psychiatry, 42*, 526-544.

Devereux, G. (1969). *Mohave ethnopsychiatry: The psychic disturbances of an Indian tribe.* Washington, DC: Smithsonian Institution Press.

Ellison, C. G., & Levin, L. (1998). The religion-health connection: Evidence, theory, and future directions. *Health Education and Behavior, 25*, 700-720

Engler, J. (1986). Therapeutic aims in psychotherapy and meditation: Developmental stages in the representation of self. In K. Wilber, J Engler, D. Brown (Eds.), *Transformations of consciousness: Conventional and contemplative perspectives on development* (Chapter 6). Boston: Shambhala.

Epstein, M. (1990). Psychodynamics of meditation: Pitfalls on the spiritual path. *Journal of Transpersonal Psychology, 22*,17-34.

Finkler, K. (1998). Sacred healing and biomedicine compared. In. P. J. Brown (Eds.), *Understanding and applying medical anthropology.* (pp. 118-128). Toronto: Mayfield Publishing Company,

First, B. M. (2006). Beyond clinical utility: Broadening the DSM-V research appendix to include alternative diagnostic constructs. *American Journal of Psychiatry, 163*, 1679-1680.

Foskett, J, Marriott, J & Willson-Rudd, F. (2004). Mental health, religion and spirituality: Attitudes, experience and expertise among mental health professionals and religious leaders in Somerset. *Mental Health, Religion & Culture, 7*, 5-22.

George, L. K., Larson, D. B., Koenig, H. G., & McCullough, M. E. (2000). Spirituality and health: What we know, what we need to know. *Journal of Social and Clinical Psychology*, *19*, 102-116.

Grabovac, D, A., & Ganesan, S. (2003). Spirituality and religion in Canadian psychiatric residency training. *Canadian Journal of Psychiatry*, *48*, 171-175.

Grabovac, D. A., Clark, N. & McKenna, M. (in press). Pilot study and evaluation of postgraduate course on "The interface between spirituality, religion and psychiatry."

Grouzet, F. M. E., Ahuvia, A., Kim, Y., Ryan, R. M., Schmuck, P., Kasser, T., Dols, J. M. F., Lau, S., Saunders, S., & Sheldon, K. M. (2005). The structure of goal contents across fifteen cultures. *Journal of Personality and Social Psychology*, *89*, 800-816.

Greyson, B. (1997). The near-death experience as a focus of clinical attention. *Journal of Nervous and Mental Disorders*, *185*, 327-34.

Hill, P. C., Pargament, K., Hood, R. W., McCullough, M. E., Swyers, J. P., Larson, D. B., & Zinnbauer, B. J. (2000). Conceptualizing religion and spirituality: Points of commonality, points of departure. *Journal for the Theory of Social Behavior*, *30*, 51-77.

House, R. (2001). Psychopathology, psychosis and the kundalini: Postmodern perspectives on unusual subjective experience In Clarke (Ed.), *Psychosis and spirituality: Exploring the new frontier*. (pp. 107-125). London: Whurr Publishers.

Hutchinson, G., & Haasen, C. (2004). Migration and schizophrenia: the challenges for European psychiatry and implications for the future. *Social Psychiatry Psychiatric Epidemiology*, *39*, 350-357.

Jackson, M., & Fulford, K. W. M. (1997). Spiritual experience and psychopathology. *Philosophy, Psychology, Psychiatry*, *4*(1), 41-65.

Josephson, A. M., Larson, D. B., & Juthani, N. (2000). What's happening in psychiatry regarding spirituality. *Psychiatric Annals*, *30*, 533-541.

Kabat-Zinn, J. (1982). An outpatient program in behavioral medicine for chronic pain patients based on the practice of mindfulness meditation: Theoretical considerations and preliminary results. *General Hospital Psychiatry*, *4*, 33-47.

Kessler, R.C., McGonagle., K.A., Zhao, S., Nelson, B.C., Hughes, M. Eshleman, S., Wittchen, H., & Kendler, S. K. (1994). Lifetime and twelve-month prevalence of DSM-III-R psychiatric disorders in the United States. Results from the National Comorbidity Survey. *Archives of General Psychiatry*, *51*, 8-9.

Kirk, K., Eaves, L., & Martin, N. (1999). Self-transcendence as a measure of spirituality in a sample of older Australian twins. *Twin Research*, *2*, 81-87.

Kirmayer, L. J. (2006). Beyond the 'new cross-cultural psychiatry': Cultural biology, discursive psychology, and the ironies of globalization. *Transcultural Psychiatry*, *43*, 126-144.

Kirmayer, L. J., Brass, G., & Tait, C. (2000). The mental health of Aboriginal peoples: Transformations of identity and community. *Canadian Journal of Psychiatry*, *45*, 607-616.

Kirmayer, L. J., Corin, E. & Jarvis, E. (2004) Inside knowledge: Cultural constructions of insight in psychosis. In: X. Amador & A. David (Eds.), *Insight in psychchosi.* (pp.197-229). New York, NY: Oxford University Press.

Kirmayer, L. J., & Minas, H. (2000). The future of cultural psychiatry: An international perspective. *Canadian Journal of Psychiatry*, *45*, 438-446.

Kirmayer, L. J., Rousseau, C., Jarvis, G. E., & Guzder, J. (2003). The cultural context of clinical assessment. In A. Tasman, J. Lieberman & J. Kay (Eds.), *Psychiatry* (2 ed. pp. 1-11). New York: John Wiley & Sons.

Koenig, H. G. (1998). *Handbook of religion and mental health.* London: Academic Press.

Koenig, H. G. (2004). Religion, spirituality, and medicine: Research findings and implications for clinical practice. *Southern Medical Journal*, *97*, 1194-1200.

Koenig, H., G. (2005) *Faith and mental health: Religious resources for healing.* Philadelphia: Templeton Foundation Press.

Koenig, H. G., George, L. K., Peterson, B. L. (1998). Religiosity and remission from depression. *American Journal of Psychiatry*, *155*, 536-542.

Koenig, H. G., & Larson, D. B. (2001). Religion and mental health: evidence for and association. *International Review of Psychiatry*, *13*, 67-78.

Koenig, H., McCullough, M., & Larson, D. (2001). *Handbook of religion and health.* Oxford: Oxford University Press.

Koenig, H. G., & Pritchett, J. (1998) Religion and psychotherapy. In H.G. Koenig (Ed.), *Handbook of religion and mental health.* (pp. 323 48) London: Academic Press.

Larson, D. B., Swyers, J. P., & McCullough, M. E. (Eds). (1998). *Scientific research on spirituality and health: A report based on the scientific progress in spirituality conferences.* New York, NY: Sponsored by The John M. Templeton Foundation.

Lewis-Fernandez, R. (1996). Cultural formulations of psychiatric diagnosis. *Culture, Medicine and Psychiatry*, *20*, 133-144.

Levin, J., & Chatters, L. M. (1998). Research on religion and mental health: An overview of empirical findings and theoretical issues. In H. G. Koenig (Ed.), *Handbook of religion and mental health* (pp. 34-47). London: Academic Press.

Lindgren, K. N., & Coursey, R. D. (1995). Spirituality and mental illness: A two part study. *Psychosocial Rehabilitation Journal*, *18*, 93-111.

Longo, D. A., & Peterson, S. M. (2002). The role of spirituality in psychosocial rehabilitation. *Psychiatric Rehabilitation Journal*, *25*, 333-335.

Lopez, S., & Guarnaccia, P. J. (2000). Cultural psychopathology: Uncovering the social world of mental illness. *Annual Review of Psychology*, *51*, 571-598.

Lukoff, D., Lu, F., &Turner, R. (1992). Toward a more culturally sensitive DSM-IV: Psychoreligious and psychospiritual problems. *The Journal of Nervous and Mental Disease, 180*, 673-682.

Lukoff, D., & Lu, F. G., (1999). Cultural competence includes religious and spiritual issues in clinical practice. *Psychiatric Annals, 29*, 469-472.

McCullough, M., & Larson, D. (1999). Religion and depression: A review of the literature. *Twin Research, 2*, 126-136.

McClain, Rosenfeld, B., & Breitbart, W. (2003). Effect of spiritual well-being on end-of-life despair in terminally-ill cancer patients. *Lancet, 361*, 1603-1607.

Miller, R. W., & Thoresen, E. C. (2003). Spirituality, religion, and health. *American Psychologist, 58*, 24-35.

Moreira-Almeida, A., & Neto, F. L. (2005). Spiritist views of mental disorders in Brazil. *Transcultural Psychiatry, 42*, pp.570-595.

Mueller, S. P., Plevak, J. D., & Rummans, A. T. (2001). Religious involvement, spirituality, and medicine: Implications for clinical practice. *Mayo Clinic Proceedings, 76*, 1225-1235.

Nelson, C. J., Rosenfeld, B., Breitbart, W., Galietta, M. (2002). Spirituality, religion and depression in the terminally ill. *Psychosomatics, 43*, 213-220

Newberg, A. B., & d'Aquili, E. G. (1998). The neuropsychology of spiritual experience. In H. G. Koenig (Ed.), *Handbook of religion and mental health* (pp. 76-94). New York, NY: Academic Press

Oman, D., & Thoresen, E.C. (2002). "Does religion cause health?": Differing interpretations and diverse meanings. *Journal of Health Psychology, 7*, 365-380.

Oman, D., & Thoresen, E C. (2003). Without spirituality does critical health psychology risk fostering cultural iatrogenesis? *Journal of Health Psychology, 8*, 223-229.

Pargament, K. I., Koenig, H.G., Tarakeshwar, N., & Hahn, J. (2001). Religious struggle as a predictor of mortality among medically ill elderly patients: a 2-year longitudinal study. *Archives of Internal Medicine, 161*, 1881-5.

Phillips, R. E., Lankin, R., & Pargament, K. I. (2002). Brief report: Development and implementation of a spiritual issues psychoeducational group for those with serious mental illness. *Community Mental Health Journal, 38*, 487-495.

Powell, H. L., Shahabi, L., Thoresen, E. C. (2003). Religion and spirituality: Linkages to physical health. *American Pscyhologist, 58*, 36-52.

Post, S. G. (1998). Ethics, religion and mental health. In H. G. Koenig (Ed.), *Handbook of religion and mental health* (pp. 22-28). London: Academic Press.

Powell, H. L., Shahabi, L., Thoresen E. C., (2003). Religion and spirituality: Linkages to physical health. *American Psychologist, 58*, 36-52.

Puchalski, C., & Romer, R. L. (2000). Taking a spiritual history allows clinicians to understand patients more fully. *Journal of Palliative Medicine, 3*,129-37

Richards, P. S. & Bergin, A. E. (1997). Religious and spiritual assessment. In P. S. Richards & A. E. Bergin (Eds.), *A spiritual strategy for counseling and psychotherapy* (pp. 171-200). Washington: American Psychiatric Association.

Seeman, E. T., Dubin, F. L., Seeman, M. (2003). Religiosity/spirituality and health: A critical review of the evidence for biological pathways. *American Psychologist, 58*, 53-63.

Sirois, F. M., & Gick, M. L. (2000). An investigation of the health beliefs and motivations of complementary medicine clients. *Social Science & Medicine, 55*, 1025-37.

Sheridan, M. J., Bullis, R. K., Adcock, C. R., Berlin, S. D., & Miller, P.C. (1992). Practioner's personal and professional attitudes and behaviors toward religion and spirituality: Issues for education and practice. *Journal of Social Work Education, 28*, 190-203.

Smye, L. V. (2004). *The nature of the tensions and disjunctures between Aboriginal understandings of and responses to mental health and illness and the current mental health system.* PhD Thesis, University of British Columbia, Vancouver, BC.

Stewart, B. (2002). Spirituality and culture: Challenges for competent practice in social care. In M. Nash and B.Stewart (Eds.), *Spirituality and social care.* (pp. 49-70) Philadelphia: Jessica Kingsley Publishers.

Tanner, A. (1993). *Bringing home animals: Religious ideology and mode of production of Mistassini Cree hunters.* Newfoundland: Memorial University

Tepper, L., Rogers, S. A., Coleman, E. M., & Newton Malony, H. (2001). The prevalence of religious coping among persons with persistent mental illness. *Psychiatric Services, 52*, 660-665.

Thielman, S. B. (1998). *Reflections on the role of religion in the history of psychiatry.* London: Academic Press.

Turbott, J. (1996). Religion, spirituality and psychiatry: conceptual, cultural and personal challenges. *Australian and New Zealand Journal of Psychiatry, 30*, 720-727.

Waldram, B. J., (1997). *The way of the pipe: Aboriginal spirituality and symbolic healing in Canadian prisons.* Peterborough, ON: Broadview Press.

Waldram, B. J., (2004). *Revenge of the Windigo: The construction of the mind and mental health of North American Aboriginal peoples.* Toronto: University of Toronto Press.

World Health Organization. (2001). *The world health report 2001: Mental health new understanding, new hope.* Retrieved October 13, 2005, from http://www.who.int/whr/2001/en/.

Zinnbauer, B. J., Pargament, K., & Scott, A. B. (1999). The emerging meaning of religiousness and spirituality: Problems and prospects. *Journal of Personality, 67*, 889-819.

Zinnbauer, B. J., Pargament, K. L., Cole, B., Rye, M. S., Butter, M. E., Belavich, G. T., Hipp, K. M., Scott, A. B., & Kadar, J. l. (1997). Religion and spirituality: Unfuzzying the fuzzy. *Journal for the Scientific Study of Religion, 36*, 549-564.

CHAPTER NINE

RELIGIOUS AND CULTURAL ASPECTS OF ISLAMIC SUFI HEALING

Marcia Hermansen

This chapter will consider shared elements of the Islamic religion that establish a set of beliefs underlying many healing practices in Muslim cultures. In addition, practices associated with Sufism – the mystical or esoteric element of Islam – are introduced in order to illustrate Islamic cultural healing and belief systems. In the concluding portion of the chapter, I reflect on issues such as historical change, cultural differences, the contemporary use of healing practices, and the role of class, gender, etc., within diverse Muslim cultural systems.

ISLAMIC HEALING: RELIGIOUS AND CULTURAL

The Islamic religious tradition spread widely to many parts of the world even in the pre-modern period. Currently, there are more than a billion Muslims living in regions as far flung as South-East Asia and sub-Saharan Africa to the Middle East and now, increasingly, in Western Europe and the United States.

Since it would be impossible in a single article to consider all of the cultural variables and techniques employed by Muslims within indigenous healing systems, this chapter focuses on the shared or unifying elements of the Islamic religion that establish a set of beliefs underlying many traditional healing practices. Specific attention will be paid to the Sufism because the Sufi interpretations and practices of Islam are more receptive to pre-existing local cultures, often incorporating these diverse elements into normative religious practices to create a synthetic approach to healing.

Islam is a Western religion in the sense that historically, geographically and doctrinally it continues elements of Judaism and Christianity. These common elements emerge within Islam's own unique sacred history, even though revelations come from the same divine source. As early as the ninth-century CE, Muslim intellectuals incorporated elements of Greek heritage and Hellenistic concepts of the soul and healing into the Islamic cultural repertoire. In fact, *Yunani* or Greek medicine is a healing tradition still practiced among the Muslims of South Asia.

ISLAMIC CONCEPTS OF PERSON AND WELL-BEING

The concept of person within Islamic theology is based the Qur'anic account of the first human ancestors, Adam and Eve. Like the Bible, the Qur'an recounts the story of Adam and his consort and their disobedience to God, yet for Muslims, the focus of the story lies in Adam's subsequent repentance, not his sin. God forgives Adam in response and gives him words of guidance (*Qur'an* 2:37). Thus, it is turning back to God and remembering the primordial connection with Him that is stressed in Islam (7:172). To be healed humanity is therefore required to fulfill the original sound human nature (*fitra*) by following divine guidance. Qur'an 95:4 states: "Indeed We [God] created humans according to the best stature." Consequently, the model of human well-being and the natural human state lies in being positive and balanced. The divine being provides natural and revealed sources that inspire and sustain this healthy state. These sources can be drawn on to restore health in the case of mental or physical illness. God is the healer and the one who suffices (*al-Shafi al-Kafi* in Arabic). This phrase is sometimes recited as an invocation and is used by Islamic mystics and healers in certain rituals. In a verse from the Qur'an, Abraham supplicates, "If I become ill then He is the One who heals me" (26:80). The Qur'an also presents God as the ultimate source of health and healing in the verse, "If God touches you with an affliction, no one can remove it but Him" (*Qur'an* 6:17).

The Qur'an indicates that God has repeatedly sent prophets to humanity to remind people of their bond of faith and to encourage them to obey divine guidance. Hence, the Islamic tradition emphasizes obedience to the specifics of the divine law (*shari'a*) as brought by the final messenger, Muhammad. In this manner, psychological and physical health may be restored from illness and well-being may be maintained through applying or invoking religious practices or symbols.

Based on the Qur'an, later Muslim scholars, especially those attuned to the philosophy and mysticism of Sufism, understood human nature as the constant tension of two major elements: the spiritual and physical or, said differently, angelic and animalistic (al-Ghazzali, n.d.). A key concept of human well-being is the necessity of balancing between material and spiritual needs, and avoiding both excessive deprivation and excessive indulgence. Attitudes of gratitude (*shukr*), patience (*sabr*), and acceptance – one meaning of the word *Islam* – are all understood to promote a healthy way of meeting circumstances that arise in one's life and maintaining the proper relationship with one's Creator.

More elaborate discussions of the soul and its maladies were developed in the Sufi manuals of the tenth- and eleventh-centuries by luminary thinkers such as al-Kalabadhi (ca. 990), al-Makki (996) and al-Qushayri (d. 1072). The Arabic word *nafs*, variously meaning soul, self, or ego, became central in Sufi concepts of the person and spiritual development. The Sufis further combined Qur'anic references to *commanding*, *blaming*, and *contented* levels of the soul (*nafs*) with Hellenistic ideas of vegetative, animal, and rational souls, thus, providing symbolic models of basic and spiritually advanced human development.

PROPHETIC MEDICINE AND QUR'ANIC HEALING

The life of the prophet Muhammad is paradigmatic for Muslims. He is "the best example" (*Qur'an* 33:21) and detailed records of his sayings, known as *hadith*, and his deeds constitute a well-trodden path known as the *Sunna* for adherents of this faith. Some of the prophet's specific healing practices are mentioned among the voluminous corpus of this *hadith* material and these continue to be used by religious healers. Because these practices came from the prophet Muhammad, they became known as *prophetic medicine*. Examples of such prophetic healing techniques include reciting verses from the divine word (*ruqya*) and then blowing on the afflicted individual. As the Islamic tradition was further articulated by the scholars (*ulema*) of generations following Muhammad, a corpus of prophetic medicine (*tibb nabawi*) developed (Ibn Qayyim al-Jawziyya, 1994). These medical practices were extrapolated from the Prophet's recommendations and habits regarding food and drink as well as his more general injunctions and healing practices. Admonishments such as, "one third of the stomach should remain empty after eating" and the numerous taboos and recommendations regarding food consumption and bodily cleanliness may be seen as constituting a preventative element of Islamic teachings regarding health and healing.

Other ways of transferring spiritual energy (*baraka)* used by Muslim healers would be writing down specific verses of the Qur'an on paper or on utensils such as saucers, then dissolving the writing material (saffron or ink) in water, and having this ingested by the ill person. Since these practices are sanctioned by the *hadith*, they are acceptable, even though they adhere to the most literal interpretations of the religion. The strong influence of these stricter definitions of normative Islamic practices arise from the influence of Saudi Arabia on global Islam since the 1980s. A category known as *Qur'anic healing* often claims the most or even the sole legitimacy among Islamic healing practices. Another means of curing is through amulets and talismans (*tawidh, talasm*) that are prepared in some Muslim cultures by religious teachers or healers. These amulets are used to repel negative energies or boost spiritual protections from positive influences surrounding an individual. Some amulets contain verses from the Qur'an, while others are numerological magic squares that may be generically reproduced or individually prepared based on the name of the client or one of his or her parents.

ILLNESS

The ritualized nature of most Islamic religious healing practices remains consistent with a concern for purity of the body, the mind, and the surrounding space. For example, advice to a troubled person to undertake the recitation of specific phrases from the Qur'an may indicate that special attention should be taken in maintaining a state of ritual purity through proper ablutions (*wudu*), performing the ritual prayers regularly, and so on. Health care institutions and providers might learn from this example sensitivity for a Muslim client's concern regarding food contents and cleanliness, since the psychological state and potential for healing is often associated with ritual purity. Words and attitudes reflect another dimension of health and purity, since improper speech, such as gossip or hostile words, interfere with the experience of Islamic religious practices such as the fast and the pilgrimage.

Islamic religious healing often involves the concept of the charisma or healing power of the Qur'an's revealed words. This positive energy can counteract negative forces arising from other persons through envy or hostility, or from projections of negative forces of evil that are embodied in the symbols of devils or *jinns*. Moreover, states of impurity or contact with unlawful substances can leave the human body and psyche vulnerable to illness. Even so, Muslim theology sees illness not as a punishment but, rather, as a test. Suffering, borne patiently, is said to eliminate the effects of sin "as leaves fall from a tree in the autumn," according to a saying of the Prophet.

ISLAMIC RELIGIOUS HEALING IN THEORY AND PRACTICE

In many contemporary Muslim societies, competing models of healing coexist. For example, Muslims in India and Pakistan who experience disease of one sort of another may consult practitioners of allopathic medicine, homeopathic treatments, *Yunani* medicine, or various *ruhani* cures (spiritual forms of diagnosis and treatment). These forms of healing may be applied simultaneously, selected on the basis of the type of complaint, or tried successively; the choice often depends upon the resources available to the client, the nature of the complaint, individual beliefs, and social location (Qidwai, 2003). Such diversity occurs commonly through Islamic cultures because various systems of indigenous curing exist alongside religious models and, of course, modern medical treatments (Dole, 2004; O'Brien, 2001).

ISLAMIC MYSTICAL OR SUFI HEALING

Coalescing and intermingling various systems of healing means that healers and experts will come together from different backgrounds: a *ulema* or religious scholar may interpret dreams or provide amulets, while elsewhere some Sufi *shaykhs* may perform these roles and provide spiritual direction. In South Asia, *hakims*, meaning wise or learned persons, are usually specialists in some system of traditional medicine such as *Yunani* medicine or homeopathy. Magical healers (*amil*) are specialists in healing through control over spiritual forces such as *jinns* or familiar spirits (*muwakkils*). In Turkey, a class of practitioner known as a *cinci* (*jinn* expert) specializes in problems attributed to the influence of malevolent spirits (Dole, 2004).

With Sufi healing specifically, the Islamic mystics developed a system of psychological theory and spiritual development drawing on Islamic roots while at times incorporating insights from local pre-Islamic customs and practices including Hellenistic systems of philosophy and medicine. Health and healing in Sufism, both within the high Islamic tradition and modern re-formations of this heritage by Western Sufis and Muslim intellectuals, address two main needs: moral healing and spiritual enhancement. Modern medical theory and global organizations such as the World Health Organization are interested in forms of traditional healing. In Sufi healing, imbalance or disease at the lower levels of physical or psychological structures need healing before attempting to progress further through the process of spiritual awakening. Physical ailments might be addressed by medicines or treatments involving touch. In some cases, these ailments are viewed as manifestations of deeper maladies of the soul that require spiritual attention to be healed.

Techniques for addressing fundamental moral defects or character flaws involve regular review and rectification of behavior and attitudes (*muhasaba*), remembrance of one's connection to God, and service to others. Classical Sufi practice includes group activities such as participating in collective rituals of chanting and, in some cases, communal living in the environment of a hospice (*khanqah*) under the direction of a Sufi master. Ideals of spiritual poverty, generosity, selflessness, and high moral standards, called spiritual chivalry (*futuwwa*), are promoted (Bakhtiar, 1993).

198 Cultural Healing and Belief Systems

Sufi healing requires insight and discernment from the practitioner or spiritual guide into the instinctive nature (*fitra*) or *qalib* of the person who needs healing. Each person requires a unique treatment, for the same procedures and healing techniques would not be effective on differing natures. The baseline for all humanity in the Islamic view lies in the proscriptions of the *shari'a*. Beyond this basic adherence to *shari'a*, the system of Sufi discipline is needed to evoke the potentials of a person's spirituality. Ideally, the enlightened spiritual guide (*murshid*) would assign practices, tasks, and cultivate experiences that most address the unique and distinctive proclivities of an individual.

Various type-psychologies are applied diagnostically by healers. For example, personal characteristics can be associated with specific divine attributes, or individual qualities can be divined through astrological mappings of the planets in a natal horoscope. Healers may employ a more esoteric model of spiritual centers (*latifa*, plural *lata'if*) that resemble somewhat the chakras of the Hindu Tantric tradition. A person's mental and physical state could reflect the influence of one of these subtle spiritual centers. A better understanding of these centers can be cultivated by the patient by contemplation, breathing exercises, or imagining the color of the center to be treated. Each center is associated with a color and, sometimes, a sound, thus aiding diagnosis by noting the colors that occur during dreams or visionary experiences (Hermansen 1997b; Schimmel 1975). Dream interpretation was commonly practiced in premodern Islam and was extensively cultivated by some Sufi orders such as the Turkish Helvetis (Ozak, 1987) Other Sufi writers held that individuals might be spiritually inspired by and, in turn, emulate the model or nature of one of the prophets or great saints of the past. This inclination was known as the *mashrab*, or the source from which such a person might imbibe inspiration.

In Sufi analysis individuals might also be characterized as predominantly *jamali* (manifesting gentle or beautiful divine qualities) or *jalali* (manifesting the majestic or wrathful qualities). In popular South Asian tradition, visitors to the shrine of a departed *jalali* saint, such as Alauddin Sabiri, must be much more cautious and reverent in their deportment lest they provoke the saint's wrath. A person displaying an imbalance of either characteristic could be assigned exercises of repeating names that signified the counterbalancing qualities as treatments.

Contemporary admirers and practitioners of Sufism in the West have found certain elements of Sufi healing to be compatible with aspects of modern psychological theory, especially the therapeutic orientations of humanistic and transpersonal psychology. For example, Robert (Ragip) Frager, an American transpersonal psychologist, is also a *shaykh* in the American branch of the Turkish Helveti-Jerrahi Sufi Order. Frager is also the head of a degree-granting institute of transpersonal psychology in Redwood, California. He compares Sufi and Western concepts of person saying that:

Traditional (Western) psychologies address one or two aspects of the soul, not wholistically. Ego psychology deals with the animal soul, outlining the main motivation for existence being that of seeking pleasure and avoiding pain. Behavioral psychology focuses on the conditioned functioning of the vegetable and animal soul. Cognitive psychology deals with the mental functions of the personal soul. Humanistic psychology deals with the activities of the human soul. (Frager, n.d.)

The closest approach to Sufism, according to Frager, is transpersonal psychology since it concerns the ego-transcending consciousness of the secret soul and the secret of secret souls (Frager, n.d.).

Frager's analysis reveals the therapeutic approach to religion typical of American engagement with Sufism. Even so, drawing parallels between the Sufi *shaykh* and the Western psychotherapist brings recognition to the usurpation of the prerogatives of traditional healers and teachers by the psychologist and psychiatrist in modern Western secular culture (Shafii, 1968). American Sufis often choose to engage with this therapeutic aspect by being or becoming therapists or, institutionally, by sponsoring conferences and forming organizations for *Sufi Psychology* (Hermansen, 2004).

Among more recent American Sufi movements, the complexities within transpersonal approaches engender a number of competing models of the transpersonal for cultivating levels of consciousness. One may distinguish between psychologies rooted in Sufi spirituality and holistic therapeutic techniques that have their origins outside the Islamic Sufi tradition. American Sufi practitioners favor the latter because these techniques are viewed as being consistent with or complementary to Sufi interests in personal transformation and healing. Examples include Jungian psychology the various transpersonal orientations of Ken Wilber, Robert Ornstein, etc., and the soul psychologies of James Hillman. All have in common the idea that human beings must find a way to live in union with a transcendent or transpersonal source of meaning and orientation. Where they locate the source and how they label it varies (e.g., how much of it is beyond and how much it is within the person). The more explicitly spiritual psychologies that see this transpersonal reality as God or the divine, the more closely they parallel the mystical philosophy in various traditional forms of spirituality, including Sufism.

THE SUFI ORDER IN THE WEST

The Sufi Order in the West was founded by Inayat Khan (d. 1927), a Sufi from Baroda, India. Khan wrote extensively on Sufism and Sufi theories of healing. In the 1970s the order was revived in Europe and the United States by his son, Pir Vilayat Khan (d. 2004). Jungian psychology, because it incorporates a spiritual dimension and involves a more compatible approach to dream work, has found acceptance in the Sufi Order as well as in some other western Sufi movements (Spiegelman, 1991). One of Pir Vilayat's Khan leading deputies, the American therapist Atum O'Kane, compares the approach of Jungian transpersonal psychology and the Sufi Order to human development, especially to the field of spiritual direction. Both approaches find a common ground in an expanded vision of the personality as an instrument for manifesting the Universal Self or divine qualities. Among the practices of the Sufi Order are meditation, breathing practices, *wazifa* (recitation of a personal litany), *dhikr* (remembrance of God through chanting and contemplation), light practices, creative imagination, and sacred music (Hermansen, 1997a). Although the Indian Sufi Orders who formed the cultural background of many of Inayat Khan's teachings practiced some of these methods of healing and spiritual cultivation, his son taught and explained them in more eclectic and scientific terms.

CLASSICAL TECHNIQUES OF SUFI HEALING

Meditation (*muraqaba*) of various kinds is described by classical Sufis. In some cases it would consist of an intense focusing of attention. In others, it would feature a form of meditation based on content or visualization. For example, the Indian Chishtis imagine the word *Allah* being written on the disciple's heart. In another form of the Chishti meditation, the disciple is to imagine sitting in the divine presence under the gaze of God. The content of the meditations might develop as a sort of series of spiritual exercises, or it might be based on the needs of an individual spiritual aspirant.

The *wazifas* of the Sufis are particular litanies for personal devotions sometimes known as *hizb* or *ahzab*. *Wazifa* means duty or practice and tends to be more personal while the *ahzab* are recitations for particular orders or specific purposes that Padwick terms "semi-magical" (Padwick, 1996, pp. 23-25). These would be memorized and recited or read on regular occasions. A famous example is the litany of the sea (*Hizb al-Bahr*), said to have been composed by al-Shadhili (d. 1258). According to one method of training this litany should be recited once a day for forty days. It is fairly long so this might take up to half an hour daily. The person who has done this becomes an practitioner (*amil*) of the *Hizb al-Bahr* who can apply it efficaciously in healing practices or for protection or influence. Much of the litany parallels the phraseology of the Qur'an, especially chapter 36, called "Ya Sin." Certain subsections of the *Hizb al-Bahr* are used thaumaturgically as spells or incantation so as to repel negative influences or to ensure other results. Similar incantation books (*a'mal*) are readily available in many Muslim societies. Shakyh Muzaffer Ozak (d. 1985) of the Helveti Order composed a manual that explains the ninety-nine divine names and provides their usefulness in healing and as incantations (Ozak, 1978). There is some debate as to whether a personal *wazifa* practice should only be assigned by an expert *shaykh* since the self-prescribed use of such powerful words might lead to instability or inappropriate outcomes.

The *dhikr* is a personal and a group practice for invoking *remembrance of God* through reciting pious phrases, especially the profession of faith (*shahada*) "there is no God but God." The Qur'an indicates that *dhikr* has a special calming effect in the verse: "Hearts find rest in the remembrance of God" (13:28). The *dhikr* also symbolically polishes the heart: according to a *hadith* report from the Prophet Muhammad, "there is a polish for everything that removes rust and the polish for the rust of the heart is *dhikr* (remembrance) of God" (Bayhaqi, II:419 #519). During the *dhikr*, the practitioner may strike (*darb*) the head or quickly breath downward towards the chest to symbolize a negation of the ego.

In terms of sacred music, there are traditions of various forms found in Muslim societies. For example, Inayat Khan was trained in the classical music of both North and South India. He wrote a number of treatises on the healing effects of music:

> What is wonderful about music is that it helps man to concentrate or meditate independently of thought. Therefore music seems to be the bridge over the gulf between the form and the formless. If there is anything intelligent, effective, and at the same time formless, it is music. Poetry suggests form, line and color suggest form, but music suggests no form.
>
> Music also produces that resonance which vibrates through the whole being. It lifts the thought above the denseness of matter; it almost turns matter into spirit, into its original condition, through the harmony of vibrations touching every atom of one's whole being. (Khan, n.d.)

Music associated with Sufism takes different forms in diverse Muslim cultures. Many religious scholars, both classical and contemporary, expressly oppose music because it induces frivolous attitudes and stirs sensual passions. Despite this opposition, music played a role in the practices and healing traditions of some Sufi orders. Notable examples of Sufi music include South Asian *Qawwali*, Moroccan *Gnawa*, the music of the Egyptian and Sudanese *zar* ritual, and the Turkish practice of musical healing through the orchestral accompaniment to the whirling of the Mevlevi dervishes. Each genre has different symbolic associations, performance traditions, and degrees of participation from the audience (Hoffman, 1995; Qureshi, 1995; Wolf, 2004).

In South Asian Sufism, *Qawwali* is performed and consists of music accompanied by lyrics composed of vernacular and Persian classical poetry. The intent of the music is to evoke ecstasy through the meaning of the mystical Arabic phrases and through rhythmic syncopated drumming (Qureishi, 1995; Wolf, 2006). Although *Qawwali* could be influenced by Hindu devotional singing, through the symbols, lyrics, and traditions that the Sufi Amir Khusrau (d. 1325) invented, plus the musical instruments, the scales, and many of the songs themselves, the music is now thoroughly Islamic. The African musical traditions seem to draw more on ideas of inducing trance to purge and purify. These traditions also involve women more often by including all of the audience in the dance. Ideas of spirits and spirit possession are interwoven with the meaning of the performance in a manner that may be thought of as purgative rather than ecstatic.

In Turkey, healing music reached it zenith in the Ottoman period. A restored fifteenth-century Ottoman hospital, now a museum in Edirne, was used primarily to treat the mentality ill. A major complaint of the time seems to have been love sickness or a sort of seasonal *weltschmerz* that was cured through a quiet and aesthetic setting, walks in well tended gardens watered by bubbling fountains, and the regular playing of appropriate melodies designed to harmonize the humors and calm agitated souls. The celebrated traveler and diarist Evliya Chelebi visited the hospital in 1640. In her account, she described musicians playing particular scales of music to treat different disorders afflicting the patients. Doctors would verify the effect by observing the patients' physical responses to the music.

CONCLUSION

I have only been able to suggest an outline of some of the frameworks and therapeutic techniques adopted by Islamic mystics. Within certain orders that stress the master-student interaction, generalized therapeutic models that can be applied without charismatic discernment were rarely developed. However, in some Sufi movements the dispersal of charisma and reduced personal contact with teachers encouraged the construction of systematic models of transformation that could be applied irrespective of the practitioner's unique needs.

The role of traditional healing practices and differing models in contemporary Muslim societies reflects a struggle to define normativity and rationality in the context of modern nation states. In the case of Turkey, modern systems of medical knowledge and treatment are identified with the project of secular nationalism while traditional and Islamic elements of healing are seen as superstitious and ineffective (Dole, 2004). In other societies, Islamist or Wahhabi traditions advocate for the elimination of certain cultural practices that draw on pre-Islamic elements.

In both classical Islamic law and in current debates, terms such as *adat* and *taqalid* (customs and traditions) indicate an allowable strata of common sense and communal practice that may be Islamicized and retained, whereas beliefs and practices stigmatized as *bid'a* or *kufr* (heretical innovation or disbelief) are strongly disparaged (Sengers, 2003). Healing through attributing ultimate power to anything other than God – to the stars, saints, or persons – would be considered *shirk,* a sinful case of *associationism* (O'Brien, 2001). Qur'anic or Islamic healing, however, would be acceptable since it is achieved through the mediation of Islamic symbols reinforcing normative belief.

In modernizing societies, consulting traditional healers is a practice normally associated with the poor or disadvantaged, who are considered more credulous and who may also lack the resources to locate or pay for treatments in medical clinics. In some Muslim cultures, certain popular healing practices favored by women, such as going into trance, visiting shrines and petitioning for cures, or effecting possession by jinns and spirits, are among the only culturally sanctioned ways for females to publicly express and release painful emotions.

The range of approaches to religious healing among Muslims raises the problematic of culture within the contemporary Islamic discourse, where Islamist ideologies reject many cultural elements in favor of legalistic, internationalist definitions of religious normativity. These legalistic models, however, may marginalize many of the beliefs and symbols involved in traditional healing practices.

A Dutch researcher on Muslim healing who practices in the Netherlands, Hoffer (1992), proposes a distinction between belief in *popular* Islam and *official* Islam, defining official Islam as the teachings propagated by the religious scholars (*ulema*) and prayer leaders (*imams*) of mosques. He characterizes popular belief as consisting of local traditions that incorporate pre-Islamic customs. I would argue that this distinction accepts the categories of Islamists (modern Muslim reformers) who are trying to assert only their version of Islam as valid. However, individual Muslims encounter religious healing in a variety of contexts, and Islamic legitimacy may be claimed for any one of these forms, including the *popular* practices.

Sufism itself has been condemned by secular nationalists as well as Salafi and Islamist religious purists during the modern period. Sufi healing methods, along with other elements of traditional medicine, have therefore been marginalized in many Muslim cultures. This suppression has occurred despite attempts to protect there methods as part of a valuable heritage or to understand their efficacy as an alternative to rationalized medical bureaucracy.

References

Bakhtiar, L. (1993). *God's will be done, volume one: Traditional psychoethics and its personality paradigm.* Chicago: Kazi Press.

Bayhaqi, A. (1986). *Shu`ab al-iman, volume two.* Bombay: al-Dar al-Salafiah

Dole, C. (2004). In the shadows of medicine and modernity: Medical integration and secular histories of religious healing in Turkey. *Culture, Medicine and Psychiatry 28,* 255-280.

Frager, R. (n.d.). *"Heart, self and soul: Concepts in Islamic/Sufic psychology"* http://www.crescentlife.com/articles/islamic%20psych/heart-self-soul2.htm Retrieved March 18, 2007.

al-Ghazzali, A. D. M. (n.d.) *The alchemy of happiness* (chap 4). (Claud Field, Trans.). http://muslim-canada.org/sufi/ghach4.html Retrieved Feb. 19, 2007.

Hermansen, M. K. (1997a). In the garden of American Sufi movements: Hybrids and perennials. In P. Clarke (Ed.), *New trends and developments in the world of Islam.* (pp. 155-178). London: Luzac Oriental Press.

Hermansen, M. K. (1997b). Mystical visions as 'good to think': Examples from pre-modern South Asian Sufi thought. Religion, 27, 25-43.

Hermansen, M. K. (2004). What's American about American Sufi movements? In D.Westerlund (Ed.), *Sufism in Europe and North America,* (pp. 36-62). New York, NY: Routledge.

Hoffer, C. (1992). The practice of Islamic healing. In A. Shadid (Ed.), *Islam in Dutch society.* (pp. 40-53). Kampen, Netherlands: Kok Pharos.

Hoffman, V. (1995). Sufism, mystics, and saints in modern Egypt. Columbia, SC: University of South Carolina.

Ibn Qayyim al-Jawziyya, M. (1994). *Natural healing with the medicine of the prophet.* (Muhammad al-Akili, Trans.). Philadelphia: Pearl Publishing.

Khan, I. (n.d.). Music: Spiritual attainment by the aid of music. In *The Sufi message of Hazrat Inayat Khan: Volume two, the mysticism of sound and music* (chap. 22). http://sufimessage.com/music/index.html Retrieved Feb. 19, 2007.

O'Brien, S. M. (2001). Spirit discipline: Gender, Islam and hierarchies of treatment in postcolonial Northern Nigeria. *Interventions, 3,* 222-241.

Ozak, M. (1978). *Ninety-nine names of Allah: The beautiful names.* (Shems Friedlander, Trans.). New York: Harper and Rowe.

Ozak, M. (1987). *Love is the wine: Talks of a Sufi master in America.* Putney, VT: Threshold.

Padwick C. E. (1996). *Muslim devotions.* Oxford: Oneworld.

Qidwai, W. (2003). Use of the services of spiritual healers among patients in Karachi. *Pakistan Journal of Medical Sciences, 19,* 52-56.

Qureshi, R. (1995). *Sufi music of India and Pakistan: Sound, context and meaning in Qawwali.* Chicago: University of Chicago.

Schimmel, A. (1975). *Mystical dimensions of Islam*. Chapel Hill: University of North Carolina.

Sengers, G. (2003). *Women and demons: Cult healing in Islamic Egypt*. Leiden: E. J. Brill.

Shafii. A. (1968). The pir (Sufi Guide) and the Western psychotherapist. In *The R. M. Bucke Memorial Society Newsletter*, *3*, 9-19.

Spiegelman, J. M. (1991). *Sufism, Islam and Jungian psychology*. Scottsdale, AZ: New Falcon.

Wolf, R. K. (2006). The poetics of "Sufi" practice: Drumming, dancing, and complex agency at Madho Lal Husain (and beyond). *American Ethnologist*, *33*, 246-268.

CHAPTER TEN

CHRISTIAN HEALING:
A REVIEW AND DISCUSSION OF EFFICACY

Simon Dein
&
Goffredo Bartocci

And he went throughout all Galilee, teaching in their synagogues and
proclaiming the gospel of the kingdom and healing every disease and
every affliction among the people. So his fame spread throughout all
Syria, and they brought him all the sick, those afflicted with various
diseases and pains, those oppressed by demons, epileptics, and
paralytics, and he healed them. (Matthew 4:23-25)

One Sunday morning in an Evangelical church in London, twenty
members of the congregation came to the front to receive healing. The pastor, a
man from Nigeria in his forties, was visiting. He claimed to have the gift of
healing. One by one each member of the congregation filed past him. He laid his
hands on their heads. Some became aroused, foaming at the mouth; they started
shaking. Many of them fell to the floor and were *slain in the spirit* – an experience
whereby the Holy Spirit overtakes them. This pastor believed that all sickness was
in the mind. He preached loudly to his audience that prayer can abolish any
sickness, even cancer. Sickness is demonic.

This brief anecdote exemplifies a phenomenon that occurs on a weekly basis in churches across the world. Many people resort to religious healing at times of sickness. But what is religious healing? How effective is it? Is it associated with any risks? This chapter is divided into two parts. After reviewing various types of Christian healing, we move on to examine questions of efficacy focusing on specific biomedical results.

The terms *religion, spirituality,* and *healing* are used in a multitude of ways in the scientific literature. Here, the term *religion* refers to an institutionalized set of beliefs in relation to the divine, whereas the term *spirituality* refers to an individual's sense of connectedness to the transcendent. The two terms are often used interchangeably, although recent authors (see Dein, 2005) have appealed for some degree of clarity. Similarly, the word *healing* is a contested and complex term. On one level it can mean a direct unequivocal and scientifically measurable cure of physical illness. The term can also refer to coping, coming to terms with, or learning to live with a condition that cannot be changed (including physical illness and emotional trauma). It can also refer to developing a sense of wholeness – emotional, social, spiritual, and physical – and signify a process of repairing one's relationship with God.

Only recently has the Western world divided medicine and religion into separate and distinct realms of knowledge. For much of Western history, performing healing was the prerogative of religious professionals. At present, religious or faith healing is often associated with supposedly superstitious populations, while biomedicine is generally the prevailing healing system in the so-called advanced Western world. Although statistics are difficult to obtain, it appears that religious healing is, nonetheless, a common activity practiced widely within the Christian tradition. While we acknowledge that religious healing is not unique to Christianity and occurs within other religious groups, we chose to concentrate on Christianity and healing because of the stark contrast between two co-existing paradigms in Western nations: faith healing and advanced biomedicine.

The Christian Church practices healing in a number of ways: through personal and group prayer; the use of laying on of hands; special services for the sick; saintly intercession; medical missions; pilgrimages to healing shrines; and, occasionally, the use of exorcism for deliverance of spirits. Many people who resort to faith healing do so in cases of otherwise incurable disease. However, the predominant view among supporters of faith healing is that medical treatment should be sought whenever necessary. For these Christians, the two systems of healing are compatible because they believe that God can heal both supernaturally and through modern medical practice. Generally, Christians are expected to seek biomedical healing rather than expecting miracles.

The miraculous acts of healing by Jesus and his disciples form a major theme in the development of early Christianity. Jesus always saw sickness as something to be healed whenever he encountered it (Matthew 4: 23-25; 8:16-17; 9:35). He held sickness to be the result of sin or the work of the devil (Mark 2:5; John 5:14), drew a direct connection between faith and healing (Matt 8:10), and saw healing as one of the signs of the presence of the Kingdom of God (Luke 9:11). Much of the Gospels relate to Jesus's healing of physical disease, mental illness, and spiritual disease involving possession by evil spirits. Often the three afflictions are intertwined. In fact, examples of healing occur sixty-five times in the Gospels, attracting public attention and inspiring faith by exposing Jesus's power.

Spiritual healing in the Gospels takes a number of forms: exorcism, healing at a distance by prayer, magical acts or gestures, and healing by touch. Healing through direct contact, such as touching Jesus' garments, is also described (Hankoff, 1992). These forms of healing continued after Jesus's death and there is no shortage of accounts of miraculous healings by religious figures. In the second-century CE., St. Ignacious was the first to describe the Eucharist as a medicine of immortality. Prudentius, a fourth-century poet and Christian apologist, celebrated the healing power of St. Cyprian's tongue. Bokenham, a medieval English friar, reported the healing power of milk from St. Agatha's breasts.

Porterfield (2005), in *Healing in the History of Christianity*, underscores the fact that healing has played a major role in the historical development of Christianity as a world religion. She contends that Christian healing had its origins in the Judean belief that sickness and suffering were linked to sin and evil while health and healing stemmed from repentance and divine forgiveness. Thus, Christianity might not have survived in the first centuries if not for the vigorous nursing that was done by the early church during epidemics. The healing of mental illness through religious practice was a key element of early Christianity. In medieval times, early medical care existed primarily in Christian hospitals and monasteries. The fact that illness and suffering were linked to sin and that healing could be brought about through repentance and divine forgiveness made religion tremendously appealing to outsiders and contributed greatly to its growth.

We now move on to discuss various forms of Christian healing. We are aware that the use of the term Christian may be contested by different groups. For instance, many within mainstream Protestantism and Catholicism would not agree that Christian Science is a form of Christianity. Also, we have been necessarily selective in our discussion due to limitations of space.

FORMS OF CHRISTIAN HEALING

CONTEMPORARY CATHOLIC HEALING AT LOURDES, FRANCE

Perhaps the most renowned site of Catholic healing is at Lourdes in France. The town of Lourdes is situated in the South-West of the Pyrenees, lying on the Pyrenean foothills. Originally an unremarkable market town, following the apparition of the Virgin Mary to the fourteen-year-old Bernadette Soubirous, Lourdes developed into a major tourist destination as a Marian city. Soubirous claimed to have witnessed this apparition on a total of eighteen separate occasions, a claim that has been supported by the Catholic Church (Harris, 1999). On January 18, 1862, Bishop Laurence, the Bishop of Tarbes, gave the solemn declaration that the apparitions were real and the site was holy, The Bishop's commission was convinced in part by Bernadette's testimony, but also because of the miraculous healings that were reported at Lourdes.

At present there are five million pilgrims and tourists who visit every season. Every year from March to October, the sanctuary of Our Lady of Lourdes is a place of mass pilgrimages from Europe and other parts of the world. Many hold that the spring water from the grotto possesses healing properties. Since 1860, an estimated 200 million people have visited the shrine, originally dedicated to the goddess Persephone. The candlelight and sacrament processions are especially impressive. Associated with the pilgrimage is the consumption or bathing in the Lord's water, which comes out of the grotto – the cave in which the apparitions took place in 1858.

Sixty-seven miracles, authenticated by the Catholic Church, have been described at Lourdes. Over seven thousand people have sought to have their cases confirmed as miracles but only sixty-seven have been declared scientifically inexplicable. These miracles involve a wide range of disorders. We can only mention a few. On May 10, 1948, a student nurse, aged thirty-one, was brought to Lourdes in a coma; emaciated and with a fluctuating fever, she suffered from tubercular peritonitis (an abdominal infection secondary to tuberculosis). She was given a tiny fragment of the Eucharist and awoke. She reported being instantly cured while lying in a wheelchair beside the spring. July 17, 1959, a man from Marseilles in France with femoral osteomyelitis with a fistula (a bone infection draining into the skin) was reputedly cured. October 9, 1987, a fifty-one-year-old Frenchman with multiple sclerosis was able to walk again.

British psychiatrist and psychical researcher, Donald West, examined the records of eleven cases of cures at Lourdes judged by the Catholic Church as miraculous (West, 1957). Although aware from previous experience that sufficient medical information is often lacking in reputed cases of faith healing, West (1957) felt that the situation at Lourdes would be different because medical files appeared comprehensive. Although the cases he reviewed were generally well documented, he showed that, even in these, the case notes lacked crucial information. A similar conclusion was also reached by James Randi (1987), who looked into some Lourdes healings. The water from Lourdes has been analyzed on a number of occasions and there is no empirical evidence that it has any curative properties in itself.

CATHOLIC HEALING IN SOUTH ITALY: PADRE PIO AND NATUZZA EVOLO

Southern Italy is renowned for reports of miraculous healings. Here we discuss two prominent figures, Padre Pio and Natuzza Evolo (Littlewood & Bartocci, 2005). Francesco Forgione was born near Benevento in Pietrelcina, South Italy to an illiterate and pious peasant family. There were many stories of miraculous events in his life. Beginning from the age of five, he experienced demonic and divine visions that continued throughout his life and led him to self-flagellation. In 1903, he entered a Franciscan Order on Mount Gargamo and took the religious name of Pio. He spent the rest of his life in that Capuchin community.[2] Throughout his life he suffered from frequent symptoms of illness, including chest pain and exhaustion. He was ordained in 1910 and went into military service in 1915 but was discharged on health grounds.

At the end of the First World War, he exhibited the full stigmata of the five wounds of Christ's crucifixion, which led to him wearing mittens in public over his bleeding hands. These stigmata continued for fifty years and, in his last year, he had circular wounds on both sides of his hands and feet. The wounds exuded bright red blood surrounded by regular layers of clotted blood, with no sign of inflammation or discharge of pus. He had a reputation for spiritual and physical miracles, which included: bilocation (the ability to appear in two places at once), levitation, prophecy, healing, the power to read peoples' hearts, the gift of tongues, and a fragrance that emanated from his wounds. He was known as an unrelenting and implacable healer. The Catholic Church adopted a rather ambivalent view of him and he was subjected to various Vatican investigations. However, in his last years he was supported by Pope Paul VII. At times, the Vatican doubted his stigmata and miracles; however, he was orthodox in doctrine and observance. He was also subject to many diagnoses by the medical establishment, particularly by the well-known father Gemelli, a physician and psychologist and the rector of the Universita Cattolica, who prior to his death denied the diagnosis of hysteria originally made in 1920.

The Italian mass media has played a large part in propagating the miracles of Padre Pio. For instance, the newspaper *Messaggero* published an article reporting on the miraculous phenomenon of bilocation that was reported by three prominent members of the modern Vatican state while they were in a normal state of consciousness and engaged in normal acts of their daily life. Because the Italian media drew attention to miracles like these, Padre Pio became popular throughout Italy; he even stands as the emblematic figure of one of the largest hospitals in Italy. Pio was consecrated as a saint by the Vatican in 2002.

A second case of stigmata and healing involves Natuzza, born in 1924 to an illiterate peasant family. As a young girl she was sent out to work as a household servant. At the age of ten, while working as a servant for a rich family, she started having visions of a priest and was admitted to a local psychiatric hospital. In 1938, she first exhibited stigmata after being discharged from hospital. She is married and has five children, one of whom is a doctor, and now lives with attendants in a purpose-built building with a chapel attached containing a statue of the Virgin as seen in one of her visions. The stigmata consist of various unique shapes: On her lower left leg there is a ring pattern, above it a rather naive picture of Christ; on the right leg there is another circular ring and above, letters standing for the Latin spelling of Jesus; on the dorsal side of the left wrist is the outline of St. Peter's Dome in Rome; and there is another ring on the right wrist with protuberances in the centre of the right and left hand palm signifying the end of the nails. Some scratches also appear on her shoulders and an unidentified mark appears in the centre of her cranium, most likely signifying the crown of thorns. She is regularly approached by people with various health problems who attribute to her the power of healing and the power of prophecy. In our own fieldwork, we found one lady who approached her because she was infertile.

The traditional theological explanation of these stigmata and those exhibited by others, such as St. Francis of Assisi, is that they reflect the individual's identification with the suffering Christ, which is so great that his wounds appear on their physical bodies. Since the time of St. Francis of Assisi, there have been some four hundred cases of stigmatics, the female-to-male ratio being seven to one (Harrison, 1995). There is much debate over whether these stigmata are self-inflicted cases of hysterical conversion or are, in fact, miracles. The factitious induction of skin marks, known as dermatitis artefacta, is well recognized.

THEOLOGICAL VERSUS MATERIALIST UNDERSTANDINGS OF ITALIAN HEALING

In Italy, explanations for the above phenomena have been largely theological. Materialist explanations have been lacking. What we can learn from cultural psychiatry is that special sets of cultural factors, combined with an individual's ability to transcend her or his individual psyche, may trigger psychobiological mechanisms. These mechanisms may facilitate the manifestation or experiences that are felt and described as pertaining to a realm *beyond the human*, that is, culturally ascribed to the divine.

In addition to the previously described miracle-working performed by holy places and by holy figures such as Padre Pio (Bartocci & Littlewood, 2004) or by non-canonic persons like Natuzza Evolo (Littlewood & Bartocci, 2005), we are witnessing a scholarly movement ruled by Vatican Universities that is aimed to remake the image of Christ from a divine entity deserving worship and theological contemplation to a powerful healing figure directly acting to alleviate mundane suffering. The re-interpretation of God's healing power portrays Christ more like a modern Asclepius than an irreproachable deity concerned only with exorcising evil spirits.

In his remarkable lecture presented at the decennial celebrations of the University San Raffaele, Cardinal Carlo Maria Martini attributed Christ's healing works to medical power rather than miraculous acts empowered by grace. In response, San Raffaele University granted the Cardinal an honorary degree in medicine and surgery – a degree that is rarely granted to Cardinals (Martini, 2006). Instead of using theological terms that portray God as forgiving but remote from his creation, Cadinal Martini depicts God as one who acts with surgical expertise in favor of his people. That is, doctors and nurses derive their healing ability from God who, in turn, acts through them. The medical doctors were interested most in Cardinal Martini's claim that scholars in medicine act as the agents of Christ's healing power: "Nowadays healing processes do not apply only to a group of skilled operators or to medical doctors but it is Christ who gave to Christianity the gift of healing peoples' illnesses eventually thanks to the intervention of nurses or graduate medical doctors" (p.59)

PENTECOSTAL HEALING

The practice of healing has a long tradition within Pentecostalism. The practice of faith healing has become revitalized in the past 150 years during the height of religious revivals. In America, it was not until the twentieth-century and the rise of Pentecostalism that divine healing once again assumed a central role in Orthodox Christian practice, linked with salvation itself. Pentecostalism as a movement began in the United States early in the twentieth-century and derived from the earlier holiness movement. The movement is composed of people who propagated the belief that the carnal nature of man could be cleansed through faith and by the power of the Holy Spirit, if one has had her or his sins forgiven through faith in Jesus. The Pentecostal movement within Evangelical Christianity places special emphasis on the direct personal experience of God through baptism of the Holy Spirit, as modeled after the Biblical account of the Day of Pentecost. It also places a new emphasis on the operation of New Testament gifts of the Holy Spirit, such as speaking in tongues, and gives prominence to divine healing and miracles (Poloma, 2003).

One high profile healer is Benny Hinn, a Pentecostal preacher and televangelist who is known for his flamboyant and highly theatrical style of ministry. He was born in 1952 in Tel Aviv to a Greek father and Armenian mother and was raised within the Greek Orthodox Church. He founded the Orlando Christian Centre in 1983. He hosts a thirty-minute show, *This is Your Day*, on various Christian television networks and organizes regular *miracle crusades*. Revival meetings and faith healing summits are held in large stadiums.

Frequently, members of the congregation are *slain in the spirit* and many claims of miraculous healings are made by his followers.

His teaching is similar to the Word of Faith doctrine, with a particular emphasis on healing. Word of Faith, or simply Faith, is a movement within Pentecostal and Charismatic churches nationwide that derives from the teachings of E. W. Kenyon, a New England Evangelical biblical teacher. Its central doctrine is that health and prosperity are promised to all believers: physical healing was included in Christ's atonement and, therefore, healing is available here and now to all who believe. Specific biblical passages are invoked to legitimize their doctrines, most notably Isaiah 53:5: "But he was wounded for our transgressions, he was bruised for . . . by whose stripes ye were healed."

Because the passage uses the present tense – we *are* healed – many of the most prominent Faith preachers teach that believers should overlook the symptoms of sickness and positively believe that they are already healed. Sickness is seen as an attempt by Satan to rob believers of the divine right to total health. Still, most advocate taking medical treatment, although some claim to be strong enough in faith to no longer need medicine. Not surprisingly, this teaching has been widely criticized. Critics point out that Isaiah 53:5 refers to forgiveness of sins, rather than to physical healing. Others also claim that the gift of healing died with the last Apostle so that the church will have to endure sickness and disease. Word of Faith ministers have also been accused of teaching that believers are little gods and even incarnations of Jesus Christ, seen by some Christians as a heresy. The Word of Faith theology also sees financial prosperity and wealth as part of Christ's atonement. Positive confession leads to positive life changes. They teach that Jesus and the Apostles were rich and, similarly, believers should accept, and even see financial success.

CHRISTIAN SCIENCE

Christian Science is a religious denomination founded in the U.S. in 1879 by Mary Baker Eddy, who herself claimed divine healing of an otherwise incurable illness. Although holding some major Christian tenets such as the omnipotence of God, the authority of the Bible, and the necessity of the crucifixion and resurrection of Jesus in human redemption, Christian Science departs from traditional Christianity by considering Jesus as divine, but not a deity, and regarding creation as wholly spiritual. As such, they hold that redemption from the flesh requires curing disease through spiritual means alone, likely the church's most controversial belief. In 1875, Eddy published *Science and Health* (Eddy, 1934), the founding text of Christian Science. She asserted that all is mind and there is no matter, that death and sickness are only illusions, and that everything emanates from God and is thus perfect. Healing comes from a true understanding of these doctrines.

Followers rely on spiritual rather than medical or material means for healing and most members refuse medical help for disease. Instead, they engage with Christian Science practitioners who provide a healing ministry. The Church teaches that God is good and comprises the only reality; all sin, evil and illness are overcome on the basis of this understanding. Practitioners heal patients through prayer, sometimes charging a modest fee. Only through study of the inspired words of the Bible can one learn to heal. Healing is understood, not as an end in itself, but as a natural way to be closer to God. From its inception, Christian Science has been embroiled in controversy and an increasing numbers of law suits have been leveled that challenge the claims and efficacy of Christian Science healing practices.

THE EFFICACY OF CHRISTIAN HEALING:

PHENOMENOLOGICAL, SPIRITUAL, AND EMPIRICAL

This chapter so far has described various types of Christian healing. We now move on to address the question of efficacy. The efficacy of Christian healing can be discussed at a number of levels: phenomenological, spiritual, and biomedical (in terms of altered biology and physiology). In his study of Charismatic Catholic healing, Csordas (1994) argued that this form of healing is necessarily effective by virtue of the phenomenological changes that ensue from it. Using theories of embodiment, he associated healing with perceived changes in the sense of self. Csordas was not specifically interested in biomedical changes associated with charismatic healing. Others have argued for the efficacy of Christian healing in terms of spiritual changes, such as increased closeness to the divine, that again disregard the physiological state of the sufferer. What changes instead is the state of metaphysical entities, such as the soul; a new sense of meaning in the person's life emerges, such as being *born again in the spirit*. Koss-Chioino (2006) used the term *spiritual transformation* to refer to this aspect of healing as the "fundamental change in the place of the sacred or the character of the sacred in the life of the individual" (p. 47). She associated healing with changes in self-perception and religious views; such changes appear to be a central component of healing in many belief systems apart from Western biomedicine.

It is important to distinguish *curing* from *healing*: Curing relates to the complete removal of physical or mental disease, whereas healing is a wider concept that refers to the restoration of wholeness to the sufferer. This requires a kind of transformation in one's understanding and experience of suffering and includes cognitive or behavioral changes as well as psychological or spiritual ones. Christian healing results in a changed perspective on suffering and undoubtedly enables the sufferer to derive a renewed sense of meaning and connectedness with the divine. However, is there evidence that Christian healing can cure disease from a biomedical perspective?

Christian healing typically takes on two forms: public Revivals – staged by famous preachers who promise dramatic and miraculous healings before the patient's eyes – and the less spectacular phenomenon of intercessory prayer. Both of these forms of healing have, to greater or lesser degree, been subject to empirical scrutiny. In order to demonstrate biomedical efficacy we would argue that three criteria must be met:

1. The illness must be one that does not normally recover without treatment. The majority of alleged cases of miraculous healings at Lourdes were later considered by doctors to be the result of spontaneous remission.
2. There must not have been any prior medical treatment that may be expected to influence the illness.
3. Both diagnosis and recovery must be demonstrable by detailed medical evidence.

Unfortunately, we would argue that these criteria have not been applied scrupulously to most alleged claims of healing, and those that have been subject to strict scientific validation fail to demonstrate any effects beyond that of a placebo, a substance containing no medication and prescribed to reinforce a patient's expectation of getting well. On this basis we contend that there is no empirical evidence that faith healing has cured organic disease. That being said, the patient's faith in miraculous healings may reinforce an expectation of getting well that produces positive results through a relaxation or placebo response.

Performing double blind clinical trials on Christian healing is a difficult endeavor: A major problem exists in establishing what constitutes an appropriate placebo in this context. Furthermore, Christian healing comprises a number of interrelated elements – prayer, ritual, laying on of hands, etc. – and it would be difficult to establish which of these is effective. However, until this level of scientific rigor is achieved we cannot conclude with any degree of confidence that religious healing has its own specific efficacy above and beyond placebo treatment.

One aspect of Christian healing that has received increasing attention in the scientific literature is intercessory prayer, a prayer to God on behalf of another person (Benson, Dusek, Sherwood & Lam 2006; Byrd, 1988; Cha, Worth, & Lober, 2001; Krucoff, Crater, & Green, 2001; Krukoff, Crater, & Gallup, 2005). Although these studies have attempted to reach the gold standard of the double blind controlled trial, they have attracted much criticism and, to date, have failed to demonstrate an effect of intercessory prayer on biomedical processes. In the past ten years, a burgeoning literature arguing for a positive effect of faith on both physical and mental health has arisen (Koenig, 1997). A poll in 1996 of one thousand adults found that 79% believed that spiritual faith can help people recover from disease (McNichol, 1996). However, some have questioned whether religious beliefs or prayer actually benefit health at all (Sloan, Bagiella, & Powell, 1999). Is it possible that religious or spiritual beliefs might in fact worsen health? This hypothesis is borne out by a well designed study of patients discharged from a British hospital. The authors evaluated the outpatient records and responses of 189 patients' questionnaires. They concluded that the health status of patients with stronger spiritual beliefs was twice as likely to be unimproved or worse (King, Speck, & Thomas, 1999).

Flamm (2004) has outlined some of the difficulties in examining intercessory prayer empirically. It is impossible to divide people into groups that received prayer and those who do not, for people outside the scope of the study could be praying for someone without the researcher's knowledge. Also, how could one assess the degree of faith in patients who are too sick to be interviewed or comatose? Since control groups are not possible, scientific experiments are not possible.

There are other problems with intercessory prayer studies. When experiments are carried out to determine the effects of prayer, what precisely is being studied? For instance, what type of prayer is being employed? Are Christian, Jewish, Muslim, and Buddhist prayers equal? Is prayer to a saint equivalent to prayer to God? What about prayers to the Virgin Mary? Are prayers to God and Jesus equivalent? What is the length and frequency of the prayer? Are two ten-minute prayers equal to one twenty-minute prayer? How many people are praying and does their religious status and religion matter? Is one priestly prayer identical to ten parishioner prayers? Does the sincerity of the prayer affect its power and how might this be measured? Most prayer studies lack such operational definitions and there is lack of consistency across studies.

We would argue that, unfortunately, studies of revivalist healing have so far failed to adopt the rigorous assessment criteria discussed above and deployed by those involved in studies of intercessory prayer. Many purported studies are simply attempts to discredit evangelical healers and are no more scientifically rigorous than the claims made by the healers themselves. Evangelists will often ask patients what the problem is and accept their lay diagnoses: For instance, someone seeking help may say he or she has a kidney problem when the issue is a backache instead. An evangelist does not verify whether the patient was indeed suffering from kidney problems, nor is the evangelist familiar with the patient's medical history, yet he or she might announce that the patient was healed of kidney problems to an entire audience. Evangelists rarely perform follow-up examinations, thus exaggerated numbers of reported healings can multiply rapidly in these environments. Many people are embarrassed to say that God has not healed them and will affirm that healing has occurred when it has not – a sure way of resolving cognitive dissonance.

Other reports of healing are precipitated by the erroneous assumption that doctors always diagnose problems correctly. In some cases, a doctor might tell a patient that he or she has an incurable illness for which death will occur within a short period of time. At the end of this period, however, the patient is alive and much better. The patient's survival may be attributed to divine healing when the physician's diagnosis may initially have been wrong.

Empirical studies of faith healing reaching any level of scientific credibility are rare in the literature. An early study by Rose (1971) examined several hundred cases of healing over twenty years and concluded that not one example of a miracle cure had been found and, therefore, he was not convinced of the efficacy of faith healing.

A comprehensive examination of contemporary healers in James Randi's (1987) book, *The Faith Healers*, describes how many Evangelistic healers use deception and fraud. As an example, he describes the work of Peter Popoff, an evangelist who would call up names of people in the audience and describe their illnesses. He said he received this information from God but it was actually obtained by confederates who mingled with the audience before his performance. Relevant data would be given to his wife, who broadcast it over a small receiver in his ear. However, Randi did not subject patients to empirical examination.

Although there is no empirical evidence for the efficacy of faith healing on organic illness, there is some evidence that the perception of being healed relates to the intensity of professed belief in the healer's abilities. If a person believes that the healer possesses some healing ability, he or she will feel better. An Australian study by Lyvers, Barling, Harding-Clark (2004) investigated the psychic healing ability of a well-known Australian psychic. Twenty volunteers suffering from chronic pain were recruited by newspaper advertisements. Half were assigned to a treatment or control condition using a double blind procedure. The comparison of pre- and post-treatment McGill pain questionnaire ratings indicated that psychic healing had no effect. However, the pre-treatment questionnaire ratings of belief in psychic healing and related phenomena were correlated with improvement in the McGill pain questionnaire ratings, irrespective of treatment condition. These results suggest that the effects of psychic healing and faith healing were attributable to the power of belief. The effects of faith healing were no greater than that of a placebo.

In another pain study, Abbot, Harkness, and Stevinson (2001) examined the use of face-to-face healing compared to simulated face-to-face healing for 120 patients suffering from chronic pain. The pain predominately was of neuropathic and nociceptive origin and resistant to conventional treatment. It was concluded that a specific effect of face-to-face or distant healing on chronic pain could not be demonstrated over eight treatment sessions in these patients.

THE DANGERS OF FAITH HEALING

There are problems beyond the lack of evidence for the efficacy of faith healing; it also has inherent dangers. For instance, it can cause patients to shun effective medical care or cause doctors who accept faith healing to diminish their medical efforts, believing that God will do all the work. In addition, faith healing could have emotional and psychological repercussions for patients. Emotional stress combined with fear of treatment failure can lead to serious depression.

Christian Scientists are probably the best known group that shuns traditional medical care. In fact, this is the only form of faith healing that is deductible as a medical expense for federal income tax purposes. The weekly magazine, *Christian Science Sentinel*, publishes several testimonies in each issue. They claim that prayer has brought about recovery from diverse conditions such as, anaemia, arthritis, corns, deafness, defective speech, multiple sclerosis, paralysis, visual difficulties, and more. No systematic, medically supervised study of the outcomes of Christian Science healing has ever been performed. However, there is evidence that devout Christian Scientists rarely consult doctors and, therefore, pay a high price for avoiding medical care.

Some evidence suggests that Christian Scientists may have higher mortality rates than Seven Day Adventists, both of whom have dietary restrictions and avoid alcohol (Simpson, 1989), but only Christian Scientists avoid medical treatment. A study comparing the mortality of Christian Scientists and Seven Day Adventists found even greater differences of two college groups with higher mortality rates among Christian Scientists (*CTC Mortality and Morbidity Weekly Report*, 1991).

CONCLUSION: WHERE DO WE GO FROM HERE?

We have discussed various forms of healing in Christianity. Evidence for an empirical effect of Christian healing on physical disease is lacking despite increasing numbers of studies and, thus, we appeal for more stringent research. But the question remains: Where do we go from here? A need clearly exists for greater rigor in the empirical study of faith healing both in medicine and in psychiatry.

Nonetheless, the issues go far deeper than raising important epistemological and ontological questions. A correct methodology for evaluating religious healing in clinical psychiatry and medicine should examine the coherence between the cultural categories that support religious healing and the cultural categories based on materialist therapeutic approaches to mental and physical illness. In order to engage better the old antinomy between spiritual credo without organic substrate and secular credo with material, it is important for scientists to absorb into the secular credo study of the epistemological compatibility of science and faith. Using new hybrid sciences such as biocultural approaches to mental and physical health, it is possible to go deeper into the science and faith debate, beyond consideration of ontological or cultural categories to neuronal functions that are activated by particular kinds of experiences. If we accept Darwin's statement that, in order to develop his theory of species evolution, he did not need a notion of God and his theory proved to be successful, why do we not accept that, in order to cure biological illness or functional mental illness, that the same notion is also unnecessary? However, we cannot oversimplify that complex realm; cultural memes are as strong as genes (Dawkins, 2006). The bioscientific approach considers that the biocultural construction of the mind has produced a sort of synaptic-God within the mind. In order to pursue research on science and faith as belief systems, it would be beneficial to be involved in studies aimed at identifying which biological mechanisms facilitate a God-construct within the human mind (Bartocci & Dein, 2005; Dawkins, 2006).

In addition, by adopting a clinical approach, there is enough data to suggest that a positive outcome for a mental illness is often obtained through a sudden crisis, a subversion, a detachment from the previous conditions of the pathological mind. While the religious scholar infers the transformation as divine intervention, from the agnostic perspective of biocultural medicine it appears preferable to call the psychic and behavioral transformation a sudden rearrangement of the synapses, rather than a supernatural conversion. Such synaptical reorientation can be achieved by the play of extramundane energy or reached by very mundane (but longer) current psychiatry therapeutic procedures. Clearly, cultural psychiatrists and anthropologists must negotiate between two positions: They must understand the emic views of the religious practitioners themselves in which all healing is the miraculous work of the Divine, while also attempting to understand this healing through biomedical mechanisms involving synaptical reorientation. From the first position, health professionals are but mediums for divine intervention and their role is relatively peripheral, but, according to the second position, health professionals play a more central and active role.

NOTES

1 See Dein (2002) for examples of healing within Orthodox Judaism.

2 The Order of Friars Minor Capuchin is among the chief offshoots of the Franciscans in the Roman Catholic Church.

References

Abbot, N., Harkness, E., & Stevinson, C. (2001). The study of spiritual healing as a therapy for chronic pain: A randomized control trial. *Pain, 91*, 79-89.

Bartocci, G., & Littlewood, R. (2004). Modern techniques of the supernatural: a syncretism between miraculous healing and the mass media. *Social Theory and Health, 2*, 18-28

Bartocci, G., & Dein S. (2005). Detachment: Gateway to the world of spirituality. *Transcultural Psychiatry, 42*, 545-569.

Benson, H., Dusek, J. Sherwood, J., & Lam, P. (2006). Study of the therapeutic effects of intercessory prayer (STEP) in cardiac bypass patients: A multicenter randomized trial of uncertainty and certainty of receiving intercessory prayer. *American Heart Journal, 151*, 934-942.

Byrd, R. (1988). Positive therapeutic effects of intercessory prayer in a coronary care unit population. *Southern Medical Journal, 81*, 826-829.

Cha, K., Worth, D., & Lober, R (2001). Does prayer influence success of in-vitro-fertilization-embryo transfer? *Journal of Reproductive Medicine, 46*, 78-87.

Csordas, T. J. (1994). *The sacred self: A cultural phenomenology of charismatic healing.* Berkeley: University of California Press.

CTC Mortality and Morbidity Weekly Report (1991). *40*, 579-582

Dawkins, R. (2006). *The God delusion.* Boston: Houghton Mifflin.

Dein, S. (2002). The power of words: Healing narrative among the Lubavitcher Hassidim. *Medical Anthropology Quarterly, 16*, 41-63.

Dein, S. (2005). Spirituality, psychiatry and participation: a cultural analysis. *Transcultural Psychiatry, 42*, 526-544.

Eddy, G. M. B. (1934). *Science and health: A key to the scriptures.* Boston, MA: Trustees under the will of Mary Baker G. Eddy.

Flamm, B. (2004, September-October). The Columbia University "miracle" study: Flawed and fraud. *Skeptical Inquirer, 4*(5).

Harris, R. (1999). *Lourdes: Body and spirit in the secular age.* London: Allen Lane.

Harrison, E. (1995). *Medieval phenomena in the modern age: The study of six contemporary cases of stigmata and reactions to them.* PhD thesis: University of Kent.

Hankoff, L. (1992). Religious healing in first-century Christianity. *The Journal of Psycho History, 19*, 387-408.

King, M., Speck, P., & Thomas, A. (1999). The effect of spiritual beliefs on the outcome of illness. *Social Science and Medicine, 48*, 1291-299.

Koenig, H. (1997). *Is religion good for your health: the effects of religion on physical and mental health.* New York, NY: The Hayworth Pastoral Press.

Koss-Chioino, J. (2006) Spiritual transformation and radical empathy in ritual healing and therapeutic relationships. In J. Koss-Chioino and P. Hefner (Eds.), *Spiritual transformation and healing: Anthropological, theological, neuroscientific and clinical perspectives* (pp. 45-61). Oxford: Alta Mira Press.

Krucoff, M., Crater, S., & Gallop, D. (2005). Music, imagery, touch and prayer as adjuncts to interventional cardiac care: The monitoring and naturalization of noetic trainings (Mantra 2): A randomized study. *Lancet, 366,* 211-217.

Krucoff, M., Crater, S., & Green, C. (2001) Integrative noetic therapies as adjuncts to percutaneous interventions during unstable coronary syndromes: Monitoring and actualization of noetic therapies (Mantra) pilot. *American Heart Journal, 142,* 760-769.

Littlewood, R., & Bartocci, G. (2005). Religious stigmata, magnetic fields and conversion hysteria: One survival of "vital force." Theories in scientific medicine? *Transcultural Psychiatry, 42,* 596-609.

Lyvers, M., Barling, N., Harding-Clark, J. (2004). The effect of belief in "psychic healing" on self reported pain in chronic pain sufferers. *Journal of Psychosomatic Research, 60*(1), 59-61.

Martini, C. M. (2006, October 13). Se Dio ci guarisce. *La Repubblica,* p. 59.

McNichol, T. (1996, April 7). The new face of medicine. *USA Today,* p. 4.

Poloma, M. (2003). *Mainstream mystics: The Toronto blessing and reviving Pentecostalism.* Walnut Creek, CA: Altamira Press.

Porterfield, A. (2005). *Healing in the history of Christianity.* Oxford: Oxford University Press.

Rose, L. (1971). *Faith healing:* Baltimore, MD: Penguin Books.

Randi, J. (1987). *The faith healers.* Amherst, NY: Prometheus Books.

Simpson, W. F. (1989). Comparative longevity on a college total Christian Scientist. *JAMA, 262,* 1657-1658.

Sloan, R., Bagiella, E., & Powell, T. (1999). Religion, spirituality and medicine. *Lancet, 353,* 664-87.

West, D. (1957). *Eleven Lourdes miracles.* London: George Duckworth.

CLINICAL ISSUES
IN CULTURAL HEALING

CHAPTER ELEVEN

QUALIFICATIONS AND STANDARDS OF INDIGENOUS HEALERS: A CROSS-CULTURAL CHALLENGE IN COLLABORATION

Jonathan H. Ellerby

As blended approaches and integrated cultural approaches to care are developed to serve cross-cultural communities, credentialing among non-Western practitioners becomes a central issue. Recognizing that Indigenous rates of mortality, morbidity, and incarceration are typically disproportionately higher than in most other groups, the matter of effective models of care and rehabilitation for Indigenous people has become a critical issue. This chapter explores the collaborative work between Western institutions and Indigenous healers. A framework for understanding the differences in credentialing in the Indigenous world versus the Western world is discussed, as well as the essential means by which Indigenous healers receive recognition for their qualification.[1]

Determining credentials and standards is currently a critical issue in the complementary and alternative healing community. Complementary and alternative medicines are forms of healing, treatment, and therapy that have originated and are sustained outside the Western allopathic biomedical model. A range of remedies and practices, such as meditation, herbal medicine, Healing Touch, and acupuncture fall within this category of medicine. Public interest in complementary and alternative medicine is growing (Barnes, Powell-Griner,

McFann & Nahin, 2004). Consumers are seeking more involvement in the treatments and preventions of their illnesses. Moreover, many people recognize the shortcomings of Western medicine and are now searching for other solutions. As a result, medical practitioners and healthcare organizations need to discern which practitioners are credible, safe, and reasonable to work with and refer to. Partnerships with practitioners who are inadequately educated, lacking in clinical experience, and unprincipled ethically must be avoided to protect the financial and legal concerns of institutions and, more importantly, to protect the community being served. This same issue figures predominantly in Indigenous communities around the world where traditional healing practices are still in use.[2]

Traditional Indigenous healing techniques include as wide a range of practices and remedies as found in other complementary and alterative medicines. Traditional medicine may include things such as prayer, fasting, purification ceremonies, herbal medicines, massage, and counseling. Particularly, credentialing is of concern in Canada and the United States where users of traditional Indigenous medicine and healing have experienced a variety of personal violations and misdemeanors ranging from deception, outright misrepresentation, and fraud, to sexual abuse (Churchill, 1994). It should not be assumed that these negative cases are indicative of the typical quality of Indigenous medicine or practitioners. Even so, the perception of Indigenous healers by an individual, community, or organization can quickly and permanently be changed by a single damaging experience. Therefore, infrequent or not, the issue of standards and credentials becomes important for all groups involved. While setting standards for Indigenous healers is a difficult and widely debated topic, this chapter presents a simple overview of the key issues and some possible steps to guiding individuals and groups.

The Need for Recognized Standards

The importance of distinguishing legitimate healers from those who are not is a complex and highly politically charged topic, yet it persists and requires attention. Non-Indigenous communities and organizations seek to ensure that the development of healthcare initiatives to support, serve, or partner with Indigenous people is done with the input of Indigenous spiritual leaders and traditional healers. Indigenous spiritual leaders and traditional healers are two separate categories of practitioner within the world of Indigenous healing and spirituality. Traditional healers use various remedies to treat illness and imbalances. Spiritual teachers, who may also often be called healers, are known for their gift of speech and philosophical instruction, similar to priests or psychologists in other cultures.

Association with fraudulent or unrepresentative healers can prove destructive to the communities involved; yet, most non-Indigenous collaborators have no means to discern if they are working with qualified people in the first place. As an example, some hospitals in Canada and the U.S. are establishing traditional healing programs involving traditional Indigenous healers to enhance the care of Indigenous clients (Young & Smith, 1992). Selecting healers is difficult for many non-Indigenous administrators. The wrong selection can put clients at risk or create schisms between the hospital and the local Indigenous community.

Discerning between qualified healers and frauds is also a critical issue for the general public. Many Indigenous people seek complementary and alternative approaches to care and traditional healers are a common choice. Indigenous people are seeking healers because they have complex health issues in their communities such as high rates of diabetes, cancer, heart disease, obesity, drug addiction, metal health conditions, and domestic violence. Many suffer from multiple conditions compounded by a lack of healthy identity (low self-concept, poor boundaries, and experiences of trauma), in conjunction with a lack of healthy association with traditional beliefs and practices. Many of these people have had little exposure to traditional Indigenous healing practices and have little capacity to distinguish one healer from the next. Charisma and availability may sometimes be the only criteria by which a healer is chosen: Such choices can prove disastrous. There are endless stories of Indigenous people who have been abused and taken advantage of by other Indigenous people who claimed to be healers. In some cases the fraudulent healers may not only be poorly trained, but also not even of the Indigenous ancestry they claim (Churchill, 1994).

Problems related to fraudulent or poorly trained healers become multiplied when these people serve non-Indigenous communities. The general inability of non-Indigenous people to distinguish legitimate Indigenous healers or healing practices from frauds and poorly trained capitalists further complicates the dynamics of credentialing and standards. Non-Indigenous weekend workshop consumers and New Age enthusiasts often base their involvement with Indigenous medicine on simplistic and sometimes romanticized ideas about the nature of Native healing. Through the attention of the uninformed public, many non-Indigenous and unrepresentative Indigenous healers have skewed the popular image of what defines Indigenous medicine. Through the force of consumer demand, the work and literature of unskilled or unrepresentative healers reinforces the work of the fraudulent healer. Unqualified healers may improperly gain credibility through popularity and local fame alone.

HISTORICAL CHALLENGES

COLONIZATION AND CONTROL

There are two essential problem areas in the conceptualization of standards and credentialing related to traditional healing and healers. The first concerns the history of colonial relationships and the second concerns the nature of the training and development of traditional healers and medicine people.

It must be noted that most forms of standardized classification in Western academia are typically used in a materialistic and reductionistic fashion to demonstrate mastery according to a scientific method (Thornton, 1998). Most Indigenous communities have experienced a long history of academic misrepresentation. Many non-Indigenous experts have documented and classified Indigenous culture, healing, and spirituality in a manner that reveals more about their own preconceptions (and misconceptions) than about the lived experiences of Indigenous people (Deloria, 1994). Western professional associations, such as in the medical, psychological, and chaplaincy communities, use credentials to ensure skill, quality, and ethics. They also use credentials to restrict and control variation, competition, and to ensure homogeneity.

Popular culture and business have also benefited through the exploitation of Indigenous healers and healing traditions. There are many authors and teachers of Indigenous culture who have benefited from wealth and popularity, while neglecting to further serve the needs of Indigenous communities or individuals they had learned from. Perhaps a surprise to some, many current pharmaceuticals – such as acetaminophen, digoxin, diosgenin, and Taxol – were derived from Indigenous remedies and pharmacopoeias. Nevertheless, the acknowledgement of intellectual property or contribution is still rare (Balick & Cox, 1997). A stark divide exists between the pharmaceutical industry, one of the most prosperous industries in the world, and Indigenous communities, the most consistently impoverished groups of people in the world.

Additionally, it is critical to recall that less than one hundred years ago Indigenous expressions of medicine and spirituality were prohibited and punishable offenses throughout the world by the same non-Indigenous governments that remain dominant today. Both the United States and Canada are examples of nations that made Indigenous healing practices illegal (Pettipas, 1994). Naturally, any process that would define and classify Indigenous healers in a documented and legalistic format, even if done by Indigenous people, could potentially serve as a tool for the control or manipulation of Indigenous people by consumers, academics, profiteers, or governments.

INDIGENOUS PARADIGMS OF TRAINING

The second major area of complication is correlating the means by which healers are trained with standards intelligible to non-Indigenous people and systems. While there are clear and long-standing traditions of education and credentialing within Indigenous communities and medicine societies, they are not as simply homogenous, or as empirically oriented, as those found in Western medicine. Consequently, it is more difficult to find mutual agreement – either between Indigenous groups or with Western professional associations – in defining credentialing standards. Indigenous medical systems and healing traditions thrive on plurality and diversity in skill, method, and specializations, and are strongly dependent on the participation and guidance of the non-corporal/spiritual world. The spiritual world is understood as a multilayered world of sentient beings that exist independent of physical form, and yet can interact with human beings through dreams, intuition, meditation, and waking visions. Some spiritual beings may be deceased ancestors, or may be supernatural forces or beings. The spiritual world plays a key role in Indigenous spirituality and healing (Kalweit, 1992).

In a simplistic summary, there are four predominant manners in which Indigenous healers are trained and recognized. These four areas may be labeled as: ancestral, apprenticeship, cumulative, and transformative. Virtually every Indigenous healer should be able to self-identify with one or more of these categories of training. Accordingly, each of these four manners of *becoming* a healer may be verified through community members and personal history. Frequently, a healer's right to practice will be earned from a combination of all four categories of training. It is important to note that each of these categories of training and credentialing may also be revoked through congruent means. An understanding of each of these areas can provide the foundations for a system of credentialing, or simply a framework for consumers and partners – organizations, researchers, and practitioners – to determine the credibility of a healer.

DEFINING THE FOUR-FOLD SYSTEM OF TRAINING AND RECOGNITION

Prior to explaining the four main categories of training and recognition, it is critical to make a few contextual notes. First, in most Indigenous healing systems, regardless of how a person is trained, there is often a wide spectrum of healing specialties that may be practiced. Much like those in the Western medical community, Indigenous healers may specialize in areas such as herbal medicine, counseling, surgery, or musculoskeletal manipulation. Some healers may have subspecialties in these areas, in which they focus on specific techniques, or even diseases such as cancer or AIDS. Therefore, a healer may be qualified to work in some areas but not others. As an example, a healer may be a well regarded ceremonialist and counselor but is unable to prescribe plant medicines. Similarly, a healer may conduct shamanic healing ceremonies, yet is unqualified to provide counseling or psychosocial support outside a ceremonial setting.

Second, many healers will not self-identify as healers, or at least not to the full extent of their wisdom or history of experience. Conversely, healers or charlatans whose motivation is profit or fame tend to draw more attention to themselves. This dynamic has created much confusion for those seeking the aid of Indigenous healers. Often the most qualified healers are hard to find and identify. On the other hand, self-promoting healers tend to be poorly skilled and motivated. All the same, one cannot assume a lack of credentials simply because a healer is assertive or boastful; personality and cultural background may also be a factor. In some traditions, it is expected that a healer will boast of his/her abilities to heal to prospective clients to increase their confidence and trust. Generally, healers who are preoccupied with remuneration and popularity are to be investigated with caution and respect.

Third, great diversity exists among Indigenous communities, making generalizations of any kind difficult. The healing traditions and systems of medicine vary from one Indigenous community to another, locally and globally. In some cases, two Indigenous nations separated by thousands of miles may have more in common than two that border one another. It is imperative that consumers and partners use generalizations as guides in a process to learn respectfully about local and specific practices and systems. Often healers within a single cultural group will demonstrate diversity, not only in specialization, but even in their therapeutic approach to the same health concern. These differences may be based on family tradition, an experience of apprenticeship, learning from another culture, or through the healing tools and gifts received from the spiritual world. Gifts from the spiritual world may include insights, talents, or aptitudes that are attributed to a supernatural source and not personal development.

Finally, these categories should not be interpreted in a reductionistic fashion, and assumed to be clear cut or universally acceptable to all Indigenous people. The categories are not mutually exclusive, but overlapping and, in some respects, interdependent. While a healer should be able to identify with one of these categories as the primary process by which she or he became a recognized healer, the most experienced, widely recognized and effective healers tend to qualify in all four of the following categories (Kalweit, 1988, 1992).

1 – ANCESTRAL

In many Indigenous communities around the world, the ability to heal is strongly associated with a person's lineage (Kalweit,1988). It is understood that the power to heal is transferable and moves from one generation to the next. This is exemplified in the book *Gift of Power*, when Archie Lame Deer discusses the exact moment he felt his dying father pass *the gift* to him (Erdoes, 1992). A traditional *Venda* healer in South Africa explained to me that a healer has to have healers in their ancestry, for it is in fact the spirit of a deceased healer that does the work of healing, not the living healer at all.

Determining a healer's relationship to their ancestry is therefore one key component to establishing credentials. Nonetheless, simply being born into a liniage of healers is not enough to establish the ability and credibility of a healer. A healer must also undergo a process of activating, developing, and controlling their abilities to heal. Techniques, tools, and ceremonies are learned through experience, practice, guidance, and spiritual sanction. These aspects develop over time.

2 – APPRENTICESHIP

Perhaps the most common manner of training and credentialing, regardless of how a healer begins their work, is through apprenticeship. Apprenticeship is much like the Western medical tradition of supervised clinical training or physician residencies. What makes Indigenous healing apprenticeships different from those in the West is that they are holistic and often deeply personal. Typically, mentors will provide guidance in lifestyle, diet, conduct, dreamwork, personal psychology, and life choices, in addition to the teaching and supervision of a therapeutic technique or ceremony. Another hallmark of Indigenous apprenticeships is their duration. While some may be short, some mentor relationships will last decades.

I worked with a healer in the Amazon jungle who had trained for more than fifteen years under a variety of *Maestros* (mentor or master). Even though he was a mature adult, he would still defer to his teacher to conduct and supervise ceremonies, and would not claim the title of master healer. Another healer whom I have worked with has studied traditional medicine in apprenticeships for more than twenty years and still maintains a relationship with senior healers in his family and community for the purpose of consultation and continued education and training.

An essential requirement for a successful apprenticeship is the approval from an external person or council confirming the apprentice's right and ability to use a particular medicine, treatment, or conduct a healing ceremony. This approval stems from a prolonged supervised training period of several years. These relationships also serve as regulating mechanisms over standards and qualifications. Most healers, regardless of age, will maintain a primary relationship with a mentor or council for the majority of their lives. The mentor-student apprenticeship is often deeply personal and one of mutual sacrifice and dependence. It is important not to confuse or misrepresent the kinds of experiences a person may have with an Indigenous healer during a short aquaintance at a workshop or ceremony as an apprenticeship relationship. Most people from Western societies are not raised with the experience of prolonged mentorship and are quick to misidentify and idealize short term relationships as apprenticeships.

3 – CUMULATIVE

Cumulative training and experience is important and common to almost all healers, but does not necessarily define credentials. Some healers are recognized by a community or a mentor based on the sheer depth and breadth of experience they may have amassed over a lifetime. Such a credential may come with old age, and/or the passing of menopause. Again, perspective between Indigenous and non-Indigenous communities about the value of cumulative knowledge and experience varies. The majority of credible healers I have met around the world, even those of senior years, will still humbly consider themselves students even after decades of training. In contrast, a Western anthropologist or ethnobotanist may be regarded as an expert on the medical and healing systems of an Indigenous community after five years of academic study.

Many traditional healers demonstrate an interest in the healing arts and related topics at a very young age. Healers often begin preliminary training and even mentorship at a young age. It is common for young people who show a predisposition to healing work to begin learning about medicine and healing as children by helping to pick medicine, by attending the ceremonies, and by witnessing the healing work of older healers in their families.

4 – TRANSFORMATIVE

The last category to be identified is complex and creates the biggest complication in the credentialing of Indigenous healers, inside and outside of Indigenous communities. Indigenous healing and medical systems are symbiotically dependent on the participation of the spiritual world and non-corporal beings. Therapeutic procedures and approaches such as cures, botanical formulas, ceremonies, and psychological insight are often directly provided to the healer by a spiritual being. Natural powers, ancestors, animal and plant spirits are all examples of non-corporal *helpers* that provide Indigenous healers with techniques and clinical acumen. Similarly, the vocation of healing work may begin with direction provided by a spirit being. As such, any person, at any stage in life or development, may suddenly be *called* to do healing work and be given a unique ability or gift to help people. Since the spiritual world follows its own logic and design, human beings can never fully predict who may be called. There remains an understanding in Indigenous communities that all people carry the potential to heal, though not all may be called to reveal or develop it.

There are means by which Indigenous medicine societies and informal community councils of healers may verify the claims of a person who professes to have been called to heal. Unless the person is already working as an apprentice or has a close relationship with a credible, qualified healer, she or he is more likely to begin work immediately because of the divine inspiration or spiritual permission she or he has received. For obvious reasons, this eagerness becomes a point of contention, yet deep respect for the spiritual world and the interface between human and spiritual beings prevents most Indigenous people from challenging those who claim to be spiritually guided to begin healing work. Nevertheless, as in any culture, there is always a concern that the strong desire and greed of some individuals may cause them to interpret events and spiritual experiences in a self-serving manner. Indigenous healing work often relies on the honesty of the healer to report what is requested or expected from the spiritual world. Since they are interpreters of spiritual realities, it becomes difficult to prove when a healer is making requests based on their desire for profit or gain. This problem emphasizes the importance of credibility among Indigenous healers. It has been argued that people who have such a strong desire to help must be able to offer some help to people, so credentials should not be an issue. Although goodwill and a desire to help mark the character of a healer, when dealing with matters of the spirit or the physical body, sheer good intentions may not be adequate to deal with the forces that may be at work.

Physical medicine can be toxic or debilitating if misused; in a similar way, spiritual medicine also has a power to influence the body and mind and, thus, if mismanaged or misused, can be harmful. Spiritual forces have a complexity and power that far exceeds the intellect, fortitude, or knowledge of most individuals, and so proper training in ritual and use of human spiritual senses are critical to ensure the safety of both the practitioner and the person seeking healing. Experience in Indigenous spiritual and healing practices reveals that spiritual forces manipulated during healing are not merely psychological or symbolic suggestions that produce a placebo-effect, but are instead actual entities and energies that impact the physical world (Young & Goulet, 1994).

CONCLUSION

TRADITION, SYNCRETISM, EVOLUTION AND INSPIRATION

The preceding analysis should not be seen as a definitive examination of the important issues surrounding credentialization. Instead, I hope to provide a guide that can be balanced with personal intuition, experience, and study. These categories could, for example, be used to develop a system of standards for individuals and organizations to use in the process of interviewing healers they wish to partner with. Asking a healer about their life and training should be done with great respect and humility. Always ask permission first, pay attention to the answer and respect their wishes. If possible, it may be preferable to find out indirectly about how a healer qualifies in each of these four areas of training and development.

In every generation there are new and evolving roles and types of healers. There are many people providing help in this world who are influenced by Indigenous medicine. Indigenous or not, there are many approaches that are influenced by Indigenous medicine that are not representative of the original tradition. Currently, a range of modalities exist that incorporate Indigenous techniques and philosophies: subtle energy healing, massage, hot stone therapy, spa services, and counseling programs. While these people or groups have their own standards and credentialing issues, the key concern of Indigenous people lies in proper representation of their traditions. If a healer or modality is not sanctioned through one of the four categories listed, or lacks the support and the validation of an Indigenous community, then the healer or methodology should not be represented as Indigenous. Counselors using shamanistic techniques in healing, for example, could call their work *shamanic*, but could not honestly call themselves shamans or their approach properly Native American. New categories are necessary to accurately represent the range of healing work being done today and to prevent the distortion or misrepresentation of Indigenous healing traditions. Terms like *earth medicine, Indigenous-based*, or *shamanic*, may create enough of a distinction to prevent practitioners and healers from incorrectly implying that they practice traditional Indigenous medicine or that they are Indigenous healers.

Indigenous healing has become a very politically and socially charged issue where the forces of ownership, representation, colonization, profit, wellness, identity, and miracles converge. Ultimately, all the perspectives presented here must be taken liberally. In many Indigenous communities, I have learned that a healer can rarely win everyone's approval: One person's healer is another's insufferable relative and vise versa. Rarely does universal agreement occur on who is an excellent healer. In a way, such preferences are no different than the bias people develop in Western medicine for favorite doctors, nurses and psychologists based on skill, personality, or a unique relationship.

In the end, healing is something that exceeds the limits of definitions. Healing is the natural gift of all human beings; each of us finds our way to receive it and to offer it in a multitude of ways that will never be fully understood or reduced to language. While there is much about healing and healers we cannot label or explain, and likely never will, there can be no denial that there are as many ways to heal as there are stars in the sky. For that mystery, we should be eternally grateful and open to the healing gifts of all people.

NOTES

[1] While I claim to be neither an expert on Indigenous culture nor of Indigenous ancestry, I draw from seventeen years of intimate experience and study with various traditional healers in Indigenous communities around the world, predominantly in the United States and Canada. Many of my dearest friends and extended family are Indigenous and I have seen first hand the impact of these issues in organizations, in communities, and on both Indigenous and non-Indigenous individuals. I offer my best thoughts with great respect and humility. I can only hope to stimulate a dialogue and perhaps some understanding between communities.

[2] The term Indigenous, in this chapter, refers to cultural groups compriseig the first or earliest known inhabitants of a region that are further distinguished by their earth-based spirituality and historical identity

References

Balick, M., & Cox, P. A. (1997). *Plants, people, and culture.* Scientific American Library.

Barnes P., Powell-Griner E., McFann K., Nahin R. (2004). Complementary and alternative medicine use among adults: United States, 2002. *.CDC Advance Data Report, 343.* Retrieved from http://nccam.nih.gov/news/camstats.htm

Churchill, W. (1994). *Indians are us?* Toronto: Between the Lines.

Deloria, V. (1994). *God is red.* Golden, CO: Fulcrum.

Erdoes, R. (1992). *Gift of power: The life and teachings of a Lakota medicine man.* Santa Fe, NM: Bear & Co.

Kalweit, H. (1988). *Dreamtime and innerspace.* Boston: Shambhala.

Kalweit, H. (1992). *Shamans, healers, and medicine men.* Boston: Shambhala.

Pettipas, K. (1994) Severing the Ties that Bind: Government Repression of Indigenous Religious Ceremonies on the Prairies, Winnipeg, MB: University of Manitoba Press.

Thornton, R. (1998). Studying Native America: Problems and Prospects, Wisconsin, WI: University of Wisconsin Press.

Young, D., & Goulet, J. (1994). Being Changed: The Anthropology of Extraordinary Experience, Peterborough, ON: Broadview.

Young, D., & Smith, L. (1992). The Involvement of Canadian Native Communities in Their Health Care Programs: A Review of the Literature Since the 1970s, Edmonton, AB: Canadian Circumpolar Institute/University of Alberta.

CHAPTER TWELVE

ABORIGINAL ELDERS AS HEALERS:
SASKATCHEWAN ELDERS SPEAK ABOUT SEXUAL HEALTH[1]

Mary Rucklos Hampton,
Kim McKay-Mcnabb,
Sherry Farrell Racette,
&
Elder Norma Jean Byrd

This chapter reports on ways that Aboriginal Elders understand healing with a focus on sexual health issues, a significant concern confronting Aboriginal youth and young adults.[2] We suggest that healing in Aboriginal communities extend beyond individuals and families to include *cultural healing*. Elders within Aboriginal communities received the teachings of previous generations through the oral history of the Aboriginal nations; they are the *keepers of knowledge*, thus serving as cultural healers. Dominant theories from psychology and related disciplines offer explanations for the causes of illness and suggest paradigms for healing problems that confront youth today (Rotheram-Borus & Futterman, 2000); however, traditional Aboriginal epistemology might suggest more effective ways of healing sexual health problems that confront First Nations, Métis, and Inuit youth of today, particularly if we frame the need for healing among Aboriginal youth as cultural healing. This chapter offers the voices of Aboriginal Elders who speak from their understanding of these issues and suggest ways of healing.

We are using the definition of *healing* offered by Katz (1993), which he derived through listening to Indigenous healers in different parts of the world. Healing is a transformative process that restores individuals and communities to meaning, balance, connectedness, and wholeness. Many Indigenous cultures regard the concept of *healing* – a process of transformation – to be a necessary alternative to the notion of *curing* – merely removing the symptoms of illness. Healing, understood in this way, frames the process of reclaiming sexual health after generations of colonization.

BACKGROUND

SEXUAL HEALTH OF ABORIGINAL YOUTH

Sexual health of Indigenous youth is a high-priority research topic globally (Aguilera & Plasencia, 2005; Eng & Butler, 1997; Foley et al., 2005). Despite this urgency, the sexual health of Aboriginal youth in Canada has garnered little attention. Based on findings from a developmental program evaluation of Planned Parenthood Regina's Sexual Health Centre, our research team discovered that Aboriginal youth in our community experience more sexual health risk factors than non-Aboriginal youth (Smith et al., 2001). For example, significantly more Métis students than other students reported being physically forced to have intercourse (Bourassa, McKay-McNabb, & Hampton, 2004). Researchers also suggest that unplanned pregnancies are a problem for Aboriginal youth and young adults (Anderson, 2002). Furthermore, the occurrence of AIDS is leveling off in the general population of Canada but is rapidly increasing in Aboriginal populations (Marsden, Clement, & Schneider, 2000; Vernon, 2001). As many as 20% of AIDS cases in Canada occur in Aboriginal populations, which also generally involve individuals who are considerably younger than in non-Aboriginal cases (Canadian Aboriginal AIDS Network). Aboriginal women, Aboriginal youth, and two-spirited people (lesbian, gay, or bisexual people) are at increased risk due to high-risk sexual behavior and alcohol and drug use (Goldstone et al., 2000; LeDuigou, 2000; McKay-McNabb, 2006; Ship & Norton, 2000).

The Royal Commission on Aboriginal Peoples identified healthy pregnancies and births as a high priority in serving the health needs of Aboriginal people (RCAP, 1998). In Saskatchewan, the most common reasons for hospitalization in the Aboriginal population are complications in pregnancy, childbirth, and the puerperium (the four-week period following childbirth) (Regina Health District, 2000a, 2000b). Furthermore, the risk of cervical cancer in sexually active women can be greatly mitigated though having regular PAP tests and follow-up treatments, yet recent statistics show that mortality from cervical cancer is up to twice as high in North American Aboriginal women compared to non-Aboriginal women (Lanier & Kelly, 1999). These findings, supplemented with information from the few studies that have included statistics on Aboriginal youth, indicate that young Aboriginals need healing in the area of sexual health (Anderson, 2002; Bertolli et al., 2004; Foley et al., 2005).

Some researchers are attempting to understand the influence of culture when delivering appropriate sexual health care (Amaro & Raj, 2000; Amaro, Raj, & Reed, 2001; Jemmott & Jemmott, 2000; Reid, 2000; Rew, 2001). Demographic profiles of Canadian population growth indicate that the Aboriginal population is increasing at about twice the rate of the general Canadian population (Frideres, 1998; Tkach, 2003). The Aboriginal population also comprises a young population of childbearing age, with one-third younger than fifteen and over half younger than twenty-five (Statistics Canada, 2001, 2002). These demographic trends, combined with the long-term positive impact of early intervention, suggest that sexual health care needs of Aboriginal youth should be a priority service delivery issue (Rew, 1997; Rotheram-Borus & Koopman, 1991). Examples of sexual health services for Aboriginal youth that draw on cultural strengths are rare (Foley et al., 2005). Effective programs that are targeted at Aboriginal youth have been shown to incorporate historical teachings, interventions that aid healing from intergenerational trauma, and traditional cultural activities (Aguilera & Plascenia, 2005).

EFFECTS OF COLONIZATION

The health disparities between Aboriginal and non-Aboriginal Peoples in Canada can be traced back directly to colonization. Access to culturally appropriate health care continues to disadvantage Aboriginal people (Foley et al., 2005; Young, 1988; 1994). The erosion of Indigenous sexual health began in the early years of colonialism when Europeans were alternately repelled and fascinated by radically different views of the body and sexuality (Stoler, 2002; Young, 1995). From the earliest contact, colonialism sought to control and exploit the sexuality of Aboriginal people, while at the same time developing racial constructs that represented Indigenous people globally as governed by their passions and lacking in intellect and self-control. Colonial strategies sought to emasculate Aboriginal men through alcohol and political manipulation, while the conquest of the bodies of Aboriginal women served as a metaphor for the conquest of land and territory (Farrell Racette, 2001; Green, 1990). During the fur trade, the sexual exploitation and devaluing of Aboriginal women was justified by depicting them as naturally promiscuous and wanton, which subsequently absolved European men of guilt or responsibility for their actions and created a representation of Indigenous sexuality that persists to the present time. In addition to a continual campaign to control Indigenous sexuality though associating it with promiscuity and shame, nineteenth-century missionaries sought to break down traditional Aboriginal family structures and replace them with Christian models.

Female power, particularly in the mother-daughter relationship, was routinely represented as a barrier to the goal of establishing a husband's authority over his wife and children (Driving Hawk Sneve, 1977). The combined strategies of eroding the respect and power of women, and degrading sexuality through shame and exploitation, laid the ground for the devastating impact of residential schools.

In 1879, Nicholas Flood Davin recommended that the Canadian government emulate the American policy of *aggressive civilization* through the creation of Industrial Schools. His rationale for this act speaks to both the strength and persistence of Aboriginal social structures and beliefs: "It was found that the day school did not work, because the influence of the wigwam was stronger than the influence of the school" (Davin, 1879, p. 1). The curriculum Davin recommended was to be the instrument that transformed boys into farmers and girls into farmer's wives. Unfortunately, Davin's recommendations to implement the highest quality of instruction in the residential schools and to maintain the trust and support of First Nations leadership were never followed through. Residential schools not only interrupted and denigrated transmission of traditional Aboriginal knowledge, they also created a legacy of sexual and spiritual abuse that impacts the generation of youth today (Aboriginal Healing Foundation, 2006; Anderson, 2000; Hanson & Hampton, 2000). Oneida psychologist Dr. Roland Chrisjohn invoked article two of the United Nations Convention on Genocide to damn the residential schools as an act of cultural genocide. The residential schools destroyed the culture of Aboriginal people by causing serious bodily or mental harm to members of the group and by forcibly transferring children of the group to another group (Chrisjohn & Young, 1997). Many aspects of the residential school experience were devastating to sexual health, particularly the practice of punishing expressions of sexuality, interest in the opposite sex, and even natural occurrences such as menstruation. The use of extreme shaming as a discipline strategy was so common that former students frequently describe themselves as incapable of feeling embarrassment because of being emotionally numb or, by contrast, consumed with rage. Girls were taught to be ashamed of their developing bodies: Nudity, even while bathing, was equated with sin.

TRADITIONAL INDIGENOUS KNOWLEDGE AND PRACTICE

A powerful way to offer culturally appropriate interventions and reverse the historical damage done to Aboriginal peoples through colonization is by drawing on the wisdom shared by Elders. A major resurgence of interest in traditional Aboriginal culture, thought, and spirituality has emerged in the last two decades (Garrett & Herring, 2001; Kulchyski, McCaskill, & Newhouse, 1999). Many post-secondary institutions are finding ways to include the teachings of Elders in their curriculum; many are including an Elder-in-residence as a way of incorporating traditional wisdom (Barnhardt & Angayuqaq, 2005; Moore, 2003; Steckley and Cummins, 2001).

Traditionally, an Elder is a highly respected older person who has knowledge of the ancient, spiritual, and cultural ways of her or his people (Kulchyski, McCaskill & Newhouse, 1991). Through their special knowledge, Elders act as bridges to spiritual experiences and teach others about spiritual matters (Cajete, 1994). Stiegelbauer (1996) has indicated that Aboriginal communities call upon the Elders for their support when making decisions about health. Because the possession of moral and ethical knowledge comes from spiritual experience in Aboriginal cultures, the Elders' knowledge has particular relevance in addressing the moral and ethical issues of sexual health. Elders traditionally offer help and guidance in a number of different ways: for example, by providing personal counseling, providing teachings, conducting ceremonies, offering healing, teaching conflict resolution, leading group problem solving, being a role model, giving a comforting physical presence, as well as continuing to learn about life themselves (Stiegelbauer, 1996).

RESEARCH QUESTIONS

Our overall research method is described best as community action research, which includes and privileges voices of Aboriginal youth, community workers, and Elders (Senge & Scharmer, 2001). We worked with a guiding Elder and ten Aboriginal community-based organizations over a five-year period to define our initial research questions, and to collect and analyze data that would be relevant for Aboriginal communities. This chapter describes focus group consultation with Elders in our community to enhance our understanding of the sexual health problems we see confronting Aboriginal youth in Saskatchewan. Therefore, the objective of our study was to ask Aboriginal Elders: Is sexual health of Aboriginal youth an area of concern? If so, why? And finally, what should we do about it? Grounded theory methods were used to analyze this information (Strauss & Corbin, 1998).

METHOD

DATA COLLECTION

Participants. Purposive sampling methods were used to recruit participants for our focus group; however, we might more accurately define this model as a *relational* recruitment method (Huberman & Miles, 1998). Our guiding Elder, who has developed relationships of care with other Elders, verbally invited the network of Elders in our area, who are active in healing work, to a focus group. We will use the definition of *Elder* provided by Steckley and Cummins (2001): those individuals who have significant wisdom in areas of traditional Aboriginal knowledge; are recognized as having that wisdom by their community and Nation; and have the capacity to transmit this knowledge to others. All Elders who participated in our research have the recognition of their communities, Aboriginal organizations, and their Nations as per Steckley and Cummins' criteria. Our research team reserved space for the focus group at a local Aboriginal gathering place and generated a printed copy invitation to these Elders. Our guiding Elder delivered these invitations to Elders and asked them to participate if they were interested. Through the respect held for our guiding Elder and the trust that exists among this community of Elders, our research team was able to be a part of this gathering of Elders. Five female Elders participated: three First Nations and two Métis women.[3] Two male First Nation Elders also participated. All participants had attended residential schools.

Focus Group. We served a traditional meal of soup and bannock prior to our focus group. Tobacco and cloth were offered and the Elders were asked for their help and guidance with our work. All the Elders were then given consent forms to sign and copies of the interview questions (Greenbaum, 1998).[4] The focus group was facilitated by all of the authors. The traditional method of the *talking circle* was used to generate conversation (Hampton & Norman, 1997). The Elders were prepared to share their experiences in order to assist others and help them gain a better understanding. Traditional talking circles would be four rounds of discussion followed by a ceremony to close the discussion, but we only had time for two rounds. In this group the Elders took the time that they needed to share and their stories were filled with honesty and emotion. It was decided at the closing that we would meet again in the future to further our discussion, which occurred the following year. Not only did many of the Elders return to share their experiences with the research team, but Aboriginal youth and high school counselors also came to this follow-up action meeting. As such, the results of the second meeting will not be reported in this research due to the confidential nature of the group sharing.

DATA ANALYSIS

The content from the focus group was digitally recorded and transcribed before being entered into NVivo for analysis (Richards, 1999) using grounded theory methods (Goertzen, Fahlman, Hampton, & Jeffery, 2003).[5] Two members of the research team generated coding categories and jointly analyzed the data. Three levels of coding were used: fourteen open coding categories that constituted the initial analytic categories and axial coding that allowed the team to see connections between the categories and generate themes. We used the NVivo program to cut and paste the fourteen open coding categories and discovered that three of these – "Definition of Sexual Health," "Life Experiences," and "Sexual Health" – contained no characters and, thus, were eliminated. The category "Healing" emerged as the largest coding category and also as the core category. Axial coding allowed us to see connections between the core category and other categories such as "Traditional Teachings" and "Residential School" and generate themes. Several unexpected findings emerged from data analysis. For example, the concept of "Staying Clean" as well as the historical importance of "Beer Parlor Days" has not been described in the literature as far as we know. Finally, selective coding was done to select quotations that best illustrated the themes. A matrix was generated (see Figure 1) that visually depicts that emerging theory. We offer here voices of Elders speaking about sexual health and healing as they see it today.

SEXUAL HEALTH IN FIRST NATIONS MATRIX

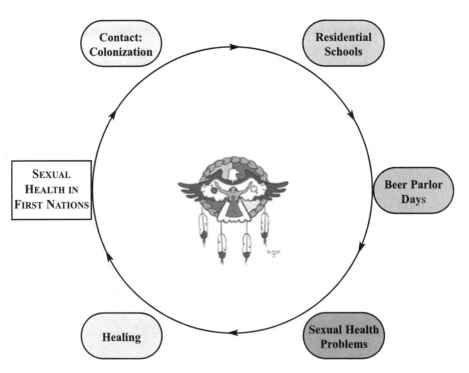

Figure 1.

RESULTS

As the Elders spoke about their experience and observations, a timeline describing sexual health in Aboriginal communities emerged (see Figure 1). There was a time when sexual health was maintained in Aboriginal communities. However, with residential schools, sexual health declined and sexual abuse, power and control inflicted on children, segregation of children by gender, and lack of access to traditional teachings left a destructive legacy for Aboriginal peoples, most notably in the association of sexuality with alcohol. Therefore, this topic must be understood within the context of colonialism experienced specifically in residential schools.

We found that it was difficult for the Elders to speak openly about the topic of sexuality and sexual health in the focus group because, traditionally, it was a subject they were not to talk about with strangers. Moreover, the experiences at the residential school added a profound layer of oppression and shame, which made the subject even more difficult for Elders to speak about. For all that, the participating Elders stated that sexual health of young people is a high priority area of concern for them. They noted that "babies are having babies," that "babies are selling themselves on the streets," and that disease is devastating their communities. Because of their concern for young people, they wished to speak out about the issue.

TRADITIONAL TEACHINGS

The Elders spoke about traditional teachings, which largely fell under the themes of "Respect," "Staying Clean" and "Becoming an Elder." Yet the overarching theme referred to the ways things were done by "The Old People" or "In Ancient Times." They remembered that sexual health in their culture was once seen as natural – a part of life.

> *MALE ELDER*: I don't recall our Indian people talking about romance. Walking down the garden path and looking at flowers, hey, that was out of this world . . . . hey, what are you doing that for? You know, they didn't have to walk with a woman to look at flowers and see the beauty of nature. They saw it when they were doing the things that their livelihood depended on, hunting and going out in the woods and just in love with nature, Mother Nature. That was love. It wasn't buying flowers and birthday cards and all that fancy stuff. I feel out of place when I do that to my wife and I'm not afraid to say that.

Most of the Elders in the focus group had been married to their spouses for forty to fifty years. They spoke about the importance of long-term, intact marriages within their traditions.

> *FEMALE ELDER*: People lived with each other for fifty-two, fifty-three, fifty-four years, sixty some of them. And no matter what they encountered in their marriages, they still sort of stuck together. I mean, I know that from my own mother and father . . . they were together for fifty-three years.

The Elders stated that sex was not something that was talked about as freely as it is today. There were boundaries; issues – and certainly behavior – of sexuality were kept private and confidential.

> *FEMALE ELDER*: And I was always told to never do your lovemaking in front of your children. That's another thing I was told and and I told my kids that too.

The theme of "Respect" emerged as a fundamental aspect of healing. For example, confidentiality was kept in issues of sexual health out of respect for others.

> *FEMALE ELDER*: Long ago sex was very confidential. And when I was a child, we didn't see anything like that at home. Even the birth of babies, even those that were born at home. Like I told you I was born in a tent, no children were allowed. They had a lot of respect, long ago, not like today. Today everything is abused.

Respect started with self-respect and extended to family and others in the community.

> *MALE ELDER*: I just want to say as my traditional teaching, as I said my dad and so on in front of me. I was talking about that respect. Today that's what I do. I don't talk first in front of my kids, my children. That's respect. I respect myself, I'm respecting them.

The concept of "Staying Clean" also emerged as an important aspect of traditional teachings. People kept *clean* sexually. This is what sexual health meant to the Elders.

> *MALE ELDER*: The families having a rough time with their kids. They're drinking and doing drugs and that's where they learn, that's where they get that disease

from. They don't know what's cleanliness, I don't say people are dirty. We get sick, looks after ourselves. That's my point of view and my Indian way I was taught. They didn't talk about it. You know my grandparents didn't drink.

One Elder stated that she fought back when a man on a local farm threatened to rape her so she would remain *clean*.

FEMALE ELDER: The workers was trying to abuse me, eh? Oh I surprise him because I took him and I just flung him right over the fence. And I thought, "you're not going to do this to me," I said, "because I've got to protect myself," so I did. He was just, "boy you're strong." I said, "you're damn right I'm strong," I said. "I'm not scared of nobody," I said. "You try to get funny with me," I said "I'll show you what a woman can do, what a girl can do." So I protected myself. I had to really fight for my protection because I wanted to be a clean person.

The Elders had no need for things like condoms since the people kept themselves clean from disease. One Elder described the first time she saw a wrapped condom.

FEMALE ELDER: I went into [an agency] one time. And I thought it was candy in the basket, so on my way out I grabbed two and while I went out I was opening the mint, and I said, 'hey how do you open this? How do you open these candies?" They said. "They're not candies." "What are they?" She asked me, weren't we brought up with anything like that. We were clean with that kind of thing. We never used anything like that. If we get pregnant, we get pregnant.

The concept of *clean* is related to "Becoming an Elder." The vision of becoming an Elder, clean and worthy of respect, was an important part of sexual health. One female Elder stated: "I wanted to be a clean person because I wanted to be an Elder some day." Another female Elder related: "I used to pray to the Creator all the time. And he's here to help me today. My mom told me I was going to be an Elder one of these times."

One participant stated that some Elders predicted the HIV/AIDS epidemic a long time ago. They predicted that First Nations people would face hard times, would stop treating themselves with respect, and, as a result, a terrible disease would come to the people.

> *FEMALE ELDER*: I grew up when my Moshum was 101 years old when he passed away. And so he taught my brother and me and my younger brother underneath us. He would tell us stories all the time. He would gather us around as young people and say . . . he even told us about AIDS coming in the future. "You know what, my grandchildren, I want you to know this," he said, "that in the future there is going to be a disease coming that people do not respect and honor the sacred gift that's given of life. And so there's going to be a disease coming, my grandchildren," he said, "and I want you to realize that, you know what? It's sacred. Life is sacred and so as a sacred person yourself, Creator put you here and please respect yourself." Respect yourself, you know?

THE SEXUAL DAMAGE OF COLONIALISM AND RESIDENTIAL SCHOOLS

When children were forced into residential schools, the passing of traditional teachings was disrupted.

> *FEMALE ELDER*: Nobody told me anything about where kids come from, when you're pregnant. I didn't know what was the matter with me. Nobody told me anything about it.

The segregation of children by gender and the shame communicated in church-run residential schools left children without the traditional sense of self-respect; it did however leave them with a strong sense of confusion and shame.

> *MALE ELDER*: I don't ever recall even in the classroom any of the teachers or anybody saying to us anything about sexual activity or sex or anything, you know. And if they did or if we start looking at the girls, "What are you doing!!! Go to your corners." They had a very negative attitude toward this kind of issue. And yet they didn't realize that any feelings that we had whether sexual or crying or laughing, they're all God-given. And they were denied. We have to learn it ourselves. And we

self-taught, you might say. You know, pick it up from this guy or that guy, what they were talking about girls, eh?

The pain that Elders carry from residential school is inter-generational. Sexual abuse that occurred in residential schools has devastated sexual health of First Nations.

> *FEMALE ELDER*: Some of the Elders that were really healthy, like the grandparents, for instance, they would be telling stories, like my grandfather told me, right? But maybe they were sexually abused so there was really feelings of not knowing what was right and not knowing what was wrong, right? And so then when they went into residential schools and they heard that from their grandparents or their Moshums or their Kokhums, you know, then that gave them mixed messages then. You know, here keep your body sacred and then when they went to residential school, they were abused, sexually abused. So what we would be doing is sending really mixed messages and really messing up young people.

Abuse inflicted at a young age in residential schools has caused much emotional scarring in First Nation individuals.

> *FEMALE ELDER*: For about nine years I lost it, when I was in boarding school. Because I was called a dirty Indian, black little Indian, a little savage. I got mixed up in that world. Savage . . . savage. Mostly it went bad through boarding school. One time me and this boy were caught talking together and they called them up. It happened I met him there, I was going to get the mop and I was talking to him, we were standing and talking. All of a sudden this door come slowly opening, there was a nun standing there. She told me, '[name],' she said, 'you go upstairs and put your nightgown on. And you, too, [name], you go upstairs into that room.' He got the strap and I got the strap just because we were talking together. It was very hard in boarding school. I was always emotional, wanting to go home but I couldn't.

BEER PARLOR DAYS.

The Elders referred to a time in the 1960s and 1970s when Indian people became citizens and were allowed to enter bars. For example, prior to 1970 it was illegal for Indian people to go into bars. After becoming citizens, the Elders stated that Aboriginal individuals could go into bars and the social context changed. In the *beer parlor generation*, individuals found that alcohol helped loosen inhibitions imposed on them from residential schools and allowed them to socialize with members of the opposite sex. They stated that pregnancies occurred and babies were born with fetal alcohol syndrome/fetal alcohol effects.

> *MALE ELDER*: When I look back at the history of my life and when that started. I don't recall that ever happening in my age, for the Elder days, right up till, shall I say, the seventies. Then because our Indian people were allowed to go into the bars and the poor . . . was a poor situation for many of our Indian babies because they went in and they started drinking, lots of them just couldn't control it and then they, as a result of drinking and all that, they got pregnant. And you can't blame them I guess, because of what happened to them as a result their youngsters are affected by the drinking, you know, those are the things today. What I have seen through the years is it began in those years before then I don't ever recall hearing of our mothers and babies before the beer parlor days, you know.

Alcohol served as a social lubricant for girls and boys who had been segregated in residential schools and did not know how to relate to each other. Pregnancies would occur when partners were drunk or drugged.

> *FEMALE ELDER*: It's sad to see this. People getting out of control, babies being born with no dads. Like he was saying about drinking. I think it was started from there and having sex and you don't know. You're pregnant and you don't know who to blame. I know a lot of my relatives, young women, they don't know who their dad is. And they're trying to find out now. And you see it is very sad.

Alcohol and the social environment in bars helped individuals deal with the pain and shame they had accumulated in residential schools.

> *MALE ELDER*: But you see, that was the extent of our sexual, shall we say, experience. And my god, as time

went on and I start to grow older, like I say, I start taking up the feeling that I had about the opposite sex. I was shy about it you know. Come in and have a drink . . . oohhhh, god, there was a woman.

The Elders feel that the legacy of colonization, residential schools, and the use of alcohol to cope and numb has left many people a with lack of true love.

HEALING

The Elders stated that the way back to sexual health is moving away from use of alcohol and drugs and back to spirituality and traditional teachings. They feel they have a responsibility to set a good example for young people.

MALE ELDER: Today I pray every night, ever more, ever since I left all the alcohol, I practice my teachings every day. And as I said, that's how I stopped drinking, and I still need help so I'm still sober today.

They stated that they will speak out about sexual health because they care about the young people: "Well, we're talking about it because we're concerned. Because we want to help them." They agree that Aboriginal communities are in a process of healing to reverse the devastation caused by colonization and need the active participation of the Elders.

MALE ELDER: It's quite a concern for many people, not only our Elders, but the HIV and all those diseases, you know. And it's not going to reverse itself and just go down like that, no way. For goodness' sakes, can you tell me and we all possess it, the sexual desires that we have.

The Elders stated that the emergence of the diseases they see today results from a society that does not conduct itself properly.

FEMALE ELDER: We never heard of AIDS or anything like this. That time was mostly polio that was all. That's what I remember, how my sister was in a sanitarium for a long time. So today sicknesses, I don't know. I don't know where it's coming from but it . . . we're sure getting a lot of it.

Many Elders expressed concern over the influence of modern, urban life on the sexual health of youth.

FEMALE ELDER: Today everything is abused. Like sex . . . I think mainly they learn from TV, books, there's a lot of that on TV. I only have basic TV now but still there's sex that comes on. Kissing and everything. And yeah, it is sad, to. It is very sad to see this, and especially when the children watch it on TV, and they even have books for that, movies and books, yeah.

The Elders also wish to give proper love to young people.

MALE ELDER: They're not my daughter, but I take them as one because if I can extend to them the love that they have and they can't express it because of the drinking and drugging, you know? That's what's holding them back. They have it. They want to give it. But the poor little thing, how do they know when the mother's trying to extend the love that they have for this child. You know, this child may cry and do all that, eh? I mean this child is crying out for the love that they want, you know, and some of them unfortunately don't have a mom, their mom passes away because of drug and alcohol. And they're left in an orphan state.

They also offer healing in circles to help people express their pain in a safe setting.

FEMALE ELDER: They need to bring out their feelings because there's so much inside here that they can't talk about and they need to bring it out. It's like when I'm talking the residential schools, nobody can heal us. We have to heal ourselves and the only way we're going to heal is by sitting in a circle.

For the Elders, the answer lies in their ability as spiritual leaders to offer the traditional teachings to young people, to practice their own spirituality, to live a clean life, and to offer spiritual guidance to youth.

FEMALE ELDER: We have to pray, you know. Keep on asking the Great Spirit to slow down this life, the way it's going. I never forget to pray, morning and night. I have a lot of sweet grass. I burn it in the morning. I raise it to the east and I have a stone there. My offering to the Great Spirit, the Creator, pray for the children who are having a lot of problems, because there's a lot today.

CONCLUSION

Our results offer insight into a specific priority health issue confronting Aboriginal youth in Canada. The Elders describe healing as a process of transformation: restoring Aboriginal individuals and communities to a state of meaning, balance, connectedness, and wholeness. Our emerging theory clarifies the multi-generational negative impact of colonization on sexual health of Aboriginal families.

Several unexpected findings emerged from our analysis of the focus group data. For example, the relationship between the historical experience of residential schools and present-day health problems became clearer. The importance of the beer parlor days in this negative cycle of disease was unexpected. As a research team, we had not previously encountered this part of the historical context behind the denigration of Aboriginal sexual health. This new information highlights the use of alcohol for coping with trauma. We also heard that the HIV/AIDS epidemic was predicted by the Old People.

Sexual health problems confronting Aboriginal youth globally have been recognized as derivative of the conditions of imbalance or disharmony created by colonialism (Aguilera & Plasencia, 2005). In response, we propose a model of healing that uses local cultural traditions in conjunction with programs proven to reduce sexual behavior in other contexts (Thin Elk, 1993).

TRADITIONAL CONCEPTS OF HEALTH AND HEALTHY SEXUALITY

Aboriginal Elders can convey traditional epistemology to younger people that suggest a way of life that can prevent disease and aid the recovery of their communities (Castellano, 2000; Ermine, 1995). We expand here on one traditional concept that was stressed by the Elders: the concept of cleanliness and living a clean life. What do Elders mean when they advocate living a clean life? Individuals are cautioned to only come to ceremonies or the drum if they are *clean*. To do otherwise is to show disrespect and risk personal spiritual consequences. Cleanliness also relates to sexual and moral conduct. The concept of cleanliness can be found in the Bible, and nineteenth-century religious texts translated into Algonkian languages contain the directive, "Be Thou Clean" (London Gospel Tract Depot, 1872). The twentieth-century adoption of contemporary sobriety strategies has also made the phrase *clean and sober* common in First Nation communities. Yet, an exploration of the philosophical concepts embedded in protocols, language, and stories of Aboriginal cultures suggests that there is an Indigenous foundation to the notion of living a clean life. Cree Elders interviewed by Freda Ahenakew used the term *living a proper life* (Ahenakew & Wolfart, 1998). Glecia Bear compared vital Cree traditions that embraced the entire community and honored a world alive with animate spirits to "the White-Man's customs where everything is dead" (Ahenakew & Wolfart,

1998, p. 79-81). A proper life involved respect, prayer, self-discipline, and hard work.

Indigenous concepts of health and wellness are active words related to a way of living that simultaneously embraces people, the natural world, and the inner worlds of the spirit and emotions. The Jesuits commented on Indigenous preoccupation with the importance of a healthy life, noting, "they have a horror of Theft, and have but little love for worldly goods, but much more for health and life." The people the Jesuits lived among were described as very modest, charitable, and good humored. When Paul Le Jeune's 1634 expedition met with disaster, he was cautioned by his companions: "Do not be cast down, for anger brings on sadness, and sadness brings sickness" (Le Jeune, 1899-1900, p. 81). Three hundred years later, Cree Elders used the healing power of the forest to promote physical and mental health after the emotional trauma of relocation to a centralized village (Adelson, 2002; Niezer, 1997). The Cree concept of *miyupimaatisiiun* (being alive well) integrated physical vigour and spiritual well-being within the Creator's constant presence in the natural world. Similarly, the Ojibwe term *Bimaadziwin* can be alternately translated as the good life, the sharing life, and the living teachings (Toulouse, 2001). These concepts of life and health were closely related to notions of the body, spirit, and life force.

Cleanliness, self-discipline, and restraint were also critically related to personal power, which might determine success in healing and hunting. Power is elusive and if not used, or used improperly, it could be taken away or lost. Ojibwe Elder, Martin Assinewe, cautioned, "For it to be effective, you're supposed to follow the rules . . . . I can't teach you the easy way, that's what we all want, my teacher is very stern" (Toulouse, 2001, p. 63). Sexuality and sexual health were also an aspect of the good life. While the Jesuits found that seventeenth century Innu had no word for *sin*, their word for *wickedness* translated as the violation of purity (LeJeune, 1899-1900). Sexual excess and gluttony were discouraged through the oral tradition. Trickster escapades with hilarious consequences resulted from unbridled sexuality and greed. More frightening narratives of Whetigo, were also cautionary tales that encouraged virtue and restraint over excess. In the Dakota oral tradition, a man who approached White Buffalo Calf Woman with unclean thoughts was reduced to ash (Erdos & Ortiz, 1984). She gave gifts and instructions to women, telling them they were equal to men because the work they do with their hands and fruits they produce through their bodies keep the people alive (Erdos & Ortiz, 1984). Women's bodies in particular deserve honor and respect for their potential for creating and sustaining life. Cree women in Saskatchewan were taught that their souls resided in their uterus and cervix:

It is a sacred area and it is an area where a woman gets her strength. In our culture a woman is considered to have a lot of power and a lot of sacredness and it comes from our monthly menstruation . . . Life comes from there and that's a woman's sense of power. I don't know how else I can explain it, but that's where we get our source of energy, our source of power, our source of strength (Wilson, 2002, p. 54).

With these ideas in mind, perhaps we can approach the Elder's words about being clean with greater understanding and appreciation, as they spoke with urgency about the growing crisis in sexual health among youth and young adults in their community.

ELDERS AS HEALERS

The Elders who shared their wisdom in our focus group did so in traditional ways; that is, similar to way other Elders have shared their words. To illustrate, Kulchyski et al., (1991) suggest that, in their teachings, Elders stress listening, observing, and waiting in an attitude of respect. Teachings frequently involve moral lessons that link behavior to a spiritual understanding. Elders teach a worldview based on the knowledge that all things are governed by natural law and are related in a sacred manner. This teaching constitutes wisdom, the precious gift that the Elders have to offer. Traditionally, Elders maintain tribal memories of the stories and social structures that ensured the good life of the community through the spirit (Cajete, 1994). The role of the Elders rests in sharing their wisdom and offering a spiritual dialogue that informs proper behavior (Tacay, 1998). They teach and we listen.

But are we listening? Elders pass on their teachings through somewhat unfamiliar oral traditions, so younger generations must creatively interpret and apply the directives of Elders by critically reflecting on their own experience (Cowell, 2002; Gamlin, 2003). Even so, Elders have been found to be particularly important to urban Aboriginal communities because their knowledge of traditional ways, teaching, stories, and ceremonies provides guidance for those who may feel disconnected from their community or their ancestral land (Stiegelbauer, 1996). The Elders who participated in our research also realize what others have suggested, that Elders not only know the teachings, but they know them so well that they are able to live by them and provide role models for their People. What they learned from their experience, they want to communicate to younger generations (Steigelbauer, 1996). Elder participants in our research have been through the residential school experience, they may have battled alcoholism. They also say it is not their fault. They have learned how to love and now want to give this message: love – unconditional acceptance and spiritual power – will heal young people of the sexual health problems they face today.

NOTES

1 This research was supported with funding from the CIHR HIV/AIDS Research Program (#HHP-56967), a component of the Canadian Strategy on HIV/AIDS We acknowledge co-investigators Dr. Bonnie Jeffery and Barb McWatters.

2 Aboriginal is defined in the Constitution of Canada to refer to all Peoples of Indian, Inuit, and Métis heritage, including non-status Indians. Other terms such as "Indigenous" or "Native" are also used to refer to First peoples or Original Residents of a land.

3 See Bourassa, Mckay-McNabb & Hampton (2004) for a definition of *Métis* and *First Nation*.

4 At the time of the signing of consent forms, a few of the women Elders indicated that they did not feel comfortable signing the forms due to their historical experience. Through a discussion we discovered that these Elders had past experiences when their families signed forms (i.e., signing of the treaties; the historical results of these signings were negative for First Nations). The Aboriginal research assistant on the team explained that signing the form was an agreement between the University and them to have a discussion and they could choose not to participate. Informed consent was discussed at this point and the Aboriginal women felt comfortable with the purpose of the evening and agreed to sign the forms.

5 Another issue occurred while introducing the use of the digital recorder to the Elders. When the research assistant asked the group if it would be okay to use the digital recorder, she was soon educated by an Elder in the group about listening. He shared a lesson that he had been taught about listening and indicated that if the Creator wanted us to remember what we needed from the evening, then we would not need to rely upon an electrical device to remember. The Elder went on to describe the historical importance of oral history and listening, but ended by stating that he knew that we needed to do this for the research. Nonetheless, his lesson about undue reliance on technology had the desired effect on the research assistant and she now has a greater respect for the words carefully listened to and remembered over those recorded but quickly forgotten.

References

Aboriginal Healing Foundation. Retrieved October 15, 2006 from. http://www.ahf.ca/english/newsletter_sept_000pdf

Adelson, N. (2002). *Being alive and well: Health and politics of Cree well-being.* Toronto: University of Toronto Press.

Aguilera, S. & Plasencia, A.V. (2005). Culturally appropriate HIV/AIDS and substance abuse prevention programs for urban Native youth. *Journal of Psychoactive Drugs, 37,* 299-304.

Ahenakew, F. & Wolfart, H.C. (1998). *Our Grandmothers' lives as told in their own words.* University of Regina, SK: Canadian Plains Research Centre.

Amaro, H. & Raj, A. (2000). On the margin: Power and women's HIV risk reduction strategies. *Sex Roles, 42,* 723-748.

Amaro, H., Raj, A. & Reed, E. (2001). Women's sexual health: The need for feminist analysis in public health in the Decade of Behavior. *Psychology of Women Quarterly, 25,* 324-334.

Anderson, K. (2000). A recognition of being: A reconstruction of Native womanhood. Toronto: Second Story Press.

Anderson, K. (2002). *Tenuous connections: Urban Aboriginal youth sexual health and pregnancy.* Toronto: The Ontario Federation of Indian Friendship Centers.

Barnhardt, R., & Angayuqaq, O.K. (2005). Indigenous knowledge systems and Alaska Native ways of knowing. *Anthropology and Education Quarterly, 36,* 8-23.

Bertolli, J., McNaughten, A. D., Campsmith, M., Lee, L. M., Leman, R., Bryan, R. T. & Buehler, J. W. (2004). Surveillance systems monitoring HIV/AIDS and HIV risk behaviors among American Indians and Alaska Natives. *AIDS Education and Prevention, 16,* 218-237.

Bourassa, C., McKay-McNabb, K. & Hampton, M. (2004). Racism, sexism, and colonialism. *Canadian Woman Studies, 24,* 23-29.

Cajete, G. (1994). *Look to the mountain: An ecology of indigenous education.* Durango, CO: Kivaki Press.

Canadian Aboriginal AIDS Network: Retrieved October 1, 2007, from http://www.caan.ca/english/links.htm.

Castellano, M. B. (2000). Updating Aboriginal traditions of knowledge. In G. J. S. Dei, B. L. Hall & D. G. Rosenberg (Eds.), *Indigenous knowledge in global context: Multiple readings of our world* (pp. 21-36). Toronto: OISE.

Chrisjohn, R. & Young, S. (1997). *The circle game: Shadows and substance in the Indian residential school experience in Canada.* Penticton, B.C.: Theytus.

Cowell, A. (2002). Bilingual curriculum among the Northern Arapaho: oral tradition, literacy, and performance. *The American Indian Quarterly, 26,* 24-44.

Davin, N. F. (1879). Report on industrial schools for Indians and Half Breeds. Ottawa, ON: National Archives of Canada, RG10,Vol.6001. File 1-1-1.

Driving Hawk Sneve, V. (1977). *That they may have life: The Episcopal Church in South Dakato.* New York: Seabury.

Eng, T. R. & Butler, W. T. (Eds.) (1997). *The hidden epidemic: Confronting sexually transmitted diseases: Report of the Institute of Medicine.* Washington, D.C.: National Academy Press.

Erdos, R., & Ortiz, A. (1984). *American Indian myths.* New York: Pantheon Books.

Ermine, W. (1995). Aboriginal epistemology. In M. Battiste & J. Barman (Eds.), *First Nations education in Canada: The circle unfolds* (pp. 101-112). Vancouver, B.C.: UBC Press.

Farrell Racette, S. (2001). Sex, fear, women, travel and work: Five persistent triggers of Eurocentric negativity. In J. Oakes, R. Riewe (Eds.), *Pushing the margins: Native and northern studies* (pp. 144-159). University of Manitoba: Departments of Native Studies and Zoology.

Foley, K., Duran, B., Morria, P., Lucero, J., Jiang, Y., Baxter, B., Harrison, M., et al. (2005). Using motivational interviewing to promote HIV testing at an American Indian substance abuse treatment facility. *Journal of Psychoactive Drugs, 37,* 321-329.

Frideres, J. S. (1998). *Aboriginal peoples in Canada: Contemporary conflicts* (5th ed.). Scarborough, ON: Prentice Hall Allyn and Bacon Canada.

Gamlin, P. (2003). Transformation and Aboriginal literacy. *Canadian Journal of Native Education, 27,* 16-22.

Garrett, M.T. & Herring, R.D. (2001). Honoring the power of relation: Counseling native adults. *Journal of Humanistic Counseling, Education, and Development, 40,* 139-160.

Goertzen, J., Fahlman, S., Hampton, M.R. & Jeffery, B. (2003). Creating logic models using grounded theory: case example demonstrating a unique approach to logic model development. *The Canadian Journal of Program Evaluation, 18*(2), 115-138.

Goldstone, I., Albert, R., Churchill, K., Schilder, A., Perry, T., Markowski, S., Hogg, R. S., & McLeod, W. A. (2000). HIV injection drug use amongst First Nations in Vancouver: Outcomes of care and neglect. *Native Social Work Journal, 3,* 145-163.

Green, R. (1990). The Pocahonts perplex: the image of Indian women in American cultures. In: E.C. Dubois & V.I. Ruiz (Eds.), *Unequal sisters: A multicultural reader in U.S. women's history.* Toronto: Routledge.

Greenbaum, T. L. (1998). *The handbook of focus group research* (2nd ed.). Newbury Park, CA: Sage Publications.

Hampton, M., & Norman, C. (1997). Community-building in a peer support centre. *Journal of College Student Development, 38,* 357-364.

Hanson, I., & Hampton, M. R. (2000). Being Indian: Strengths sustaining First Nations peoples in residential schools. *Canadian Journal of Community Mental Health, 19,* 127-142.

Huberman, A. M., & Miles, M. B. (1998). Data management and analysis methods. In N. K. Denzin & Y. S. Lincoln (Eds.), *Collecting and interpreting qualitative materials* (pp. 179-210). Thousand Oaks, CA: Sage Publications.

Jemmott, J. B., & Jemmott, L. S. (2000). HIV behavioral interventions for adolescents in community settings. In J. L. Peterson & R. J. DiClemente (Eds.), *Handbook of HIV prevention* (pp. 103-124). New York: Plenum Publishers.

Katz, R. (1993). *The straight path: A story of healing and transformation in Fiji.* New York: Addison-Wesley Publishing Company.

Kulchyski, P., McCaskill & Newhouse, D. (1991). *In the words of Elders: Aboriginal cultures in Transition.* Toronto: University of Toronto Press.

Lanier, A. P., & Kelly, J. L. (1999). Knowledge, attitudes, and behavior of Alaska Native women regarding cervical and breast cancer. In: D. Weiner (Ed.). *Preventing and controlling cancer in North America: A cross-cultural perspective,* (pp. 71-83). Westport, CT: Praeger.

LeDuigou, C. (2000). A historical overview of two-spirited people: A context for social work and HIV/AIDS services in the Aboriginal community. *Native Social Work Journal, 3,* 195-214.

LeJeune, P. (1899-1900). Relations of what occurred in New France in the year 1634. In: R. Thwaites (Ed.), T*he Jesuit relations and the allied documents: Travel and explorations by the Jesuit mission in New France 1610-17* (Vol. 6, p. 135). Quebec, PQ: The Burrow Brothers.

London Gospel Trace Depot. (1872). *"Wokumayan: Be Thou Clean,"* Micmac Pamphlet. CIHM microfiche series FC 19C36no. 34732.

Marsden, N., Clement, K., & Schneider, D. (2000). "Honouring and caring for Aboriginal people and communities in the fight against HIV/AIDS" Healing our Spirit BC First Nations AIDS Society – providing prevention, care, treatment and support services for Aboriginal Peoples in British Columbia. *Native Social Work Journal, 3,* 127-141.

McKay-McNabb, K. (2006). Life experiences of Aboriginal women living with HIV/AIDS. Canadian Journal of Aboriginal Community-Based *HIV/AIDS Research, 1,* 5-28.

Moore, P. J. (2003). Lessons on the land: The role of Kaska Elders in a university language course. *Canadian Journal of Native Education, 27,* 127-139.

RCAP: Report of the Royal Commission on Aboriginal Peoples. (1998). Ottawa, ON: Canada Communications Group.

Regina Health District (2000a). *Aboriginal Health Initiative Report.* Regina, Saskatchewan.

Regina Health District (2000b). *Aboriginal Profile: Regina Health District.* Regina, Saskatchewan.

Reid, P. T. (2000). Women, ethnicity, and AIDS: What's love got to do with it? *Sex Roles, 42,* 709-723.

Rew, L. (1997). Ethnic differences in perceived health status: Preliminary findings. *Journal of Pediatric Nursing, 12*, 223-227.

Rew, L. (2001). Sexual health practices of homeless youth: A model for intervention. *Issues in Comprehensive Pediatric Nursing, 124*, 1-18.

Richards, L. (1999). *Using NVivo in qualitative research.* Thousand Oaks, CA: Sage Publications.

Rotheram-Borus, M. J., & Futterman, D. (2000). Promoting early detection of human immunodeficiency virus infection among adolescents. *Archives of Pediatrics and Adolescent Medicine, 154*, 435-441.

Rotheram-Borus, M. J., & Koopman, C. (1991). HIV and adolescents. *The Journal of Primary Prevention, 12*, 65-82.

Senge, P., & Scharmer, O. (2001). Community action research: Learning as a community of practitioners, consultants, and researchers. In P. Reason & H. Bradbury (Eds.), *Handbook of action research: Participative inquiry and practice* (pp. 238-249). Thousand Oaks, CA: Sage.

Ship, S. J., & Norton, L. (2000). "It's hard to be a woman!" First Nations women living with HIV/AIDS. *Native Social Work Journal, 3*, 73-89

Smith, P., Daniel, J., Hampton, M. R., Jacques, M., Jeffery, B., & McWatters, B. (2001). *Renewing partnerships and commitment: Community sexual health, services, education, and recommendations.* University of Regina, SK: Sample Survey & Data Bank Research supported by Health Canada, HTFSK 334.

Statistics Canada (2001). *Aboriginal peoples of Canada: A demographic profile.* Catalogue no. 6F0030XIE2001007.

Statistics Canada (2002). *Health of the off-reserve Aboriginal population.* 83-003-SIE.

Steckley, J. L., & Cummins, B. D. (2001). *Full circle: Canada's First Nations.* Toronto: Prentice Hall.

Stiegelbauer, S. M. (1996). What is an Elder? What do Elders do? First Nation Elders as teachers in culture-based urban organizations. *The Canadian Journal of Native Studies, 16*, 37-66.

Stoler, A.L. (2002). *Carnal knowledge and imperial power: Race and the intimate in colonial rule.* Berkeley, CA: University of California Press.

Strauss, A., & Corbin, J. (1998). *Basics of qualitative research: Grounded theory procedure and techniques.* Newbury Park, CA: Sage.

Tacay, D. (1998). What are we afraid of? Intellectualism, Aboriginality, and the sacred. *Melbourne Journal of Politics, 25*, 189-193.

Thin Elk, G. (1993). Walking in balance on the Red Road. *Journal of Emotional and behavioral Problems, 2*, 54-5.

Tkach, M. (2003). *Aboriginal Census Information: Impact and Implications or Saskatchewan.* Statistics Canada: Government Relations and Aboriginal Affairs.

Toulouse, P. R. (2001). *Bimaadziwin (the good life) Sharing the living teachings of the People of Sagamok Anishnwbeck: Implications for education.* Vancouver, BC: University of British of Columbia.

Vernon, I. (2001). *Killing us quietly. Native Americans and HIV/AIDS.* Lincoln, NE: University of Nebraska Press.

Wilson, T. M. (2002). *Onion Lake First Nations women: Knowledge, attitudes, and health beliefs of cervical cancer and cervical cancer screening.* Edmonton, AB: University of Alberta Press.

Young, R. J. C. (1995). *Colonial desire: Hybridity, theory, culture and race.* Toronto: Routledge.

Young, T. K. (1988). *Health and cultural change: The Indian experience in the Central Subarctic.* Toronto: University of Toronto Press.

Young, T. K. (1994). T*he health of Native American: Toward a bicultural epidemiology.* Toronto: Oxford University Press.

CHAPTER THIRTEEN

THE CIRCLE OF HEALING AND THE SQUARE:
A MODEL FOR THE INCLUSION OF CULTURALLY BASED HEALING
APPROACHES WITHIN ALLOPATHIC MEDICAL PRACTICE

Robert Morgan,
Lyn Freeman,
&
Rebecca Shaw

We are at a moment in time when opportunities to re-arrange and expand our concepts of treatment and healing present themselves in a multitude of ways in laboratories, institutions of learning, and culturally based communities. It appears that momentum is growing to reverse the recent trend from a managed care process, notorious for limiting treatments to those deemed medically necessary and non-experimental, toward a system that is more inclusive of mind, body, and spirit. The change is happening, albeit slowly, and there are still some major hurdles. This chapter identifies some of those challenges and offers a unique resolution that blends Native healing with allopathic and alternative strategies to form a holistic service delivery plan.

We have observed that a large number of allopathic patients are, often at their own expense, also using the services of alternative practitioners. Often, they do not inform their allopathic physician of their non-allopathic treatments. We have found that this reluctance to inform their physician of their alternative treatment is often based on their belief that their choice of care would not be respected. This suggests to us that it is an ideal time to develop a new approach to healing that lessens barriers of qualifications, profit, and control. We believe there is a way to unify the technological advances of modern medicine with culturally based traditional practices. Medical models could maximize delivery of a wide spectrum of allopathic and traditional medical practices in a manner reflective of the needs of individuals across the country. Local regulatory and financial realities might affect the manner in which coordination of medical practice can be implemented, in whole or in part.

ALASKA: A NEW MODEL OF COOPERATIVE MEDICINE

Alaska has proven an ideal place to evolve a new model of cooperative medicine. It has served as a melting pot where forms of culturally based medicine have clashed with the allopathic model. In the end, allopathic and traditional healing knowledge have come together as a new tapestry of healing – a cloth created from the threads of each others' healing concepts. As Alaskan Natives have gained control of their medical institutions financially and legislatively, they are making valiant efforts to integrate culturally based treatment models with allopathic medicine. The purpose of this integration is to alleviate many of the social ills that have developed in Alaskan villages since first contact with non-native cultures.

The integrative treatment model proposed in this chapter was conceptualized by one of the authors (Morgan) and is based on decades of work as a consultant/practitioner in the allopathic, integrative, and tribal medicine areas. The model is simple in design. It offers a means of developing a working partnership between differing healing and medical systems. It holds promise to renew the practice of medicine as a healing art and to imbue a sense of pride in its practitioners. It is a replicable model that can serve as a basis for similar efforts in culturally based communities throughout America.

In Alaska, this model is commonly referred to as the *Circle of Healing* (Morgan, 1999). However, a more appropriate descriptor would be the *Hoop of Healing*, as it emerged from Black Elk's vision for a re-emergence of a strong *Hoop of Life* (Neihardt, 1932). The realization of his vision lies in the unification of many hoops – many nations – into a great effort to bring about healing of the earth, and the life upon it. This could come about through shared knowledge and respect for the wisdom and spirit of indigenous people of the earth, bringing balance to all cultures. Sharing wisdom with respect and using our gifts together for the sake of healing the human race forms the basis of the Circle of Healing (Morgan, 1999; Morgan, Richards, & Frank, 1995).

Jason Harmon, a naturopathic physician, contributed the following paragraph to the *Circle of Healing*:

As we enter the 21st century, we face great challenges in medicine and modern health care. We carry a legacy of a fragmented and divided approach to health and healing in this and many of the world's countries. We have experienced over the last 100 years, phenomenal growth in advances of science and medical breakthroughs. With this growth, a wider chasm has developed in relation to science and medical breakthroughs. With this growth, a wider chasm has developed in relation to traditional, holistic, and western allopathic medicines. Managed health care and pharmaceutical profit potential has in many instances dictated current day medical evolution. The results have been discouraging for patient and doctor alike. With this realization comes the acknowledgment that we must come together and work for a united approach to health and healing. (p. 4)

It is our sincere wish that the concepts we have developed will enhance a return to a more patient-centered practice of medicine that will apply all available and appropriate knowledge to the treatment and concurrent healing of people.

THE HISTORY AND PRACTICE OF TRADITIONAL HEALING

The question why funds and efforts have failed to resolve medical, social, and economic issues for *Indian country*, was discussed with Walter Austin (personal communication, 2005), a prominent Tlingit Elder, teacher, and story teller. He explained: "The problem is our white brothers sometimes develop their answers before they understand the question. They rely upon their training and knowledge they get from textbooks. They treat the symptoms. It creates a lot of jobs." As a professional community, we have not spent enough time to understand the root causes of problems that result from the destruction of many of the Alaska Native and American Indian communities.

Addressing some of the devastating tragedies that the Native communities have endured in Alaska will allow the reader to understand the Circle of Healing model better. Much of the following historical information was obtained by personal communication with various traditional healers and Elders within Native communities. In traditional Native style, much of the information has been passed on verbally by the healers and Elders from generation to generation through storytelling and talking circles. Only some of the historical information has been passed on through written accounts of personal experience (Hildebrand, 2005; Napoleon, 1996).

A series of events set the stage for the decimation of Native culture, changing its indigenous population from a state of independent self-sufficiency to one reliant on the culture and largess of an occupying force (Eby, 1995). Before contact, the indigenous people of Alaska depended on their own knowledge of anatomy, herbal medicine, and healing practices for health maintenance. Early records indicate that the Alaska Native cultures had a fairly sophisticated medical system in place that included: surgery, weapon removal, amputation, ligation, opening of the abdominal cavity, acupuncture, bloodletting, considerable skill in breech birth deliveries, massage, and the use of herbal medications and hot packs. After contact, the Western-trained medical practitioners became an increasingly important source of health care, especially for combating epidemic diseases introduced to Native populations by Euro-Americans (Napoleon, 1996).

At the time of the Great Death, when smallpox and other diseases swept Alaska in the early 1900s, the dominance of Western medicine increased. Simultaneously, traditional beliefs and practices were discouraged by church, educational, and governmental groups. Native cultures were viewed as deficient, even pathological, without virtue or value. Policies were constructed by government to *civilize* Native Americans, to separate them from their culture and convert them to Euro-American traditions and religion by whatever means necessary. An independent and proud people became dependent. The Native social system, ideally suited to its peoples, was destroyed and replaced by another social system that was ill-suited to the social, physiological, and psychological needs of the Alaskan Native (Napoleon, 1996).

Residential schools were built to *civilize* Native children, some of whom were literally kidnapped from their communities and families. The implication was that there was nothing these children could learn from their language, culture, or families that would be of value to them during their journey into a new world. These young people, once they were deemed acculturated into the so-called civilized world, graduated and were sent back to their villages. They arrived home devoid of the years of training provided by Elders, medicine people, and their families. That training consisted of the moral laws for living, namely, how to contribute to the community and to become a strong positive factor in the family. These young people became the parents of the future, yet they lacked the traditional understanding of what it meant to be Native and a responsible parent. This process of deculturalization, at a formative time in life, appears to have laid the foundation for many of the social, psychological, and physiological ills that have plagued Alaskan Native families since that time (Napoleon, 1996).

Even so, the Alaska Native peoples are beginning to implement culturally based healing efforts to lift the people from a dependent existence, clouded with shame, into an equal state of opportunity and health. Tina Melin, a traditional community mentor from Kotzebue Alaska, stated:

> The people of this region have expressed their desire to take responsibility for their own health and happiness. We are not alone in suffering from illnesses of the mind, body and spirit that are manifested in painful and destructive ways such as alcohol and drug abuse, violence and suicide. There are many historical, spiritual, social, cultural, and environmental factors that have contributed to this suffering. Our health care system and government programs, although with good intentions, have not always provided the help that is needed. The healing must begin within each individual. Only then will our families and communities find relief. The people of this region wish to put their heads and hearts together with guidance from our Creator to attempt to get to the root of the cause of suffering. They are working to acknowledge the truth to help ease the suffering and overcome these barriers to wellness. They have their own legitimate ways of knowing how to do this. Those of us who are a part of the Health Care System need to work together with them and wish to look to our Creator first, their ancestors, the Elders, the young people, each other, and their environment and cultural values. They wish to remember the healthy ways of the days of old blended in with the new. They wish to acknowledge historical trauma and understand it and overcome it. They wish to work through the sadness and grief of the loss of so many loved ones over the years and hit it head on. They wish to regain and strengthen their cultural identity and pride. They wish to help themselves and each other to get on that path to health and stay there. (Tina Melin, personal communication, 2000)

Much of the physical, spiritual, and psychological healing that is occurring has come from the re-emergence of traditional healing practices. These practices were driven underground for several hundred years (Walter Austin, personal communication, 1989; Rita Blumenstein, personal communication, 1999), but somehow managed to survive the dominance of Western science. This resilience indicates the strength of these traditions in the face of the negative attitude of Western educators, lawmakers, and law enforcement, and the hostility previously shown by certain religious groups: "It was amazing that any of the indigenous ceremonial and healing practices in North America should have survived the zeal of the missionaries, the scorn of the unthinking, and the curiosity of anthropologists" (Attneave, 1974, p. 6).

It seems that the revival of indigenous healing practices can not only be attributed to a lack of allopathic medical services, but also, more importantly, to the absence of a culturally congenial and holistic approach to modern medicine. A holistic approach has been conceptualized by transcultural psychiatry and psychosomatic medicine but has not been applied in practice.

In 1977, Mohawk Elder Ernie Benedict explained the difference between allopathic medicine and traditional Native healing practices. White man's medicines, he noted, tend to be very mechanical. The person is repaired physically, but is not psychologically or spiritually better than before. Benedict explained that it is possible, with proper medicine in the Native way, to become a better person after going through a sickness (personal address, Eagle Project, Thunder Bay, Ontario, August 7, 1977).

Beginning in 1950, medical care for Alaska Natives was provided by Indian Health Services, an agency of the federal government (Eby, 1994). In 1994, a process called *compacting* began in Alaska. This process refers to the arrangement whereby local tribal groups are allocated funds to provide medical services. Federally controlled tribal funds allocated for health services are transferred to tribes that determine how funds will be utilized. With an ability to mold healthcare into a model most beneficial to Indigenous peoples, tribal corporations began to offer a combination of traditional healing, complementary and alternative medicine (CAM), and allopathic medicine at the Alaska Native Medical Center along with varying outpatient clinics throughout the state. All the same, allopathic medicine remained the dominant model and, as a result, the blending of these systems of healing has not always gone smoothly. For example, consider Eby's (1995) work:

Allopathic medicine sees the body as a machine composed of many parts which break down and need fixing. It is probably understood as a physical entity, largely independent of the mind. Medicine perceived individuals as essentially similar and prone to illness, caused by specific vectors, which can be catalogued into specific disease categories. The central drive and medical interaction is towards diagnosis, with one of a specific list of disorders, which is then usually corrected with chemical or physical manipulation, medications, and surgery. The doctor-patient relationship is also structured so that it is focused around the drive towards a diagnosis. Once a diagnosis is arrived at, the chemical or procedure of physical intervention, deemed most appropriate by the physician, is arranged and the patient is left to comply or not. The perception, on the part of most physicians and patients, is that the knowledge and decision-making process, underlying the prescribed intervention, is too technical and complex for the patient to understand. The time factors in most medical offices usually limit conversation to information directly related to the presenting complaint, the specific body part, the presenting individual patient, and the categorization of that information into already created definitions of illness. In a drive towards efficiency, this is all the doctor and patient perceive as relevant, or that there is time for. The process is rather linear and specific and places the control of the treatment rather directly into the hands of the physician. (p. 2)

Since making this statement, Dr. Eby, medical director of Southcentral Foundation, has continued to diligently work for the creation of facilities and programs where the patient partners with an integrated treatment team of conventional, tribal, and complementary medicine professionals.

In rather direct contrast to this, traditional healing generally assumes that disease is part of a larger energy field that cannot be treated in isolation from non-organic and spiritual-based belief systems that affect patients' ability to bring themselves into a state of balance. From this perspective, disease relates directly to the patients' lifestyle, personality patterns, and body constitution; people fall ill because, in most instances, they fell out of harmony with the forces of nature in some way. The purpose of the treatment must be to reintegrate the individual with the harmony of nature, while family members and neighbors are asked to join together to assist in this process.

These concepts were in place among the varying cultures in Alaska before contact with Europeans occurred; moreover, specific treatment procedures were in place to treat instances of injury and disease (Rita Bleumenstein, personal communication, 1999). There was widespread knowledge regarding proper nutrition, medicinal use of local plants, midwifery, setting broken bones and realignment of dislocated joints, as well as various forms of energy healing, including the laying on of hands and the directing of spiritually healing force from practitioner to patient (Rita Bleumenstein, personal communication, 1999; Tom Farqurar, personal communication, 1999).

Generally, traditional healing focused on the person and her or his community, rather than on a discrete biomedical sickness. The emphasis was on health, not disease. Disease was perceived as something not to be merely conquered and removed from life, but to be respected as a natural part of the person and of life itself. The tribal doctors were seen as servants of the people who were, by nature of their gifts, obligated to share their expertise rather than using it to accumulate power. These instances illustrate the major differences between allopathic and traditional healing practices.

In most Native communities, it was understood that healing came from a spiritual source and was given to the people. In this sense, it was a renewable resource: The more the healing was received, the more there was to give. In general, healing assistance was continually available for all. When healing is viewed as a gift that must be shared, it becomes empowering and seeks to move people to their own power, helping to self-liberate themselves from obstacles to their well-being. Traditional healing seeks to make things whole among people, cultures, and communities.

A current re-emergence of ceremony long forgotten is underway. An increased respect is being given to healing practices that have lived underground, safe from the destructive winds of change. A people who have suffered through decades and, in some cases, centuries of cultural confusion and deprivation, underscored by frustration, discouragement, and defeat, are finding themselves empowered and regenerated once again. They are taking the reins of their own healing. The erosion of Native mental health – propagated by the loss of traditional culture – is being reversed by surge of spiritually based energy. This has resulted in feelings of renewed hope and challenge.

While rates of alcoholism, suicide, sexual abuse, post-traumatic stress syndrome, diabetes, and related disease are still inordinately high, gains are being recorded. Awareness is growing that one-on-one treatment in Alaska's Native communities has had the effect of patching pinholes in an overflowing dam. The recovery of old songs and ceremonies that were all but forgotten reflects a rise in cultural pride and a hope for the future in many villages. Interest in resurrecting Alaskan Native languages is also growing. More and more villages are returning to Native healers in combination with public health, to address the problems of disease and social disintegration. The governance of hospitals, clinics, and social agencies by Native corporations and tribes has become a model of healing and demonstrates a path to follow for many native communities that have held little hope for the future over the past decades.

EMERGENCE OF TRADITIONAL WAYS

Beginning in the mid-nineties and continuing to the present, some of the major health providers in the state fostered the initiation and implementation of combined traditional and allopathic techniques. Traditional peoples have always known intuitively what science has only recently come to understand about nurturing or damaging health.

Research in psychoneuroimmunology, imagery, and healing has revealed the power of the mind to heal or inflict illness; the potent influence of family and community on morbidity and mortality; and the effects of belief and prayer on health outcomes (Freeman, 2004b, 2004c, 2004d, 2004e, 2004f, 2004g). Some allopathic practitioners have argued that staying current with changes within their own specialized field is difficult enough without also having to cope with the cultural influences, such issues of prayer and spiritual belief, in the communities they serve. They feel that the lack of calculable control in adopting traditional practices unnecessarily complicates the task of healing people. The use of herbal remedies provides a poignant example of this issue. Many traditional herbal remedies have been demonstrated to be efficacious for medical treatment in clinical trials (Freeman, 2004a). However, because herbal products cannot be patented, and herbal strength varies based on location, weather, and gathering techniques, allopathic medicine has raised concerns about these time-honored methods of healing, referring to them as *dirty drugs*. Many of our most powerful medicines are based on chemical compositions discovered from herbs. Nonetheless, pharmaceutically produced medications are a standard of care for allopathy because their strength and purity can be controlled in a laboratory.

Southcentral Foundation developed a traditionally based program of care that functions alongside allopathic medical dentistry, optometry and family medicine programs. Complementary care practices of acupuncture, acupressure, chiropracty, and naturopathy are also offered. A resource library in traditional healing practices is in its developmental stages and programs of treatment that involve certified tribal doctors and community based traditional healing programs are now functioning.

The Native hospital put procedures in place for bringing traditional healers into the treatment arena as co-professionals. Also, programs are underway to examine traditional healing herbs and to evaluate and categorize their properties and treatment efficacy. Herbal healers are working directly with patients referred to them by medical practitioners. Energy healers from Siberia and Alaska are demonstrating their techniques at professional conferences and are working directly with patients. These are but a few examples of a return to the traditional ways of healing.

With the advent of compacting, Native corporations have taken responsibility for many treatment programs that previously were under the supervision of the Indian Health Service and the government. They have begun to examine ways in which traditional healing practices can be effectively used in concert with modern medicine.

In many instances, it appears that traditional practices are being welcomed, as long as they do not involve putting anything in the body or taking anything out. Furthermore, it is felt that patient care should be managed and controlled by an allopathic professional. These concerns are understandable when one views them through the lens of allopathic medicine. This hierarchy can be viewed in a very different manner, however, when considered in light of the historical treatment of Alaska Natives and the consequences of that treatment.

THROUGH DIFFERENT LENS: THE CIRCLE AND THE SQUARE

Traditional indigenous peoples see disease as a problem that cannot be treated in isolation from the patient's lifestyle, personality, and body constitution. People fall ill because they have fallen out of harmony with the forces of nature. Disease is not an enemy to be eradicated but, rather, is a natural part of life, a transforming energy to be respected and used for personal evolution. The purpose of traditional healing is to restore the individual to harmony. Family, neighbors, and the entire community are important participants in helping the patient recover. Because of the different views of disease held by the allopathic and the traditional healing communities, we can conceptualized allopathic medicine as a *square* and traditional ways of healing as a *circle*.

Allopathic medicine – the square – has been highly successful in developing techniques and treatments specific to various disorders. Allopathic medicine is defined as a rather linear system that requires research findings, supervision, case notes, and strict management of its procedures to ensure effectiveness, safety, and evidence of worth. The positive benefits of allopathic medicine are accepted by traditional peoples and viewed as lifesaving. Allopathic medicine requires proof in the form of research and clinical trials; treatment is based on diagnosis and all treatment must be documented. Other methods of healing that are intuitive, based on ceremony or spiritual practices, or differ from allopathic methods, are rejected until such time as they are tested and found valuable by Western standards.

In most Native communities, the symbol of traditional healing is the circle, representing the spiritually based nature of healing and the acceptance of other systems. Traditional ways of healing that withstand the test of time are passed down from one generation to another, their benefit tested, so to speak, by history. The records of traditional healing outcomes reside within the oral tradition. The idea that they are unacceptable until tested according to Western standards seems irrational to traditional peoples.

In comparison with allopathic medicine, spiritually based traditional healing – the circle – is permeable and malleable. It embraces a wide variety of practices that have emerged and been observed to be successful in engendering a healing response. Traditional healing welcomes and embraces any practices that have demonstrated their worth to people by engendering healing in the individual, the family, and the community.

To extend the metaphor further, attempting to place the circle within the square might result in changes in the nature and viability of traditional healing, as the structure of the square imposes its structure and control upon the circle. On the other hand, placing the square inside the malleable circle would most likely vitalize and enhance both traditional healing practices and allopathic medicine, as the marvelous technology and treatment processes of allopathic medicine work in partnership and inclusion with the ancient art of traditional healing.

THE EXPANSION OF TRADITIONAL HEALING PRACTICES

WITHIN NATIVE HEALTH SERVICES

A formal traditional healing program has functioned in a limited way in Anchorage for more than a decade, centered around Southcentral Foundation and the Alaska Native Medical Center. In the Fall of 2001, Southcentral Foundation added a second Primary Care Building to its complex. This building was designed to assure equal incorporation of allopathic, traditional healing/tribal doctor, and complementary medical care. For more than a decade, a great many forward-looking members of the Native community, as well as allies in the Euro-American, Asiatic, and Afro-American communities, have contributed to the development of workshops, conferences, courses, and papers that have served as building blocks for an inclusive way of conceiving and developing integrative medical practices. These integrative health services address social and spiritual needs of Native Peoples as well as physical care via allopathic and traditional medicine.

In 1995, a survey was developed to study the traditional Native healing practices as historically and currently practiced in Alaska. The survey revealed the following philosophy:

While Native Americans suffer from the same types of physical and mental disorders as other Americans, the problems and severity of these disorders appear to be greater, the availability of services lower, the cultural relevance of treatment plans more challenging, and the social context more disintegrated than in most parts of American society. Failure to address these issues will result in more severe emotional problems for future generations of Native Americans, individuals, families, and communities. (Southcentral Foundation, 1995, p. 7)

The following communication from a traditional healer, Grandma Jean, was written for the *Circle of Healing* document in an effort to explain the nature and the purpose of a traditional healer's work in the contemporary world:

My name is Jean; everyone knows me as Grandmother Jean. As to the healings, I don't do them, Great Spirit does them. I use my body as a vehicle for the energy to move through, but it's just something that I was born with. I inherited it from my grandmother and my great grandmother, who were both Cherokee. They passed this ability down to me, just the same way you would inherit the ability to have creative energy; talents like singing, writing, or dancing. We inherit certain spiritual abilities like healing or teaching. Teaching is spiritual because to teach is to relay spirit wisdom. When you teach, you help to guide and direct the person. These things are not learned in any school. Everything is learned by doing, by hearing. I am now an Elder, it's important to understand that what I do is to quiet my heart so that it's steady and stable, tranquil and serene. The healing is simple because the energies go through me, having been called with prayer and sincerity. You need to be able to open up your spirit, open up your heart, receive that energy . . . and allow it to go through you. You don't heal. Creator heals. You're merely a vchicle. I am a citizen of the world: I am, by the creator's choice, a Cherokee. I am a woman by his choice as well; and I know who I am. I'm blessed because I walk . . . . I walk my medicine path and my peace path. I walk with assurance that I'm being guided to walk. I do the work of giving thanks and knowledge and thanking everything that is part of the world, not just the people. You see, you yourself have to be healed before you can help people with healing. I'm just doing what I can to help others. Just the same way I was helped. In this lifetime it's very important to know when to take and when to give. Knowing that gives you a very strong feeling because now you are using a part of yourself that before was not being used. Before, you weren't sensitive enough to use it . . . to help people in time of stress, fear, sickness, worry, despair, and confusion. So, I don't say that I'm a healer, I merely walk my path. (Morgan, 1999, p. 46)

ALASKA'S FIRST CERTIFIED TRIBAL DOCTOR

Rita Blumenstein was the initial candidate for the position of Tribal Doctor. She had practiced herbal medicine and energy-based healing since childhood and had an established reputation in the native community, as well as in national and international healing circles. Her name was submitted to Southcentral Foundation for appointment after the Elders Council approval process. There was some debate in the organization as to whether to use the title Tribal Doctor or some other title, such as Physician's Assistant.

The Elders stipulated that the title Tribal Doctor was necessary so that the selected traditional healer could operate as an equal partner with medical doctors when working with patients. After some debate, the title was accepted and, for the first time, there was an officially certified Tribal Doctor in Southcentral Foundation. Rita Blumenstein became the first certified Tribal Doctor in the State of Alaska. Most importantly, a certification process was established that required any tribal doctor candidate to be vetted in the same manner as had occurred for Rita Blumenstein.

For patients identified through an established referral process, Dr. Blumenstein developed a treatment schedule and saw patients on an individual and group basis. She facilitated group therapy and trained and consulted with therapists on how to work with patients from a traditional as well as a psychological point of view. Rita presented community workshops, participated in development of the traditional healing program, and attended community and national conferences as a consultant and a participant.

Many traditional healers/tribal doctors use energy healing such as the process of transferring through them the healing power to the patient. Some found that the required record keeping, filing, and other political machinations in clinical groups interfered with their ability to serve as a conduit for healing the patient. It was discovered that this process worked best by having the tribal doctor accompanied by an administrative assistant who kept records.

In addition, it was observed that the accepted means of evaluation used to establish efficiency of clinical procedures were not effective and may not apply to all traditional healers/tribal doctors. We (Morgan and Freeman) are now exploring the development of culturally sensitive procedures for evaluating the effectiveness of tribal doctor treatments. At a later stage of our research, we will suggest steps that should be taken to develop a model that is compatible with Western models of evaluation, yet is sensitive to traditional practice and culture.

THE CIRCLE OF HEALING MODEL

The concept of the Circle of Healing is a work in progress. We have chosen, in the Native way, to give it to the universe. We invite participation in its enhancement, through suggestion and application, in whatever way fits the needs of particular populations. While the Circle of Healing concept derives from our efforts to improve medical services to the Native community, it is our intention that it be utilized in all situations where alternative groups of people have been underserved as a result the shortcomings of allopathic medical practices. We are also cognizant, particularly in view of the many health crises occurring globally, that it is adaptable to instances where allopathic medical services are strained by circumstances and wider community involvement in mass treatment is desirable.

Proponents of traditional healing believe that sharing knowledge and respect for the wisdom of the indigenous people of the Earth and spirit that surrounds us, brings balance to cultures driven by technological advances and greed. Shared wisdom and respect along with unity in the cause of healing forms the basis of the Circle of Healing. This model is especially important to Alaskan natives who believe its concepts may be the fulfillment of prophecy. Prophecies from the Hopi and other tribal nations speak of a spiritual fire that would be lit in the North – that is, Alaska – that will result in the healing of the peoples. These prophecies, passed down as oral tradition, are often shared among Alaska Native People (Personal communication, Walter Austin, Tlingit Elder, August, 1995).

The Circle of Healing model has five-components:

1. Utilizes a tri-disciplinary diagnostic team of traditional, allopathic, and CAM medical and health providers.

2. Presents all options for healing to the patient for consideration, actively involving the patient in the healing process.

3. Provides a guide, known as a Pathfinder, to act as patient interpreter and support system.

4. Implements a patient-driven healing path (plan) based on patient and tri-disciplinary team recommendations.

5. Provides follow-up care for intervention and prevention.

The Pathfinder position is critical within this model. Pathfinders are individuals who have skills as caseworkers and who possess knowledge of traditional healing practices as well as allopathic and CAM methods of healing. In essence, Pathfinders are the persons responsible for assuring clear communications and follow-up among the patient, medical team, family, and community.

THE PATHFINDER

The Pathfinder position was initially envisioned in 1992 when searching for a culturally appropriate title and job description for clinical and non-clinical professionals working within the Native health agency. This term has existed at many times and in many places and it seemed appropriate to our emphasis on culturally appropriate medical practice. The term was adopted for non-clinical intake staff in the Behavioral Health Department for a period of some years.

When the Southcentral Foundation staff began deciding on the nature and function of the new primary care building that would house and unify allopathic, integrative, and tribal medicine, it became clear that the Pathfinder position, as outlined in the following job description, would be necessary to properly implement and direct the unification as we conceived it. We see this as a core position to the Circle of Healing concept in the areas of diagnosis, treatment planning, and patient involvement.

Often, vital information is not shared between patient and medical care professionals. Poor communication leads to an iteration of appointments that fail to address the underlying psychological or medical issues. The Pathfinder attempts to improve patient/physician communication, the quality of treatment and reduce repeat visits or misguided medical tests.

THE CIRCLE OF HEALING PROPOSAL

The Circle of Healing includes four phases of diagnosis, treatment, and healing: the preventive phase, the outpatient phase, the inpatient phase (when necessary), and the aftercare phase. All four of these aspects have to be kept in mind when the treatment facility first makes contact with the patient and reviews the nature and level of patient physical, mental, and spiritual dysfunction. The following guidelines illustrate the implementation of these concepts:

1. We must strengthen the level of cultural and health science-based community services that are available for families suffering from dysfunction. In this manner, we may be able to control the numbers of patients coming to outpatient or inpatient services.
2. We must implement an effective process for reviewing medical history and self-development with the patient. We must assist the patient in understanding how to access their own cultural strengths and their family capabilities as part of the treatment/healing process. We must help patients build a level of awareness of treatment services available in the three disciplines so that we may effectively involve them in their treatment/healing process. In this way, we will dramatically improve the possibilities of that patient avoiding remission and extended hospitalization.
3. We must become effective at the outpatient level (Primary Care Center) in helping the patient develop a healing path. In this way, we will lessen the number of patients who go into inpatient or hospital treatment. For those who do enter hospital treatment, we must be able to prepare them for treatment so they can make more viable use of their time and of the treatment offered at that facility.
4. We must develop a coordinated team effort at the outpatient and hospital sites that includes all three medical disciplines (tribal medicine, allopathic and integrative medicine). We must initiate an interdisciplinary consultation, at entry, that lays out a treatment regime and educates the staff as to the history of these patients and the nature of their needs. This includes an integrated diagnosis and consultation program within the structure of these three disciplines. In this manner, we may be able to utilize the treatment time more effectively. We will

develop a healing program that patients will carry with them from the hospital into aftercare. Prevention, in this sense, will be a more viable concept, as the patient will be going home to a family who is more prepared to receive them and work with their treatment. The patients will be aware of how to utilize medications and how to conduct themselves physically, emotionally, and spiritually in a manner that will strengthen their healing response. They will be better prepared to use proper dietary techniques and exercise techniques to that end and will be prepared to work with their families in developing a balanced approach to the problem solving.

This Circle of Healing approach illustrates the interrelationship of all four phases of prevention, outpatient, inpatient, and aftercare. It demonstrates that all of our health service approaches are in fact interrelated and can more effectively achieve their goals with appropriate intercommunication and planning.

ROLE OF THE CIRCLE OF HEALING PATHFINDER

Initial contact with a group of patients, entering or reentering the Circle of Healing Program requires that the Pathfinder:

1. Review with the patient their medical history to date and the patient's view of the level of remediation/healing that has taken place as a result of these experiences.
2. Review with the patient their complete treatment history and suggest areas in which services in integrative, traditional, and allopathic care may supplement or replace their existing program. These recommendations will be developed after an initial intake meeting with the patient and concurring consultation with the Circle of Healing treatment team.
3. Participate in treatment team meetings, which will evaluate the patient's immediate health needs and suggest further traditional, integrated, and allopathic approaches that appear to be realistic supplements to the patient's present care plan.
4. Possess and demonstrate the ability to apply a high level of knowledge regarding a wide spectrum of treatment opportunities, in the integrative, traditional, and allopathic service areas.

5. Create a climate of empathy and mutual respect with the patient and demonstrate a level of caring to encourage the patient to utilize treatment recommendations and participate fully in the development of their individual healing plan.
6. Assume an objective position in consultations and meetings with traditional clinical staff regarding the patient's needs.
7. Serve when necessary as the patient's representative in reviewing and re-developing the existing treatment model.
8. Demonstrate experientially developed skills in the planning and further development of the Circle of Healing Model.
9. Maintain the required treatment records in a form consistent with the agency.
10. Provide staff consultations, appropriate supporting research, and effective analysis of the patient's healing history.
11. Through a cultural base and academic work experience, interpret, and understand the patient's medical history. Further, the Pathfinder elicits from the patient personal strengths that could be developed as part of the treatment-healing plan that may have not been evidenced through prior contact. This may have occurred because of a lack of cultural interpretation or a lack of trust and willingness on the patient's part to participate in previous diagnostic meetings.
12. Participate in ongoing review of patient satisfaction and quality assurance related to activities provided through the Circle of Healing.

The focus of the Pathfinder is holistic in nature, with emphasis placed on a valid and comprehensive view of the patient's treatment experience to date in order to develop an effective healing plan in concert with the patient.

The Pathfinder then meets for the second time with the patient to discuss the proposed plan. They receive the patient's inputs and questions, answer to the best extent possible, and supply the patient with specific information on the disciplines being recommended. This information is provided in written form or delivered by assisting the patient in using the Internet available at the Circle of Healing Resource Library. Ideally, a medical information site will be developed within the program that will include computers, medical, and library resources; a listing of community and international cultural events and approved community sites for family and individual support services.

Preferably, a training program should be available to assist the patient in utilizing this resource. The internet could be used to access a description of the effects of medications prescribed, to make connections to medical and support groups, or to contact sites exploring innovative procedures. It could also allow and encourage the patient to search for and, if appropriate to their healing plan, incorporate culturally based treatment, ceremony, and community activities into their healing plan. This process would ideally be reviewed with the Pathfinder or a similarly trained provider on a regular basis. The Pathfinder would also set up the initial appointments for the patient onsite and/or deliver recommendations for initial treatment at offsite locations.

As treatment progresses, the patient would be free to call the Pathfinder, report on progress or lack of progress in their program and request supportive information as to how to proceed with their treatment/healing process. Over several years, the patient would develop a level of wellness that would cut down on their need for outpatient or inpatient contacts and make them a health resource for their family.

CLINICAL IMPLEMENTATION OF THE CIRCLE OF HEALING

There are many operational problems to be faced when a system tries to develop an inclusive process for tribal, complementary, and allopathic medicine. Those considering such a project are advised to proceed carefully and include team representatives in their planning. These should include, but not be limited to, traditional healers/Tribal Doctors, consumers of complementary and allopathic medicine, tribal leaders, and others who may have developed insight through their life and/or academic experience. Of primary importance, is to place all participants on an equal footing regardless of qualifications.

SUGGESTED ROLE OF THE TRIBAL DOCTOR WITHIN THE CIRCLE OF HEALING PLAN

The Tribal Doctors may practice a wide variety of treatment techniques, all of which are explained to the patient during diagnosis and are used only with their permission. Tribal Doctors vary in their specialty areas and techniques; some of the techniques utilized are briefly explained below in the hopes that this will help to clarify Tribal Doctor practices.

HEALING HANDS. The Tribal Doctor may employ a technique that is similar in procedure to treatments involving healing hands – an energy-based form of medicine – and massage. These may involve breathing exercises and other techniques to relax and balance the body including cold or hot packs to release tension, relieve pain and increase blood flow; manual massage, superficially or at a greater depth according to diagnosed need; trigger point pressure release to relax contracted muscles; and concurrent tension and deep muscle massage. Tribal Doctor Rita Bleumenstein described the practice of healing hands in this manner:

> The hands are tools that the mind depends upon when it wants to get anything done. The laying on of hands has a wide range of meaning. The priest of old and the priests of today consecrated the laying on hands, which means laying on the *Hands of God*. It is a very holy act in the churches. Ministers are ordained by the laying on of hands. Special gifts are conferred to individuals with the laying on of hands. The human hand is the antenna of the mind. It is the hand that conveys the healing thought of the healer to the sick person. By this method, healing vibrations are picked up by the tissue, nerves, and cells and they quickly transfer the imprinted thought of health to other parts of the body. If you have a telephone but do not speak into the speaker, the message will not be heard on the other end of the line. If you have a sick fellow man but do not transfer your healing power of hands through special *speaker places* on their body, the sick body cannot respond and cannot take the message. (Rita Bleumenstein, personal communication, September, 2006)

RELAXATION TECHNIQUE. The Tribal Doctor frequently employs relaxation techniques as a means of assisting the patient to develop a receptive attitude to treatment and healing techniques. Relaxation techniques can include directed listening to relaxing music while in a physically receptive posture, breathing exercises, and other relaxation strategies to give the patient tools for self-management. The Tribal Doctor may use imagery techniques in a directed way to deeply relax various areas of the body. Relaxation techniques are a major component in tribal medicine, in that they prepare the patient to experience the healing effect of various traditional approaches, use them effectively and with more openness for their own healing journey.

STORYTELLING. Storytelling is an ancient art that served as the purveyor of wisdom prior to the advent of written language. As practiced now by traditional storytellers, it teaches listening skills, morality, cultural awareness and pride, and problem solving by intimation and example. While it may not address a patient's concerns directly, it does encourage the patient to seek and discover answers to concerns through interpretation and assimilation of the storyline. Tribal Doctors frequently use abbreviated storytelling approaches for a similar purpose with patients.

CLEANING AND BLESSING. Cleaning of one's body, mind, and spirit through a process of smudging (smoke cleansing) with sage, sweet grass, cedar, labrador tea, and fungi is practiced throughout the native communities in Alaska. This practice has ancient roots in ceremony and community practice and prepares the patient to enter treatment in a balanced and open way. The procedure dispels negative energy in all participants and surroundings while improving positive energy and receptivity. The blessing is given as recognition of the positive things that have been given to us and as a continuation of the healing process. It also helps direct the energy of the participants on a positive path and weakens negative thought.

NUTRITIONAL COUNSELING. The Tribal Doctor may suggest traditional and allopathic foods for the patient's diet if they are physician approved and supportive of the patient's treatment. Tribal Doctors, through their training as traditional healers, may have vast knowledge of the healing properties of various indigenous plants, minerals and animals. They have historically used these to treat many physical and mental impairments. The availability and utilization of these nutritional additives is in flux at the present time, as the movement to partnership between allopathic, integrative, and tribal medicine strengthens in a growing number of hospitals and clinics.

TRADITIONAL COUNSELING. Traditional counseling, as practiced by Tribal Doctors and culturally based counsels, differs in some major ways from the allopathic model. Traditional counseling focuses on the person and the context of their family and community rather than on a reported dysfunction. The emphasis is on health, not disease. The Tribal Doctor can assist the patient in recognizing their own healing source and, thus, access that power to heal. With the assistance of their counselor, the patient can move in the sense of self-liberation from obstacles to well-being.

EXERCISE. The Tribal Doctor may prescribe a variety of exercise options that the patient may include in the treatment plan. These may include a variety of procedures specific to the conditioning of certain areas of the body or they may be directed, more generally, to release tension, improve circulation, and so on. Traditional activities that lift the mood and improve general bodily function may be suggested, such as ceremonial dance, drumming, wilderness hikes, gardening, and berry picking, if they seem culturally appropriate.

DREAM INTERPRETATION. The Tribal Doctor assists the patient in the interpretation of their dreams as they might relate to ideas or experiences that are blocking the healing process. The patient is helped to realistically explore dream content and, where relevant, use it to develop an increased awareness of healing approaches that they may access on their healing path. The Tribal Doctor uses caution in this procedure, so that dream content is not overemphasized so as to make it irrelevant to the healing process.

THE TALKING CIRCLE. The traditional talking or healing circle, based on practices used by Alaskan Natives and American Indians generations ago, puts its emphasis on involvement, partnership, and consent of all parties. Traditional values are stressed, such as sharing, humility, respect for others, cooperation, responsibility, spirituality, and similar attributes. The circle focuses on the basic positive responsibility for one's own healing. Patients or participants are seen as human beings capable of bringing their lives into balance. The talking circle is an excellent technique to help patients find similarities with their own concerns and enhance their journey of self-discovery by listening to the issues of others. Talking circles generally follow a similar format and serve as a successful teaching and healing procedure in classroom, community, and clinical settings.

PRAYER. With the patient's request, the Tribal Doctor will join with the patient in prayer. The Tribal Doctor will also, when appropriate and at the patient's request, pray for the patient's healing. These prayers are non-denominational, unless the patient specifies otherwise. The Tribal Doctor will, upon request, participate in opening and closing prayer at a variety of conferences, workshops, and municipal, and tribal gatherings. Prayers are made in talking and healing circles as a matter of course, unless the setting or participants direct otherwise. The process of prayer has strong traditional roots and is seen as a strong component in any treatment/healing process.

SONG AND DANCE. As part of the patient's treatment-healing program, the Tribal Doctor may prescribe attendance at tribal ceremonies and, where possible, involvement in traditional song and dance. Frequently, these types of activities assist the patient in moving from depression, improving social attitude, developing a positive sense of their culture, and gaining other self-development skills that can be a major support for the patient's healing journey. Tribal Doctors may participate in the planning and implementation of these activities as consultants and presenters to insure a traditional and culturally appropriate procedure. Music, dance, and ceremony have always functioned as a major component of the traditional healing process.

JOURNEY/IMAGINATION. The Tribal Doctor may utilize a procedure with the patient that demonstrates a way to use imagination as a tool in the healing process. The patient is assisted through a process that helps them visualize a situation of wellness in themselves and/or to visit a time when trauma occurred in their life that may underlie their present mental or physical difficulties. The patient is shown a way to begin to resolve those earlier traumatic situations and find the seeds of healing. Each Tribal Doctor has a unique way of using this procedure in a healing situation. The process is fully explained to the patient prior to initiating the procedure.

THE MEDICINE WHEEL. The medicine wheel teachings allow the individual to reflect on an expanded and holistic worldview. Harmony and balance in life – emotionally, spiritually, and physically – are dynamic lessons about the personal traits that are important to each patient and work as teaching tools to promote awareness, self-esteem, and pride in one's identity and culture. An adaptation of the talking circle format can be used to involve all participants and promote respect for oneself, others, and the environment.

ENERGY HEALING. Tribal Doctors have historically believed that their gift of healing comes from a positive spiritual source and that they are merely carriers and transmitters of healing energy. Most feel that it is a gift to be shared and, when appropriately transmitted, has liberating effects and removes obstacles to well-being. This energy transfer usually occurs through a treatment similar to that described as healing hands and has the goal of moving the patient to a sense of balance and a position of wellness. In the past, practices similar to energy healing have carried a religious connotation. Most Tribal Doctors now practice these procedures with strictly non-denominational intent and only with the patient's full understanding and acceptance.

OTHER SPECIALTIES. There are many other specialty areas practiced by Tribal Doctors. They include, but are not limited to, bone setting, circulation, obstetrics, modified acupuncture, and healing of historical trauma. The type of practice conducted by the Tribal Doctor will of course depend upon their experience, training, and connections. Dr. Bleumenstein presents the experience like this:

> We all can heal – mainly ourselves. We all can help others to heal themselves. Doctors, practitioners, pharmacists, surgeons, and healers can only give the supply needed so that you can become whole. To become whole, to be healed, is a work of the individual. Just as every art, it requires knowledge and practice. (personal communication, September 2006)

INTEGRATED TREATMENT PLANNING

The Tribal Doctor's treatment goal, as a participating partner in the allopathic, complementary, and tribal medicine clinical team lies in assisting the person being treated by utilizing the opportunities that this cooperative team approach offers. By doing so, we hope to dramatically improve the possibility of a patient avoiding remission and extended hospitalization. Tribal Doctors see themselves as servants of the people, obligated to share their knowledge and expertise to assist the patient, their family, and their community in maintaining a condition of wellness.

A suggested procedure would be to have a Tribal Doctor who possesses the appropriate skills and is comfortable with the procedure perform an initial visit or visits in an outpatient or inpatient location. The Tribal Doctor will then, preferably prior to other technically based evaluations, suggest a diagnosis with treatment recommendations. Allopathic physicians, who are comfortable with the process, may use the Tribal Doctor's diagnosis and recommendations in developing their concept of what tests to order, explorations to initiate, and treatments to prescribe. In most clinical settings, as they exist today, this procedure would be best initiated as a pilot project, probably as a clinical study funded by a grant.

The role of the Tribal Doctor should be advisory as well as direct. Recommendations should be made based on cultural perspectives of health/healing and traditional remedies (ceremonies, contact with other native practitioners). The Tribal Doctor may perform diagnostic measures and offer therapeutic interventions such as prayers, healing hands, songs, and supportive counseling. The Tribal Doctor should also serve as a consultant to staff to increase understanding and awareness of traditional values, beliefs, and practices. This can be accomplished by one-on-one interaction or by group presentations on items of interest. The Circle of Healing concept has been implemented in various ways in communities across the nation. This expansion has occurred primarily with the adaptation or adoption of certain of its concepts to support similar efforts with and external to Native American communities.

WHAT WE HAVE LEARNED

Our efforts to develop and implement an integrated system of treatment for our Native communities have taught us many things. In particular, this work has directly familiarized us with some of the failings as well as the successes of allopathic medicine in serving the perceived needs of indigenous and minority populations. It has also suggested changes in our medical and social system that should be addressed if we wish to create a more viable path to healing for our patient populations. The opportunity to initiate changes in our treatment, legal, and business practices and open the door to more inclusive procedures is being driven by the need to salvage systems that are breaking under the weight of limited human and budgetary resources.

The Circle of Healing approach demonstrates an opportunity to *fix* the broken system. It requires, however, a visceral change in the manner in which treatment programs are developed, managed, and implemented. It requires more emphasis on prevention and awareness of what exists within the patient and in the community to support the evolution of treatment into true healing. Traditional/indigenous practices have been tested by peoples for thousands of years, although indigenous forms of medical research have a different structure and purpose than our current-day allopathic models. The wisdom and the results of that healing knowledge are available and should be utilized in a more productive and inclusive way.

POTENTIAL SYSTEMIC DIFFICULTIES IN

IMPLEMENTING THE CIRCLE OF HEALING

There may be many operational problems to be faced when a system tries to develop an inclusive process for tribal, complementary, and allopathic medicine. The legal system has to be altered to be more accepting of the healing profession's ability to explore alternative approaches to healing and to redevelop litigation procedures that block such approaches. Organized health providers have to adjust the profit model to recognize that healing is a more practical approach with respect to budget and to income than a system that encourages the quick fix and, as a result, recidivism. The various professions should develop research assessment tools that are compatible with Western models of evaluation, yet sensitive to traditional practice and culture. This sensitivity is particularly important when evaluating the efficacy of traditional/indigenous treatment/healing techniques. Training should be afforded to all clinical staff to demonstrate the wide range of services offered by tribal medicine and the manner in which non-linear approaches to diagnosis, treatment, and healing have proven effective in a multitude of situations.

Other services equally beneficial to the healing process, but currently seen as auxiliary to the medical process, should be evaluated for inclusion. These include, but are not limited to, healing circles, traditional musical presentation for groups of patients, direct training in traditional practices for staff, and storytelling. The Tribal Doctor services outlined here should be implemented following a brief training program to acquaint nursing and medical staff with services and to clarify and maximize their potential for patient treatment.

Eventually, as the clinical climate becomes more supportive, the Tribal Doctor program may include massage, bodywork, and energy transfer healing. Initially, the agency may implement practices that are currently considered safe in our contemporary world of excessive litigation. At every step of the way we should be sure that these changes align with the goals of the institution, the community, and the patient. Where these goals clash, efforts should be made by teams representing broad interests to bring about a convergence of these goals. While these operational considerations will be necessary to support a partial implementation of traditional healing practices into a health service agency, the eventual goal must be full operational partnership among the three medical disciplines: tribal, allopathic, and complementary.

As with any innovative approach, there will be aspects of traditional practice that may conflict with medical and malpractice and, indeed, religions/cultural concerns. The eventual goal should be the development of a culturally based process of evaluation and education that will lead to amelioration of those concerns. This goal should accomplished through a process of continuing education and training to explore the strengths and weaknesses of the three medical disciplines and move to discard the ineffective, while incorporating the effective in a working partnership.

Tribal Doctors may initially have limitations imposed by the system on the practice of their skills in the present medical climate. Such limitations may include restrictions on prescribing medications, herbs or supplements, and poking or body piercing. The Tribal Doctor program should supplement and enhance the services that can be provided in the areas of consultation, diagnosis, and treatment. In addition, a Tribal Doctor consortium should be developed that will, among other services, provide a Tribal Doctor exchange program. This will be in addition to the variety of treatments available, on request, by the medical staff and the patient population.

It will be important to fully explore the needs of the agency seeking to implement the Circle of Healing. This will begin by explaining the professions that may be least understood by the allopathic medical professional, namely the Tribal Doctor and the Pathfinder. An appropriate continuing education/training program using the talking circle model would assure all participants a voice in the proceedings as equals coming from their own level of professional strength, whether their training and experience was acquired in the halls of academia and the allopathic clinical setting or, in an equal but more culturally based way, through inheritance, mentoring, anecdotal history, spiritual evidence, and experience in the field.

CONCLUSION

The Circle of Healing model recognizes and embraces all forms of medical treatment utilized by individuals in various cultural communities. Our Circle of Healing model was structured to include allopathic medicine, tribal medicine, and many alternative approaches such as acupuncture, acupressure, naturopathy, Ayurvedic and Chinese medicine, and other activities that have shown positive potential for healing and health. These activities include, but are not limited to, community gatherings, ceremony, prayer, music, and drumming, all integrated through the talking circle.

The Circle of Healing model looks beyond the treatment concepts of allopathic medicine to strengthen the healing process for the individual and community. Of primary importance, the Circle of Healing seeks to stimulate patients to recognize themselves as the primary part of their own healing process. Finally, the Circle of Healing suggests the benefits of adopting traditional practices into current-day medicine. The Circle of Healing model seeks to enhance treatment approaches and to support individual clients in their efforts to live out their lives in a healthier way, while becoming a source of wellness for others.

References

Attneave, C. (1974). *Beyond clinic walls*. Birmingham, Alabama: University of Alabama Press.

Eby, D. (1995). *The Maori of Aotearoa/New Zealand and the Alaska Natives of the United States: A comparative analysis of health policy and planning issues*. Unpublished masters thesis, University of Hawaii.

Freeman L. W. (2004a). Herbs as medical intervention. In K. White (Ed.), *Mosby's complementary and alternative medicine: A research-based approach* (pp. 439-479). St Louis, MO: Mosby Publisher.

Freeman L. W. (2004b). How Relationships and Life Events Affect Health: Human Studies. In K. White (Ed.), *Mosby's complementary and alternative medicine: A research-based approach* (pp. 99-143). St Louis, MO: Mosby Publisher.

Freeman, L. W. (2004c). Imagery. In K. White (Ed.), *Mosby's complementary and alternative medicine: A research-based approach* (pp. 275-305). St Louis, MO: Mosby Publisher.

Freeman L. W. (2004d). Physiological Pathways of Mind-Body Communication. In K. White (Ed.), *Mosby's complementary and alternative medicine: A research-based approach* (pp. 1-35). St. Louis, MO: Mosby Publisher.

Freeman L. W. (2004e). Research on Mind-Body Effects. In K. White (Ed.), *Mosby's complementary and alternative medicine: A research-based approach* (pp. 37-67). St Louis, MO: Mosby Publisher.

Freeman L. W. (2004f). Spirituality and Healing . In K. White (Ed.), *Mosby's complementary and alternative medicine: A research-based approach* (pp. 519-553). St Louis, MO: Mosby Publisher.

Freeman L. W. (2004g). Therapeutic Touch: Healing with Energy. In K. White (Ed.), *Mosby's complementary and alternative medicine: A research-based approach* (pp. 555-567). St Louis, MO: Mosby Publisher.

Hildebrand, I. (2005). *Ritchie Boy: The life and suicide of a young Alaska Native*. New York: Universe, Inc.

Morgan, R. (1999). *The Circle of Healing*. Unpublished manuscript.

Morgan, R., Richards, B., & Frank, J. (1995). The healing of our people. Unpublished manuscript.

Napoleon, H. (1996). YU'UA'RAQ' *The way of the human being*. Mimeographed, Hooper Bay, AK. Unpublished manuscript.

Neihardt, J. (1932). *Black Elk speaks*. New York, NY: Washington Square Press.

Southcentral Foundation (1995). *Healing Our People: A Project Report. Anchorage, AK: Southcentral Foundation*. Unpublished manuscript.

CHAPTER FOURTEEN

RELATIONAL CREATIVITY AND HEALING POTENTIAL:
THE POWER OF EASTERN THOUGHT
IN WESTERN CLINICAL SETTINGS

Ruth Richards

Aspects of Buddhist philosophy and psychology, and Eastern thought generally, are finding their way increasingly into Western life, culture, and health care (see Baker, 1997; Freeman & Lawlis, 2001; Kaptchuk, 1983; Macy, 1991; Ricard & Thuan, 2001; Rothberg, 2006; Tart, 1994; Tarthang Tulku, 1984, 1994; Thich Nhat Hanh, 1975, 1997; Varela, Thompson, & Rosch, 1992). Moreover, this influence is affecting our most profound understandings of health and of life itself. Varela, Thompson, and Rosch (1992) in their influential book *The Embodied Mind*, which links cognitive science with Buddhist thought even contended that: "the rediscovery of Asian philosophy, particularly of the Buddhist tradition, is a second renaissance in the cultural history of the West" (p. 22). In considering clinical psychological experience and parallels with artistic creative process and Buddhist ideas, this chapter explores how we see and relate to each other and our world. What we experience together may be deeply healing, while bringing us richness, immediacy, and joy, and, at times, advances in personal and spiritual development.

Many Westerners were brought up as strong individualists (see Jordan, Kaplan, Miller, Stiver, & Surrey, 1991; Pilisuk & Parks, 1986) standing separate from the rest of life and poised to control. Yet, some of us today are no longer experiencing ourselves as independent agents. As Vietnamese Zen Master Thich Nhat Hanh (1988) put it, both metaphorically and literally: "the sun my heart" (p. 66). Without the sun we would die. Likewise, we would die without air or water. In the same way, we die without love and nurturance, as evinced by the heartbreaking deaths of neglected babies who have rarely been held while left for long hours in certain institutions (Eisler, 2007). Our newer Western science, from physics to systems theory (e.g., Bohm, 1980; Loye, 2007; Macy, 1991; Ricard & Thuan, 2001), illustrates the various complex connections found between what we might call entities and processes throughout the natural world, thus underscoring our profound interdependence.

Many of us, too, who once thought we were in touch with the world around us through our minds and bodies, have been learning that what we see, or think we see – including our experience of *self* – is a tiny constructed perspective on a vast and profound mystery. What we encounter is conditioned by personal and cultural experience and limited by our human faculties (Combs & Krippner, 2007; Richards, 2001, 2007a; Thich Nhat Hanh, 1974, 1988). We may find we are not present at all – perhaps lost in thoughts about the past or future – when walking through a garden, listening to our friend, or attending a child's performance. Our experience is shaped by a web of expectations, memories, wants, fears, and movement toward grasping and aversion. These thoughts bias what we encounter and often create unnecessary suffering. As with the Zen of archery (Herrigel, 1953), there is the possibility of being present, open, and aware to everything we experience, from simply saying "hello," to being deeply present with another. Worlds can open, delivering health in the truest sense.

This chapter considers these themes along five major themes: (1) relational clinical encounters on an inpatient psychiatric unit; (2) parallels to *everyday creativity*; (3) empathy and mutuality as creative processes; (4) learning we are more connected than we imagined; and (5) increasing our relational capacity.

RELATIONAL MODEL ON A PSYCHIATRIC INPATIENT UNIT

The best way to begin exploring these themes is with my experience at a psychiatric inpatient hall of a hospital on the East Coast of the US. Some years ago, I worked there daily as a clinical psychiatrist along with psychologists, social workers, psychiatric nurses, and mental health workers. The clinical experience depicted below is intended to introduce relational healing that opens the patient to realms of greater meaning and spiritual significance. I now recognize that much of what guided our work was consistent with aspects of Eastern thought across cultures, including Buddhist ones, such as attention to interconnection, impermanence, a greater underlying unity, authenticity, deeper awareness of the present moment, limitations of a dominant ego identification, a natural compassion, and, indeed, ultimate wisdom, which can manifest from our greater knowing (see Ajaya, 1983).

South Hall (a fictitious name created for the hospital ward to ensure client confidentiality) was an inpatient unit based on the *relational* model, in which relationships and the cognitive and emotional experience of intersubjectivity are considered central to identity and personal development. The practices of this unit were developed by clinician-scholars at the Stone Center at Wellesley College (Jordan, 1997; Jordan & Dooley, 2000; Jordan, Kaplan, et al., 1991). Although, in many Western cultures, relational qualities are more encouraged in women than men (Gilligan, 1982), they are vital to both men and women to experience development, health, personal well-being, and some of life's greatest satisfactions (Pilisuk & Parks, 1986; Siegel, 1999). Furthermore, relationships can heal best where the pain lies the deepest.

Our inpatient clients on South Hall were women who had endured situations so difficult that hospitalization had become necessary: some had histories that included trauma, depression, anxiety, psychotic episodes, and substance abuse. A number of women were trying to cope with the painful experiences of post-traumatic stress disorder (PTSD), which is marked by exposure to an overwhelming and potentially life-threatening danger that evokes an extreme response, such as fear, helplessness, or horror, and typically followed by a number of disturbing, arousing, or numbing sequelae. The trauma they had experienced might have involved early sexual abuse, physical abuse, or neglect and, for some, their early situation had been reactivated by current events in their lives. For certain women, especially at the beginning of their stay, there were episodes of disruption, acting out, and, occasionally, uncontrolled anger as well as potential violence. The distress of these women could be stimulated by a range of interpersonal contacts leading to fear, distrust, anger, lack of control, and perhaps flashbacks from earlier trauma. Anger at people who reactivated earlier issues included staff, who, at times, misunderstood a person's suffering or needs.

Below, I share a some of vignettes that foreground the themes of relational healing. To protect client confidentiality some details have been changed or presented in broad terms. Specific quotes from one woman, however, who will be called Martha, are shared with her enthusiastic permission. She wrote them, read them aloud at a weekly hall meeting, and then distributed typed copies for further sharing.

VIGNETTE. I remember one reportedly suicidal woman who escaped in desperation from a locked part of the hospital and tried to run off. These inpatient settings were locked for safety and she had been confined against her will.

Security forces were sent after her for fear of self-harm. She was found and transferred to us at South Hall. Later, she was able to share her story, including what had brought her to the hospital; calm and controlled, she was able to talk about what she feared and needed for herself. She said her distress at being hospitalized had much to do with feeling trapped and "managed" by others, while also feeling deeply ignored.

How can the success of South Hall be gauged? When an inpatient is out of control and a danger to him or herself or others, and when other measures did not work, chemical or physical restraints were used. What was remarkable on South Hall is that, use of these restraints was *significantly* lower there than in any other part of the hospital. It is not that our patient population was so much healthier: Other halls had a similar population. I believe that the difference was that on South Hall people talked with and listened to each other.

How Important is Connecting?

Imagine being in a hospital, frightened and, more importantly, alone. In some Eastern cultures, such as Vietnam, the word for *I* includes within its definition the relationship to others (see Jordan, Kaplan, et al., 1991). By contrast, in many Western cultures people have often been raised according to a model of *separation-individuation.* Erikson's (1950) developmental levels, as an illustration, celebrate this separation, which is achieved only after one moves from trust to autonomy to initiative to industry and, finally, identity. Even so, the importance of relationships, for women at least, has more recently been acknowledged (Gilligan, 1982; Jordan, 1997; Jordan, Kaplan, et al., 1991).

Relationship is important to the earliest brain development in male or female infants, as well as to normal growth and development in the years that follow (Eisler, 2007; Siegel, 1999). Furthermore, interpretations of Charles Darwin's theory of evolution have been skewed. The general principle of survival of the fittest was modified for the human species in the *Descent of Man* and Darwin's private notebooks to leave room for cooperation, ethical conduct, and love (Loye, 2007). The importance of relationships should not be surprising for social creatures, and the costs in health and well-being if connection is lacking should not be underestimated (Pilisuk & Parks, 1986).

Some psychiatric inpatients also feel very alone, different, and extruded from society at first. To make matters worse, some do not feel treated as a whole person. Imagine if a woman is identified primarily as "Nancy with depression" or "Shiela with PTSD." A clinical diagnosis can become central to identity in the hospital: Some of our women clients bemoaned this openly. In one therapy group, patients were deliberately asked to reintroduce themselves, including their loves, their passions, their strengths, what they wanted to do with their lives. People opened up, expressing relief they could be more fully human, and more fully themselves. Some people had started to think of themselves as only "Nancy with depression."

Clinicians also focus too often only on the problem and not the person, on what is going wrong, and not what has been going right (Richards, 1997). A deficiency model of understanding has been a problem of Western psychology in general. In Eastern models of healing (see Baker, 1997; Kaptchuk, 1983) and new Western adaptations (Freeman & Lawlis, 2001; Schlitz, Amorok, & Micozzi, 2005), a whole person view is the norm, with the focus on establishing new harmony and balance. Happily, in the West, the fields of humanistic psychology (Schneider, Bugental, & Pierson, 2001; Taylor & Martin, 2001) and the new positive psychology introduced by Seligman and others (see Peterson, 2006) have been instrumental in bringing a broader perspective to studies of humans and human possibility. Humanistic and transpersonal psychologies, in particular, have been influenced by Eastern traditions and look toward a broader and unknown human potential (Schneider et al., 2001).

Nonetheless, it is important to understand that labels and medications have their place in a hospital and at times these can be lifesaving. Proper uses as well as the design of interventions can open doors for the greater acknowledgement of humanity, personal healing, and growth. One needs to beware of situations where an approach can deaden clinicians to the reality in front of us and to the real person who is there.

VIGNETTE. Consider another woman who was very much helped by connection. She experienced relief from extreme anxiety through calming medication and could begin to talk, though it was still very hard for her. A fleeting and vague awareness she had of early sexual abuse was becoming more definite. Life events had started to trigger flashbacks and, terrified, she had ended up in the hospital. Her memories were mainly body memories that she felt in her physical being rather than being remembered as verbal or visual. Despite her fear, she took the risk to talk with her clinician; she dared to look more consciously and closely about what she was experiencing rather than try to push it away.

Being with a responsive other immediately had a calming effect. She gradually opened up – to herself as well as to others – in a variety of ways, including expressive arts and group therapy. She, and other women, found comfort in meeting each other, discovering that they were not alone, and that others had similar problems. They also got to know each other more fully as complex people with complex lives. Making progress meant developing trust in those who were helping when sharing problems and secrets. This woman knew the answers were not going to be easy, but gradually found that facing them with concerned others brought a new and surprising strength. She came to feel whole and more integrated. Finally, she connected with a community that supported her growth.

Healing can occur when someone else deeply hears, understands, and shares one's pain. The fear or anger can fade and trust can grow; the person no longer feels so alone (Jordan, Kaplan, et al., 1991; Pilisuk & Parks, 1986; Solomon & Siegel, 2003). There is evidence that some early brain misdevelopment due to trauma can be modified (Solomon & Siegel, 2003) toward a very promising new integration. Below, I will consider some guiding principles on South Hall that we followed and shared with our clients. First, however, consider the pain of not connecting in contrast to its benefits.

Here is a courageous response to feeling unheard from the woman we will call Martha. She felt treated at times like an object within a mechanical "protocol" and shared this beautifully, in speech and in writing, in a weekly community meeting. Although the staff did many good things, Martha said that

> those good things are too often overshadowed, squashed, by the intensely earnest and well-meaning focus of so many of the groups and staff on "giving" the patient "tools" to fix her life. This should be only one facet . . . please do not let the work here fall back on nostrums and patent techniques. (personal communication)

It was vital and empowering, that Martha could speak up and be heard. This empowerment was what we hoped for: people risking the truth, saying that which went unspoken, in a setting that openly acknowledged that we all could speak up without dire consequences. Giving feedback was good. In this complex hospital system, we could all stand to learn from each other. We all had much to give as well as to receive. Interactions were not just *one-way*, with faultless treaters supposedly *fixing* the treated. In addition, the staff were quite explicit about saying it is okay to have conflict. All people experience conflict. We all can have anger. The real question lies in what we do about it? Can we learn to have *good conflict*?

FIVE RELATIONAL QUALITIES

On South Hall, we used five relational qualities as guidelines and teaching tools, developed at the Stone Center at Wellesley College (Jordan, 1997; Jordan, Kaplan, et al., 1991). The five relational qualities are: "Engagement," "Authenticity," "Empathy," "Mutuality," and "Empowerment." These categories have since evolved into seven *markers* of a good connection through subdividing mutuality into two different aspects, and adding another marker, "Being Changed by and Appreciating Diversity" (Jordan & Dooley, 2000; see also Jordan, 1997). The original five, however, will suffice for the present discussion. I discuss the five qualities, with particular focus on empathy and mutuality, which are the heart of the later discussion.

Attention to these qualities was not about following a formula – the way Martha feared – but about risking not knowing and really being present. In striving for connection, clinicians were committing to something larger than comfort. Although we were not always great sages, saints, or Buddhist bodhisattvas in our ability to stay present or depth of wisdom, the staff did care and we did try to commit to staying present.

ENGAGEMENT: REALLY BE THERE! This principle is about attending, moving together. It raises the issue of mindfulness of not just one's own body and mind, but also about others and what they are experiencing (Rothberg, 2006; Tart, 1994; Thich Nhat Hanh, 1975). It is about noticing, which goes hand in hand with caring. We cannot be with someone if we are also watching television or reading the paper. The other person may feel alone.

AUTHENTICITY: BE HONEST! This is about moving toward another, sharing the truest sense of oneself and one's inner experience. Here, our mindfulness of self is crucial (see Thich Nhat Hanh, 1975), and it can at times bring up material we do not usually consider or want to know. There is risk in sharing and trusting another. It is interesting that mindful awareness practices can lead to greater mental attunement, which may be central to a more integrated brain and to improved well-being (Siegel, 2006). There is also evidence that emotional disclosure can lead to improved physical as well as psychological health (Pennebaker, 1995). Engagement and authenticity are vital, yet difficult preliminaries, to yet further relational growth.

EMPATHY: TRULY BE WITH THE OTHER. The reader may already know more about this than she or he thinks. Empathy occurs when a coworker helps a colleague through a stressful time, when a mother comforts her infant, when a couple finds out how much they have in common, or when a trusted mentor guides a student. Empathy is the capacity to receive and experience what another is saying, thinking, feeling, that is, to live their story as well as our own. Empathy involves both intellect and feelings. It requires emotional maturity and strength (Jordan, 1991). Being empathetic allows one to feel with the other while also bringing in an outside perspective. Regarding this process, a Zen Master, Thich Minh Duc, said "you listen, open the heart, dissolve boundaries," yet, he added, it is not an indiscriminate merging, but both "in and out" (personal communication, September 30, 2005). Mindful awareness practices are said to increase our human capacity for empathy (Siegel, 2006).

Modern neuroscience is now showing the presence of *mirror neurons.* These neurons "act in similar fashion when an individual performs an action and observes another individual performing it" (Viamontes & Beitman, 2006, p. 229). Thus, humans have a neurological analogue for the bridge between self and other, a model for feeling another's emotions, intent, and motives.

MUTUALITY: AN EMPATHETIC SHARING TOGETHER. Mutuality encompasses respect, mutual responsiveness, willingness to change, and a commitment to the relationship. In short, empathy becomes a reciprical experience. This encounter entails new lessons and some surprises, including surprises about the self. The process enlarges the understanding of each person involved. A mutual encounter is a discipline requiring openness, risk, synergy born of trust and willingness to learn, all of which arises from a shared commitment to a larger good than an individual's agenda, ego issues, or idea of self. The relationship becomes the priority and risks are taken for it. The conversation moves beyond defensive maneuvers or wishes to be seen a certain way.

In a Vietnamese Buddhist account, an ancient ruler asked a Buddhist monk how to rule well. He was told: "If you take the pain of others as your own, you will become a good king; *you don't need to look for the Buddha*" (Thich Minh Duc, personal communication, September 30, 2005).

EMPOWERMENT: ENERGY AND PURPOSE! One outcome of following the above principles is a feeling of new energy and a capacity for action that comes from not going off on one's own or prevailing over others in our competitive society to, instead, connect with others, seeing one's impact on others and committing to care for one another. Janet Surrey (1991) calls the capacity for this ability *response-ability.* One is even more effective and empowered when thus connected. Effects of working together can occur from the personal to the social and even to the global.

An anecdote about the Dalai Lama reveals the energy that can be tied up in feeling separate, alone, and lonely, rather than being directed to relationships. An interviewer, planning to ask the Dalai Lama how he dealt with loneliness, first asked him if he ever got lonely (Dalai Lama & Cutler, 1998). "No," said the Dalai Lama, quite simply. "No?" asked the interviewer, astounded. He just could not believe it. The Dalai Lama explained that he immediately looks at each person from a positive angle and, as such, creates an affinity, a connection, with each person. Thus, fear and apprehension are replaced by openness: The fear that by acting in a certain way we might lose respect or love of a person fades.

When asked by the still amazed interviewer how the average person could do this, the Dalai Lama recommended *compassion*, explaining: "once that thought becomes active, then your attitude towards others changes automatically . . . (it will) reduce fear and allow an openness . . . you can approach a relationship in which you, yourself, initially create the possibility of receiving affection or a positive response" (p. 69). He went on to explain that even if the other is unfriendly, a certain flexibility still exists that can prevent a person from becoming closed off, indifferent, or irritated. He recommended one take the initiative toward a positive response rather than waiting for it.

This story may remind us that we create many barriers, and create them in advance before we even know the other, in part through our own fears and suspicions of our inadequacies. This is suffering that in Buddhism we need not have. When one can see all others as human, as suffering, as doubting, as the same as us, and fundamentally connected – or know this in a profound way, as the Dalai Lama surely does – then one can take a positive step toward letting the barriers fall away. One can be greatly relieved and empowered by being connected instead of isolated, working *with* rather than *against*, committed to something together.

PARALLELS TO EVERYDAY CREATIVITY AND ARTISTIC PROCESS

How does this relational discussion connect with creativity? Think of empathy and mutuality, and of the openness required, the originality of exploration, and the co-evolution of ideas and of lives. Such, openness is central both to Western and Eastern conceptions of creativity, as well as spiritual growth (Richards, 2007b; Sundararajan & Averill, 2007). For example, compare *everyday creative process* – originality of everyday life – during the discovery phase of creativity to mutuality and empathy. Everyday creative work can be defined in terms of two criteria: newness and meaningfulness. (Richards, Kinney, Benet, & Merzel, 1988; Richards, 1998). In an in-depth longitudinal study for her doctoral dissertation, Cynthia Selby (2004) showed that psychotherapeutic work can be creative – both innovative and meaningful – for client and for therapist.

On South Hall, women dared to recapture, represent, and eventually transform an early trauma experience. This process can be creative and brave (May, 1975). The women did some open-ended searching of past history, memories, and fears, followed in the best cases by major insight and reframing. The clinicians helped guide and catalyze the work, making their own creative contribution.

The creative process (versus the creative product) is about the dynamic-doing of our creativity. It is about presence, awareness, mindfulness and openness. Creativity requires moving beyond preconceptions, beyond ego, to whatever the insights lead and, then, seeing new possibilities (Richards, 2007b). At best we live fluidly in the moment, flexibly improvise, and think in new and unusual ways. Remember that everyday creativity is not only about art. If it is done in a fresh and novel manner, everyday creativity can be about *anything*, from office work to counseling, from home repairs to raising kids (Richards, 1998).

This focus on process emphasizes that it's not what you do, it's how you do it. This focus can sometimes take us to the greatest heights. As Zen Master John Daido Loori (2005) says of creating: "The creative process, like a spiritual journey, is intuitive, non-linear, and experiential. It points us toward our essential nature, which is a reflection of the boundless creativity of the universe" (p. 1).

From a more Western context, Maslow (1968, 1971) distinguishes self-actualizing creativity from special talent creativity. Self-actualizing does more for us than give us isolated creative products; it can take us somewhere special. Also, important personal growth can occur along with fuller realization of one's human potentialities.

Self-actualizing creators work in response to *being needs*, not *deficiency needs*; thus, they are not trying to make up for some inner lack but, instead, are pleasant, innovative, spontaneous, present, and even childlike in their enthusiasm. They adhere to *being* values, such as truth or goodness. Their work – be it teaching, art, or scientific discovery – is devoted to some greater purpose beyond one's personal needs. Thankfully, what Rhodes called *deficiency creativity* eventually can transform to *being creativity* (Richards, 1997; Richards 2007b; Zausner, 2006). Our creativity can help us open, heal, and take us higher.

The expressions of Eastern creativity often are not about individualistic uniqueness but, rather, are focused on deeper and authentic expressions of profound truth (Ricard, 2003; Sundararajan & Averill, 2007). Zen arts, such as painting, calligraphy, and gardening (Loori, 2005; Ross, 1960) and Tibetan sacred dance, performed by monks, express spiritual truth. As Ricard (2003) portrays it.

> From a spiritual point of view, true creativity means breaking out of the sheath of egocentricity and becoming a new person, or, more precisely, casting off the veils of ignorance to discover the ultimate nature of mind and phenomena . . . . sacred art is an element of the spiritual path. (p. 32)

Hence, the master dancer or artist manifests traces of a profound transformation, beyond words yet still expressing health writ large (Kaptchuk, 1983). Chopra (1997) says, "Ultimately, the true healing begins when we discover within ourselves that place where we are linked with the larger forces of the universe" (p. 8). I offer that creativity can also come from our deepest and most compassionate work with other people or ourselves.

WHAT IS IT LIKE TO BE CREATIVELY INVOLVED?

Imagine, for example, working on an everyday project, a poster or a display, and becoming totally involved in the effort. Time changes, the world disappears, the difference between you and what you are doing fades. Everything works, and you know you can do it. You are totally present in the moment. You are *absorbed*. Such experience has been compared to an active meditative experience (Franck, 1993) and may involve altered states of consciousness (Richards, 2007b). You, the creator, are on task, working with real inner clarity and purpose. If something is missing, it is probably not what is needed. Worry, outside pressures, inner anxiety fade and take with them the ego, that part of self that grasps at things, pushes them away, or distorts to serve an idea of self (Csikszentmihalyi, 1990, 1996).

Flow is one notion for the absorbed and active phase of this creative process. The reader has perhaps heard the term *flow* (Csikzentmihalyi, 1990) or *optimal experience* as applied to creative activity. Flow shares features with what Zen Master Sekida (1977) called *positive samadhi*, manifesting "a total involvement with some object or activity" (p. 42). Frederick Franck (1993), author of *Zen Seeing, Zen Drawing: Meditation in Action* and other books on art and spirituality, presents creating art as a form of active meditation.

Does empathy, then, bear any similarity to this? Imagine being in deep conversation with a loved one. You are together with her or him, you are present, and focused nowhere else. At best, you hear and sense deeply where your loved one *is* in that moment. It is emotional and also intellectual: It seems all encompassing. It is complex and evolving, a creative personal encounter, that changes, improvises, and responds flexibly in each moment. Empathy is characterized in terms of an attunement and responsiveness to the inner intellectual and emotional experience of another (Jordan, Surrey, & Kaplan, 1991). Yet, a sense of separateness and difference also exists, yielding perspective from without. As noted earlier, these experiences may alternate.

What is the goal? In art the goal is to create, at times, a wondrous experience. In relationships the goal may be making connections – also a wondrous thing – but just whose goal it is, and how it is achieved, may play a crucial part in this enjoyment. Something important occurs when one moves beyond the individual to experience greater concern for the relationship.

One can learn from creativity and the artistic process. In making art, creators may forget themselves, and become one with the portrayed. William Butler Yeats put it beautifully in his poem "Among School Children":

O body swayed to music, O brightening glance

How can we know the dancer from the dance? (p. 233)

I wonder if we have not all at one time or another encountered this merging of subject and object, of seer and seen. If an artist is painting bamboo, the artist *becomes* bamboo. The artist and the audience are right there with each shoot, each twig, each segment – we can see it, smell it, be it. In the catalog notes to an exhibit of a bamboo series by Wu Chen (1350 AD) we read: "This album might be called, 'Twenty portraits of the artist as a bamboo'" (Pope, 1961, p. 152). Or consider the following from a book on Chinese brush painting, telling us how to proceed (Cassettari, 1987):

Paint with love and kindness for the materials and the subject portrayed, becoming one with both. (p. 7)

If the distinction between artist and subject disappears and the rendering reflects a deeper knowing, what is captured? A trace? A moment? A wisp of life? A deeper authentic truth? (Richards, 2001; Sundararajan & Averill, 2007). In one story, a wandering novice asked Master Ching Hao about portraying beauty. He said, "The important point is to obtain their true likeness, is it not?" Ching Hao answered,

> *It is not*. Painting is to paint . . . . Likeness can be obtained by shapes without spirit; but when truth is reached spirit and substance are both fully expressed. (as cited in Ross, 1960, p. 91)

He further cautioned that the artist who tries to express spirit through ornamental beauty will make dead things. The bamboo artist is not naming, categorizing, or drawing botanical concepts removed from the actual bamboo. It is much more intimate and real. Turning to relationships, we can ask how fully are we are present with the living and breathing person before us.

EMPATHY AND MUTUALLY VIEWED AS CREATIVE PROCESS

EMPATHY AS CREATIVE PROCESS

If we really attend and experience a person and their life directly, we tune in deeply. Temporary relaxation of our sense of separateness, of our ego boundaries, leads us to be truly there with the client. Yet, at other times, in empathy and in clinical work in general, we maintain our boundaries and focus on our own perspective and expertise (Jordan, Surrey, & Kaplan, 1991). We can bring our own perspective and also dare to actually feel the other's pain. When identification is too limited, we may have only a kind of distanced, intellectualized understanding. If our own perspective is weak, we may overly merge with their pain, become swept away and unable to manage. Nevertheless, if we keep balance, we can know the other, maintain perspective, and give a creative gift. Such an experience is very much like the creative process, what Kris (1952) called regression in the service of the ego.

When empathizing clinically, there is the additional question: What is our commitment? Our goal? A working or helping relationship is not always as pleasurable as painting bamboo. Are we willing to empathize, even if the pain is overwhelming or when people are very different from us? Some severely ill people on South Hall especially wanted to know: Can you clinicians take it? Will you stay with me? And am I really okay, or am I unacceptable, terrible, even intolerable?

VIGNETTE. Consider one survivor of Hurricane Katrina. After being in housing that collapsed, this woman and others ended up bussed to the New Orleans Convention Center. At first, they had hope. But day after day the trucks passed by without bringing any food or water. Nothing at all. This was not the fault of the Convention Center, which had opened its doors to be of service. It was a problem of multiple systems failure, in city services, and in governmental agencies that should have helped more and sooner.

This woman saw more and more people brought to the Convention Center, but still no aid arrived. Frighteningly, some young men with guns showed up. Fortunately they used the guns to keep rather than destroy order: Ironically, these scary men were the only ones helping. Several people died right next to the woman from medical causes, exposure, and lack of provisions. Over several days the number of dead only grew. Some people tried to *escape*, but an exit from town across a nearby bridge was blocked. This woman and others with her were terrified that they had been "sent there to die."

I told this very story at a talk on empathy in New Orleans almost a year after Katrina in a lecture hall at this same convention center where so many had suffered and feared they would die. The city was still devastated; huge areas of the Lower Ninth Ward and elsewhere remained in ruins, abandoned without power. According to one study of fourth-graders, almost half of the children met the threshold for psychiatric referral for problems including depression, aggression, and frightening memories (DeParle, 2006).

In the Convention Center where I delivered this talk, I read in even greater detail from the story of the woman who felt trapped and abandoned. There were people present in the audience who had worked in the Katrina relief effort. Other conference attendees were just there for the talk, but were struck by the suffering and desperation that had occurred where they now sat in safety and comfort a year later. At least one attendee was openly weeping. I just wish the woman in the story could have seen this and known how many people were with her now, hearing her story, at that moment. It can mean everything when we can be with people at the worst of times. Some of our Saybrook students found this as well: Our graduate students went to work in Katrina relief right after the hurricane.

Empathy is not easy. Clinicians at South Hall also heard and did not turn away from the heartbreaking stories of the women before any other help was given; the relief to the client can be tremendous. Being with them as another human being, we shared their human pain. We entered their world and held their hand at the hardest of times. Perhaps they also entered our world and held ours.

Will we not burn out? How do we continue? How long can we keep it up? And what about the instances when the other may be angry and resentful, instead of welcoming and grateful? Such resentment occurred on South Hall with certain women. Just by our role identification as clinicians and staff, we were automatically seen by certain women who had just arrived as jailers and bossy officials without heart, telling people what to do. How then does one hang in there?

Rothberg (2006) writes about how Joanna Macy, who leads workshops about Buddhist thought, responded to the strength it takes to face the pain of the world: how hard it is, and how to transform this hardship, and nourish ourselves to continue. First, there is opening up consciously in groups to the pain and difficulty of the challenge: facing war, poverty, oppression, environmental degradation, or other overwhelming problems. The pain is then faced by *turning* to a broader and deeper sense of interdependence and awareness, followed by "the practical 'going forth' into the world and one's life, informed by wisdom and compassion" (p. 87).

The Buddhist bodhisattva, the Christian saint, other sages, and beneficiaries across traditions may offer an open hand and endless compassion but can we ourselves do this? Perhaps we will do better if we deeply appreciate that we are part of the whole, such that our help may come more naturally, and our connection and sustenance from those who walk with us be more automatic.

MUTUALITY AND CREATIVE PROCESS

Mutuality and creatively is a *dual commitment*. How great is one's commitment to creativity in relationship, whatever may happen as one changes with another? This commitment was certainly tested in the Katrina example I mentioned. Those who went to aid the relief effort were fundamentally changed by those they helped.

Many people search for mutuality in their intimate relationships, with husband, lover, or children. They want to share deeply, be close, and grow together. How often, though, is this wish only one-sided or perhaps largely misplaced? We may be willing to learn, to grow, to help, to change as needed; we may realize this is about us together, the system we represent, something greater that we co-create together; we may see how important it is, but it can be scary.

Now consider mutuality as a creative art form – a give and take – this time a mutual painting on a joint canvas. There is flexible co-creation, new sharing and understanding. One is both *receptive* to the other and *active* in turn. There is openness, a willingness to hear and an almost magical joint painting of a new context that includes the truth of both parties. It may also include things we do not necessarily want to see or know. Yet, to honor the relationship, we ourselves may need change.

VIGNETTE. "I'm so sorry," the parents say to the rebellious teenager, "we were wrong about that. We will think more about it next time, from your point of view." Well, the abashed parents (and I include myself here, among the many other parents who have done this) sometimes wish they had said this, but did not always do it. They did not maintain the common good above all. They did not do creative and responsive listening or interact with an open mind (Pritzker, 2007). Where was the commitment? Perhaps, we were too committed to *being right*.

Comparing this to our creative painting of bamboo, this time the bamboo not only asks us to draw it differently, but to draw *ourselves* differently as well! We are, after all, changed by what we do. It is all part of the same picture, and we are drawing together in the same evolving context. We change, we learn, we do it differently. It is more of a dance, a sculpture in motion, a composition including all of the painter, the subject and the painting. All as one. The result may be harmony and beauty.

Can we handle this in relationships? Can we put our interactive process above some fixed and individualized goal? There are rich rewards when we can: growth, peace, love, and healing. Jordan (1991) says the following of mutuality. We may not always achieve what she describes, but can at least keep it as an ideal:

> When empathy and concern flow both ways, there is an intense affirmation of the self and, paradoxically, a transcendence of the self, a sense of the self as part of a larger relational unit. The interaction allows for a relaxation of the sense of separateness; the other's well-being becomes as important as one's own. (p. 82)

How often do we have allegiance to something greater than our own self-interest? Can our concern become larger? Can our capacity grow for compassion and wisdom (Tarthang Tulku, 1984; Thich Nhat Hanh, 1988 , 1997)? How far might this go? Our lover, our family, our friends, a greater good for all? Could this even extend to all beings?

FOUR IMMEASURABLE MINDS

We can draw from the Buddhist tradition, while noting there are many other resonant wisdom traditions. When we understand another person, then we truly can begin to care and to love. When we love, feeling heartfelt compassion when another suffers and experiencing joy when they benefit becomes natural. As our capacity for empathy and compassionate action grows, we move toward equanimity, wishing benefit and happiness for all beings.

The four divine abodes, or four immeasurable minds are: lovingkindess, compassion, sympathetic joy, and equanimity (Thich Nhat Hanh, 1997). According to Thich Nhat Hanh (1997), they are named abodes because, "if you practice them, they will grow in you every day until they embrace the whole world. You will become happier, and everyone around you will become happier too" (p. 1). These abodes resonate with wisdom from many traditions, such the Christian maxim, "Do unto others as you would have others do unto you."

Recall what the monk said to the ancient king, especially the second part of this: "If you take the pain of others as your own, you will become a good king; *you don't need to look for the Buddha*" (Thich Minh Duc, personal communication, September 30, 2005).

LEARNING WE ARE MORE CONNECTED THAN WE IMAGINED

In a society valuing independence, relational qualities may be devalued. This presents particular problems for women and others who value a more connected orientation. The strong independent qualities tend to be linked with men, and the more relational, cooperative, sensitive, and intuitive qualities with women. Language may be used to frame this as a devaluation (Stiver, 1991). Consider someone who is called dependent, emotional, and *wishy-washy*. This description sounds very negative, but might not these attributes be reframed as collaborative, sensitive to feelings, and able to deal with complex positions?

Different cultures have different values. For instance, in China, sensitivity to the most subtle emotional nuance can be a sign of great personal and cultural refinement (Sundararajan & Averill, 2007). Highly creative people tend to combine both masculine and feminine characteristics, resisting being boxed in by such stereotypes. They can be both assertive and sensitive, logical and intuitive. This balance has been called *androgyny* (Montuori, Combs, & Richards, 2004). The valuing of both qualities is necessary and holds great advantage.

Nonetheless, the mainstream view is dominant. After I spoke on relational healing at the Ahimsa Annual Conference in Berkeley, a gentleman came up and shared something he had written informally and brought to the meeting (Gladstone, personal communication, October 8, 2005). He wrote:

Our present way of life encourages us to be self-centered and self-protective. As children in school and as adults at work, we are urged to look out for ourselves, to compete rather than cooperate. "Success" means getting ahead of others and leaving them behind . . . . In order to go beyond superficial reform efforts we need to understand deeply our interdependence with others and with all of life . . . . Every religion recognizes interdependence in some way, often expressed in terms of love – "God is love," "love one another," "love your enemies," etc. This loving attitude is a necessary partner to understanding interdependence. Let us open our hearts and minds to this.

Resonances between Buddhist interdependence and the new sciences are becoming more obvious (Bohm, 1980; Ricard & Thuan, 2001). A diverse body of evidence reveals the interdependence of all things, from atoms to galaxies. At the quantum level, physicist David Bohm (1980) says that two events cannot be thought about, one separate from the other. Even a pair of electrons that are many light years apart can affect each other mutually and instantaneously. Here is how Einstein saw our interconnection:

A human being is part of the whole . . . a part limited in time and space. He experiences his thoughts and feelings as something separate from the rest – a kind of optical delusion of his consciousness. This delusion is a kind of prison for us. (as cited in Dossey, 2002, p. 15)

Psychologically, development of mind and brain depend on others, our surroundings, and our world. For example, which parts of our brain develop and the expression of certain genes, depends upon early experience, the world around us, and life experience (Siegel, 1999, 2006). Empathy, from the earliest moments, helps us connect us with each other. We need to be able to *read* each other. To illustrate, Goleman (1995) points out, that people with the highest IQs are not necessarily the most happy or successful. The importance of what he calls *emotional intelligence* to our lives is more and more being recognized.

For an empathetic person *inside* and *outside* may mix, an understanding more consistent with Eastern views. What you or I *see* isn't out *there*. It is a complex construction. My mind-brain, including the perceptual apparatus, and my entire history of personal and cultural education and expectations interacts with, encodes, selects, chooses, frames, and presents what I think is the external world and me. Thus, distinctions of inside and outside fade away in a worldview based on interdependence; It is all of a part of the whole (Siegel, 1999).

In a different look at our interdependence, Thich Nhat Hanh (1988) writes, in the beautiful book *The Sun My Heart*:

There are other things, outside of our bodies, that are also essential for our survival. Look at the immense light we call the sun. If it stops shining, the flow of our life will also stop, and so the sun is our second heart, the heart outside our body . . . . Plants live thanks to the sun . . . . . And thanks to plants, we and other animals can live . . . . If the layer of air around our earth disappears even for an instant, "our" life will end . . . . There is no phenomenon in the universe that does not intimately concern us, from a pebble resting at the bottom of the ocean, to the movement of a galaxy millions of light years away. The poet Walt Whitman said, "I believe a leaf of grass is not less than the journey-work of the stars." (p. 67)

How deeply can we actually experience our interdependence? If we understand our interconnection deeply and intuitively rather than intellectually, could our concern for ourselves come to automatically include concern for each other? Might a blow to you be a blow to me? If so, would I ever attack you? After all, if my foot hurts, would I not bandage it, rather than cut if off? Might our empathy, at best, even herald a reawakening of some understanding buried deep within us?

VALUING AND BUILDING RELATIONAL CAPACITY

If we do not always have empathetic understanding, we may still know when it is absent. Martha, the young woman who spoke out at a community meeting South Hall, addressed the five qualities of relational process. At the time, we called this approach *self-in-relation* (Jordan et all, 1991). Martha said,

> Self in relation is not something you do. It's something you are. You can't come in to work and "do" self-in-relation with your patients . . . . Engagement, empathy, and authenticity aren't qualities you "practice" in certain groups but not in others. They aren't elements you "give" someone by saying "the right thing." . . . They are qualities of *being.*
>
> There are no five "things" to do or say . . . that will give meaning to my life. No "affirmations" or "steps" to be followed. . . . What can make a difference is not something I need to "learn;" it is something I need to *encounter*: Authenticity. Empathy. Engagement. Mutuality. It is something I need to be met with. It is something that needs to be welcomed in me by others. And I do find these things here, some . . . I resist the effort to be a predictable outcome – it diminishes me, and those who work with me. You cannot work with me by following a set of directions, a branching tree model, or flow chart. . . . *BE* with me, and create space for me to *BE* with you.

INCREASING OUR CAPACITY FOR EMPATHY

If engagement, authenticity, empathy, mutuality, and empowerment are so important, how does one make them a more intrinsic part of how one lives, and who one is? Certainly there are resources, including many theoretical and practical ones from places such as the Stone Center at Wellesley College (Jordan, 1997; Jordan & Dooley, 2000; Jordan et al., 1991). Beyond that, a number of research studies indicate that awareness and mindfulness training can help one develop empathy.[1] Empathy can be increased either through programs for meditation or contemplation.

There are other and more active ways to enhance mindful awareness, mutual empathy, and presence in the moment: for instance, through the arts, relationships, work, enjoying a sunny day, or performing sacred dance. Again, it's not so much what we do, it's how we do it (Loori, 2005; Ricard, 2003; Richards, 2001, 2007a; Ross, 1960; Rothberg, 2006).

CONCLUSION

The five relational qualities, specifically empathy and mutuality, supported by openness, presence, and the immediacy of living in the present moment, helped by commitment to larger goals beyond our personal agendas, can help bring about healing, comfort, and peace. They can also lead to greater flexibility and mutual understanding and can be viewed as a form of creativity. In a relational context, these qualities can also enhance caring and appreciation of our deeper interconnection. This can be invaluable in clinical environments and throughout daily life. Aspects of Eastern wisdom resonate with these relational qualities and are helping many make a shift toward a worldview based on stronger relationships and mutual concern.

Happily, we can cultivate and facilitate relational qualities and sensitivities, even though this cultivation is not always easy in a culture of individuality. This work requires practice and discipline, but we can develop these as we live our lives, interact at work, at play, and through meditative disciplines.

What adds to our life satisfaction is an active creative engagement with life and with other people, as well as being part of something greater. It even leads to healthy aging and, perhaps, longevity (Adams-Price, 1998; Adler, 1995; Csikszentmihalyi, 1996; Seifert, 2007). This is health: staying vividly alive, taking risks, challenging ourselves, enjoying the moment, engaging meaningfully with people, and living beyond ego by committing to others and to the best of ourselves.

NOTES

[1] See Murphy and Donovan (1999) for a comprehensive bibliography on meditation.

References

Adams-Price, C. E. (Ed.). (1998). *Creativity and successful aging: Theoretical and empirical approaches.* New York: Springer.

Adler, L. P. (1995). *Centenarians: The bonus years.* Santa Fe, NM: Health Press.

Ajaya, Swami. (1983). *Psychotherapy East and West: A unifying paradigm.* Honesdale, PA: Himalayan Institute.

Baker, I. (1997). *The Tibetan art of healing.* San Francisco, CA: Chronicle Books.

Bohm, D. (1980). *Wholeness and the implicate order.* New York: Routledge.

Cassettari, S. (1987). *Chinese brush painting techniques.* London: Angus & Robertson.

Chopra, D. (1997). The art of healing (Preface). In I. Baker, T*he Tibetan art of healing.* San Francisco, CA: Chronicle Books.

Combs, A., & Krippner, S. (2007). Consciousness and creativity: Opening the doors of perception. In R. Richards (Ed.). *Everyday creativity and new views of human nature: Psychological, social, and spiritual perspectives.* Washington, D.C.: American Psychological Association.

Csikszentmihalyi, M. (1990). *Flow: The psychology of optimal experience.* New York: Harper-Perennial.

Csikszentmihalyi, M. (1996). *Creativity: Flow and the psychology of discovery and invention.* New York: Harper Collins.

Dalai Lama, & Cutler, H.C. (1998). *The art of happiness: A handbook for living.* New York: Riverhead Books.

DeParle, J. (August, 27, 2006). Orphaned. New York Times Magazine, 48, pp. 26-27,

Dossey, L. (2002). How healing happens: Exploring the nonlocal gap. *Alternative Therapies, 8,* 12-15 and 103-110.

Eisler, R. (2007). Our great creative challenge: Rethinking human nature-and recreating society. In R. Richards (Ed.). *Everyday creativity and new views of human nature: Psychological, social, and spiritual perspectives.* Washington, D.C.: American Psychological Association.

Erikson, E. (1950). *Childhood and society.* New York: W.W. Norton.

Franck, F. (1993). *Zen seeing, Zen drawing: meditation in action.* New York: Bantam.

Freeman, L. & Lawlis, F. (Eds.). (2001). *Mosby's guide to complementary and alternative medicine: A research-based approach.* St. Louis, MO: Mosby.

Gilligan, C. (1982). *In a different voice: Psychological theory and women's development.* Cambridge, MA: Harvard University Press.

Goleman, D. (1995). *Emotional intelligence.* New York: Bantam.

Herrigel, E. (1953). *Zen and the art of archery.* New York: Vintage.

Jordan, J.V. (1991). The meaning of mutuality. In Jordan, J.V., Kaplan, A.G., Miller, J.B., Stiver, I.P., & Surrey, J.L., *Women's growth in connection: Writings from the Stone Center* (pp. 81-96). New York: Guilford.

Jordan, J. V. (Ed.). (1997). *Women's growth in diversity: More writings from the Stone Center*. New York: Guilford.

Jordan, J. V., & Dooley, C. (2000). *Relational practice in action: A group manual*. Wellesley, MA: The Stone Center.

Jordan, J. V., Kaplan, A. G., Miller, J. B., Stiver, I. P., & Surrey, J. L. (1991). *Women's growth in connection: Writings from the Stone Center*. New York: Guilford.

Jordan, J., Surrey, J. L., & Kaplan, A. (1991). Women and empathy: implications for psychological development and psychotherapy. In Jordan, J.V., Kaplan, A.G., Miller, J. B., Stiver, I. P., & Surrey, J. L., *Women's growth in connection: Writings from the Stone Center* (pp. 27-50). New York: Guilford.

Kaptchuk, T. J. (1983). *The web that has no weaver: Understanding Chinese medicine*. Chicago: Congden and Weed.

Kris, E. (1952). *Psychoanalytic explorations in art*. New York: Columbia University Press.

Loori, J. D. (2005). *The Zen of creativity: Cultivating your artistic life*. New York: Ballantine.

Loye, D. (2007). Telling the new story: Darwin, evolution, and creativity versus conformity in science. In R. Richards (Ed.), *Everyday creativity and new views of human nature: Psychological, social, and spiritual perspectives*. Washington, D.C.: American Psychological Association.

Macy, J. (1991). *Mutual causality in Buddhism and general systems theory: The dharma of natural systems*. Buffalo, NY: State University of New York Press.

Maslow, A. (1968). *Toward a psychology of being*. New York: Van Nostrand Reinhold.

Maslow, A. (1971). *The farther reaches of human nature*. New York: Penguin.

May, R. (1975). *The courage to create*. New York: Bantam.

Montuori, A., Combs, A., & Richards, R. (2004). Creativity, consciousness, and the direction for human development. In D. Loye (Ed.), *The great adventure: Toward a fully human theory of evolution* (197-236). Albany, NY: State University of New York Press.

Murphy, M., & Donovan, S. (1999). *The physical and psychological effects of meditation: A review of contemporary research with a comprehensive bibliography, 1931-1996* (2nd ed.). Sausalito, CA: Institute of Noetic Sciences.

Pennebaker, J. W. (Ed.). (1995). *Emotion, disclosure, and health*. Washington, D.C.: American Psychological Association Books.

Peterson, C. (2006). *A primer in positive psychology*. New York: Oxford University Press.

Pilisuk, M., & Parks, S. H. (1986). *The healing web: Social networks and human survival*. Hanover, NH: University Press of New England.

Pope, J. (1961). *Chinese art treasures: Catalog for selected groups of objects exhibited in the U.S. by the Government of the Republic of China*. Lausanne, Switzerland: Skira.

Pritzker, S. R. (2007). Audience flow: Creativity in TV watching with applications to teletherapy. In R. Richards (Ed.), *Everyday creativity and new views of human nature*. Washington, D.C.: American Psychological Association.

Ricard, M. (2003). *Monk dancers of Tibet*. Boston: Shambhala.

Ricard, M., & Thuan, T.X. (2001). *The quantum and the lotus: A journey to the frontiers where science and Buddhism meet*. New York: Crown.

Richards, R. (1997). When illness yields creativity. In M. Runco & R. Richards, R. (Eds.), *Eminent creativity, everyday creativity, and health* (pp. 485-540). Stamford, CT: Ablex.

Richards, R. (1998). Everyday creativity. In H. S. Friedman (Ed.), *The Encyclopedia of Mental Health, Vol. 1* (pp. 619-633). San Diego, CA: Academic Press.

Richards, R. (2001). A new aesthetic for environmental awareness: Chaos theory, the natural world, and our broader humanistic identity. *Journal of Humanistic Psychology, 41*, 59-95.

Richards, R. (Ed.). (2007a). *Everyday creativity and new views of human nature: Psychological, social, and spiritual perspectives*. Washington, D.C.: American Psychological Association

Richards, R. (2007b). Twelve potential benefits of living more creatively. In R. Richards (Ed.). *Everyday creativity and new views of human nature*. Washington, D.C.: American Psychological Association.

Richards, R., Kinney, D., Benet, M., & Merzel, A (1988). Assessing everyday creativity: Characteristics of The Lifetime Creativity Scales and validation with three large samples. *Journal of Personality and Social Psychology, 54*, 476-485.

Ross, N.W. (Ed.). (1960). *The world of Zen*. New York: Vintage.

Rothberg, D. (2006). *The engaged spiritual life: A Buddhist approach to transforming ourselves and the world*. Boston: Beacon Press.

Schlitz, M., Amorok, T., & Micozzi, M. (2005). *Consciousness and healing: Integral approaches to mind-body medicine*. New York: Elsevier.

Schneider, K., Bugental, J. F. T., & Pierson, J. P. (Eds.), (2001). *Handbook of Humanistic Psychology* (pp. 21-27). Thousand Oaks, CA: Sage.

Seifert, L. S. (2007). *Chasing dragonflies: Life and care in aging*. Cuyahoga Falls, OH: Clove Press, Ltd.

Sekida, K. (Ed. and Trans.) (1977). *Two zen classics: Mumonkan and Hekiganroku*. New York: Weatherhill.

Selby, C.E. (2004). *Psychotherapy as creative process: A grounded theory exploration.* (Doctoral Dissertation, Saybrook Graduate School.)

Siegel, D. J. (1999). *The developing mind: How relationships and the brain interact to shape who we are*. New York: Guilford.

Siegel, D. J. (2006). An interpersonal neurobiology approach to psychotherapy. *Psychiatric Annals, 36*, 248-256.

Solomon, M. F., & Siegel, D. J. (Eds.). (2003). *Healing trauma: Attachment, mind, body, and brain*. New York: W.W. Norton.

Stiver, I. (1991). The meanings of "dependency" in female-male relationships. In Jordan, J. V., Kaplan, A. G., Miller, J. B., Stiver, I. P., & Surrey, J. L. (Eds.), *Women's growth in connection: Writings from the Stone Center* (pp. 143-161). New York: Guilford.

Sundararajan, L., & Averill, J. (2007). Creativity in the everyday: Culture, self, and emotions. In R. Richards (Ed.), *Everyday creativity and new views of human nature*. Washington, D.C.: American Psychological Association.

Surrey, J. (1991). Relationship and empowerment. In Jordan, J. V., Kaplan, A., Miller, J. B., Stiver, I. P., & Surrey, J. L. *Women's growth in connection:Writings from the Stone Center* (pp.162-180). New York: Guilford.

Tart, C. T. (1994). *Living the mindful life: A handbook for living in the present moment*. Boston: Shambhala.

Tarthang Tulku (1984). *Knowledge of freedom: Time to change*. Berkeley, CA; Dharma.

Tarthang Tulku (1994). *Mastering successful work*. Berkeley, CA: Dharma.

Taylor, E., & Martin, F. (2001) Humanistic Psychology at the crossroads. In K. Schneider, J. F. T. Bugental, & J. F. Pierson (Eds.), *Handbook of Humanistic Psychology* (pp. 21-27). Thousand Oaks, CA: Sage.

Thich Nhat Hanh (1974). *Zen keys*. New York: Doubleday.

Thich Nhat Hanh (1975). *The miracle of mindfulness: A manual on meditation*. Boston: Beacon.

Thich Nhat Hanh (1988). *The sun my heart*. Berkeley, CA: Parallax Press.

Thich Nhat Hanh (1997). *Teachings on love*. Berkeley, CA: Parallax Press.

Varela, F. J., Thompson, E., & Rosch, E. (1992). *The embodied mind: Cognitive science and human experience*. Boston: MIT Press.

Viamontes, G.I., & Beitman, B.D. (2006). Neural substrates of psychotherapeutic change. Part I. The default brain. *Psychiatric Annals, 36*(4), 225-236.

Yeats, W.B. *Collected poems, 1889-1939*. Retrieved March 23 from 2007Worldbooklibrary.com/eBooks. .

Zausner, T. (2006). *When walls become doorways: Creativity and the transforming illness*. New York: Harmony.

CHAPTER FIFTEEN

HEALING FROM ADDICTION WITH
YOGA THERAPY AND ALCOHOLICS ANONYMOUS

Angelina Baydala
&
Amanda L. Gorchynski

A diversity of theories exist that explain compulsive substance use. Volkan (1994) provides a survey of the range of psychoanalytic ideas on addiction. Early psychoanalytic literature suggests that compulsive drug use begins with self-medication to dissolve inhibitions and rigid defenses (Fenichel, 1945). Ego psychologists argue that compulsive drug users are unable to tolerate frustration or strong emotions and using substances may enable a sense of emotional control by calming strong feelings such as rage, hostility, shame, guilt, anxiety, and loneliness (Federn, 1952). Interpersonal formulations focus on the unique difficulties that persons with addictions may have with relationships. Users may experience relations with a drug in such a way that the separate loving and hating characteristics of formative relationships are reproduced (Kernberg, 1980). Moreover, drug use also may be a way of attempting to control the changeable nature of relationships (Winnicott, 1989). Overall, from a psychoanalytic perspective, it seems that compulsive drug use is an attempt to compensate for and manage difficult experiences with self and others. By extension, Alcoholics Anonymous (AA) and yoga therapy view addiction as a condition of interpersonal disconnection and, also, a psychospiritual problem where healing requires turning over one's personal need for control to a non-personal intelligence with enormously greater organizing power.

In the last thirty years, a significant increase in research has occurred identifying strategies for preventing and treating alcohol-related problems (Heather & Stockwell, 2003). In this chapter, we relate insights into the nature of addiction recovery by describing the dynamics involved in treating alcohol use disorders through a combination of the traditional Twelve-Step program of AA and classical Indian practices of yoga. Members of the Kripa Foundation and Father Joseph Pereira, founder of Kripa, offer addiction treatment services throughout India combining the principles of AA and yoga. Not only does yoga add a systematic physical discipline to the process of recovery, but the contrast and counterpoint provided by using two different traditions may also allow for more flexible interpretation of the principles involved in each system.

We begin the chapter by outlining the belief systems of classical yoga and AA. Selections from a qualitative analysis of an interview with Father Joe are included in the description of these belief systems. This interview was analyzed and coded using traditional grounded theory analytic approaches (Denzin & Lincoln, 2000). After describing principles of yoga and AA, we present the results of the grounded theory analysis. One overarching model emerged from the analysis – *The Caring Model* – with four distinct themes: "Complementary Medicines," "Existentialism," "The Clinics," and "Returning." The model and themes are presented in narrative form, depicting the story of Father Joe and the Kripa Foundation. This structure also serves as a template for reviewing research literature pertaining to the components of the Kripa Foundation and its treatment methods. We end the chapter by considering how each belief system – AA and yoga – offers a dimension of healing that makes their pairing seem particularly well suited to addressing issues of addiction.

CLASSICAL YOGA OF PATANJALI

The word *yoga* has its roots in the Sanskrit word *yuj*, which can be translated as to yoke but also means to unite, to team, to sum, and conjunction (Feuerstein, 1997). In its spiritual sense, *yoga* means to control the mind and the senses. This usage dates to the second-millennium BCE but an account of classical yoga was written down in concise aphorisms early in the Common Era, likely around the second-century CE, by Patanjali in the *Yoga-Sutras*. In the second line of the Yoga-Sutras Patanjali writes: "Yoga is to still the patterning of consciousness" (Hartranft, 2003, p. 2).

In the classical system of Patanjali's yoga, practice brings consciousness to a place of stillness wherein it can reflect *purusa*. *Purusa* translates from the Sanskrit as pure awareness, transcendental consciousness, or soul (Iyengar, 2005). *Purusa* is the witness of all experiences and is sometimes also known as "the seer" (Feuerstein, 1997, p. 236). Hartranft (2003) explains,

> Pure awareness . . . is not stuff of any sort and is therefore free of cause and effect. It was never created and never ends, existing beyond time. Even to use the word it or assert that "it exists" lends pure awareness a seeming substantiality it does not possess. Because it is immaterial, it has no location, movement, or other natural properties; nor does it have anything in common with consciousness or thought, other than the role of observing them. It is literally intangible, impersonal, and inconceivable. (pp. xxi-xxii)

Through the practice of yoga, the tendency of mind to focus on objects of awareness and to identify or relate to these objects is replaced with the silence of awareness itself. Amidst the turbulence and fluctuations of nature, or *prakriti*, at the core of being, there is an awareness not limited by space or affected by time. Iyengar (2005) states that "spiritual realization is the aim that exists in each one of us to seek our divine core. That core, though never absent from anyone, remains latent within us" (p. 3). Yoga is a discipline that allows pure awareness at the core of nature to reveal itself.

In gaining a sense of pure awareness, one is able to recognize the root of unease. Without yogic practice our "ordinary physical and mental life conceals the fact that our thoughts and actions are almost always tinged with wanting, aversion, egoism, or fear of extinction" (Hartranft, 2003, p. xv). Therefore, with yogic practice, one is able to cease identification with the fluctuations of consciousness and recognize the attachments that are inherent to the process of identifying with things, places and people, or other object relations. When one is able to recognize pure awareness as a significant force within oneself, then one need not invest in attachments to gain a meaningful and secure connection with oneself. Releasing the ego and desires to be subsumed into pure awareness brings about peace and contentment.

The eight limbs of *ashtanga* yoga represented in *The Yoga-Sutras of Patanjali* compose the system of beliefs and practices that lead to this awareness. Here, we will only be able to briefly outline this system; however, classical yoga is subject to extensive interpretation and provides rich material for lifelong study (see, for example, Feuerstein, 1989; Hartranft, 2003; Iyengar, 2002). Like petals of a flower, the limbs develop simultaneously and not consecutively. The maturity of each limb contributes to conditions for *purusa* to permeate all aspects of life. The eight limbs in Sanskrit are termed: *yamas, niyamas, asana, pranayama, pratyahara, dharana, dhyana*, and *samadhi* (see Figure 1).

THE EIGHT LIMBS OF PATANJALI YOGA

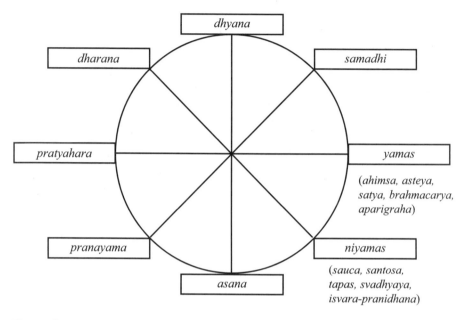

FIGURE 1

Overall, the *yamas* are restraints that regulate a person's relationship to others and to one's attitude to the world; whereas, the *niyamas* are internal observances that cultivate one's relationship with oneself. The *yamas* and *niyamas* develop moral attitudes such as friendliness, compassion, delight, equanimity, and non-attachment. *Asana* is the development of bodily alignment and steadiness, pranayama involves extending the breath and the remaining four limbs – *pratyahara, dharana, dhyana,* and *samadhi* – work with levels of meditation.

There are five yamas: *ahimsa, satya, asteya, brahmacarya,* and *aparigraha. Ahimsa* means non-harming, cultivating thoughtfulness, consideration, friendliness and kindness, in short, welcoming everyone and every situation. *Satya* can be translated as truthfulness; however, there are conditions of truthfulness that must be observed so as not to violate the first principle of non-harming. While the practitioner strives to honor and speak the truth, this practice must be done in a considerate manner. *Asteya* is the discipline of non-stealing, not taking things which do not belong to one and may include more abstract things such as not stealing time, not breaking promises, or transgressing boundaries. The fourth *yama, brahmacarya,* is the discipline of having impeccable behavior, especially sexual behavior. It means containing and directing libido to cultivate sexual relations that bring about non-attachment and a connection with *purusha*. The fifth and final *yama* is *aparigraha*, which translates as an absence of acquisitiveness or grasping. Restraining from being opportunistic and not taking advantage of situations or people is important for this discipline, that is, taking only what is necessary.

Conversely, the *niyamas* are observances that guide how one relates to oneself on the path toward realizing pure awareness. The five *niyamas* are: *sauca, santosa, tapas, svadhyaya,* and *isvara-pranidhana*. The first *niyama, sauca,* represents purification and cleanliness of the inner and outer parts of oneself. The body and mind are kept fit, clean and freely functioning through *asana* and *pranayama*. *Santosa* is about contentment, which is a consequence of modesty and being happy with what is and with what one has. Although it is necessary to do our best, *santosa* is the discipline of having and releasing desires. Instead of clinging to a particular outcome, the practitioner strives to accept any and all possible outcomes. This growth process requires reflection and learning. *Tapas* refers to the intensity of disciplined practice – the heat and energy that can be contained and then directed within oneself. The discipline of *tapas* includes, for example, consciously eating wholesome food, attending to posture and practicing breathing to keep wastes circulating out of body and mind. The *niyama* of *svadhyaya* involves self-study. This is the practice of getting to know oneself through reflection and, consequently, better understanding the yogic disciplines. Visualization and awareness are used in *svadhyaya* resulting in the capacity for neutral, detached observation. The final *niyama, isvara-pranidhana,* is dedication to the ideal of pure awareness, offering the fruits of one's actions to the universe and to life.

Although the *yamas* and *niyamas* are moral disciplines, they are not observed out of a fear of God or a sense of sin. They form a path for realizing *purusha* and the delightful connectedness of being. The *yamas* and *niyamas* address lifestyle and social attitude, the ways we relate to ourselves and to others and how we deal with problems (Desikachar, 1999). However, it is very difficult to practice a change of attitude directly and the remaining limbs of yoga – *asana, pranayama, pratyahara, dharana, dhyana,* and *samadhi* – facilitate this transformation. *Asanas* are the bodily postures that result in "profound physical steadiness and effortlessness in meditation" (Hartranft, 2003, p. 124). Eliade (1958) emphasizes that it is most important for *asana* practice to become effortless and perfectly still, overcoming the natural striving of the ego and the body. Eventually, a space emerges between the body and awareness, such that consciousness is not drawn into being troubled by the body. This is the first stage of distinguishing awareness as separate and yet linked to the conscious body. These practices bring about a state of mindfulness making one aware, as Desikachar (1999) says: "of where we are, where we stand, and how we look at things" (p. 97). The sometimes painful consequence of this awareness is recognition of mistakes, after which it becomes possible to consider actions in light of the *yamas* and *niyamas*, redressing the situation if possible and resolving to follow alternative courses of action in the future.

Pranayama, the fourth limb, is the regulation of breath. Through the practice of *pranayama*, refined respiration and tranquility are brought about. A powerful connection exists between breath and mental states. Thus, *pranayama* slows, extends, and regulates the breath of the body to affect the mental state. When one settles the breath, then one is also able to settle the mind, linking steady awareness with fluctuating states of consciousness. Regulating the breath refines and slows respiration, focuses attention, and deepens relaxation.

The remaining four limbs involve states of attention and mediation. *Pratyahara*, the fifth limb, is the withdrawal of the senses. This focusing of attention inward occurs naturally during *asana* and *pranayama* practice. While the mind remains able to respond to the senses, it becomes still and uninfluenced by them, distancing itself from sensations and perceptions. The sixth limb is *dharana*, single pointed concentration. The perceiver, the act of perception, and the perceived are yoked together in a progressive process of *interiorization*. This process is accomplished through attention on a single object or field of consciousness (Hartranft, 2003, p. 13). Focusing the mind's attention in one direction means mental energy is not scattered across fields of awareness. *Dhyana*, the seventh limb, is meditative absorption – the immersion of the subject into the object. Once concentration and an uninterrupted flow of concentration occurs, so too does *dhyana*.

The final limb, *samadhi*, is integration. When perceiving, perceived and perceiver become integrated, the restless mind stills, reflecting *purusha*; then *samadhi* can arise. This is a state of alert restfulness. Again, one does not produce this state, but the ego is surpassed such that the mind ceases to distinguish itself from the rest of creation. This state arises spontaneously from the continual practice of the limbs of yoga. By practicing *yamas*, *niyamas*, *asana* and *pranayama*, the remaining limbs spontaneously arise and develop. Once *samadhi* is attained, *samyama* can occur. This is a sustained state of still reflection wherein, with regular practice, reflections become clearer and clearer as insights become more profound.

YOGA THERAPY

Linking *purusha* and *prakriti* together is the ultimate aim of yoga. However, the disciplined practice of the eight limbs can lead to significant psychological and physical health. A review of the literature on yoga and depression seems to suggest that there is a future for yoga as a therapy for the treatment of mental disorders, including addiction.

The benefits of yoga have lead researchers to propose its use in treating depression (Pilkington, Kirkwood, Rampes, & Richardson, 2005), and stress-related mood states (Shetty, 2005), which are associated with substance use disorders. Moreover, meditative awareness may be beneficial for addictions relapse prevention (Kavanagh, Andrade, & May, 2004). A *meta-analysis* of mindfulness-based stress reduction, among such groups as psychiatric patients and people who suffer from depression or anxiety, provides evidence that such practices are beneficial (Grossman, Niemann, Schmidt, & Walach, 2004). Shetty (2005) found that the use of meditation can be a good supplement, or possible alternative, to pharmacological approaches.

Saraswati (2000) also writes about the value of meditation. He explains how everyone searches for love, appreciation, and security but people look outside of themselves when, ultimately, the source of these experiences can consistently be found within. By searching *prakriti* for ultimate fulfillment, people lose contact with an inner source of contentment, leaving them dependent on the exegeses of an unsteady reality. Sometimes an attempt to decrease negative feelings and gain a sense of control leads to the use of substances. In contrast, by becoming self-aware and learning to be objective, rather than obsessive, people are able to obtain the will and vitality to "alter the mental state of desiring and craving" (Saraswati, 2000, 13).

Generally speaking, physical exercise has been shown to increase positive attitudes and mood states of people who are in treatment, and possibly help prolong sobriety (Read et al., 2001). Brownell, Marlatt, Lichtenstein, and Wilson (1986) found promising results using exercise for relapse prevention. They suggest that the benefits come from an increase in self-esteem, self-efficacy, or a general change in patterns of lifestyle gratification. This rationale is similar to Bandura's (1991) theory of self-efficacy wherein efficacy, or the ability (and knowledge of the ability) to bring about desired results, is related to psychological well-being.

Although self-efficacy theory may explain the case of novice yoga practitioners becoming more accomplished, the true aim of yoga is to surpass the egoic self to realize the immutable awareness at the heart of being. The yogic practice creates a strong mind, spirit, and body and these components may help to maintain sobriety. *Asana* and *pranayama* provide a systematic discipline for caring for the psychospiritual, physical body. The *yamas* and *niyamas* also create a sense of belonging, happiness, and caring within a community. When people struggling with substance use disorders begin to treat others well, isolation dissipates, connections with others are made, and through these relationships a healthier sense of self develops. When the different limbs of yoga are practiced and integrated in this way, there can be significant healing.

ALCOHOLICS ANONYMOUS

The practices of yoga hold promise for healing addictions, but the most prominent method of addressing addictions in North America is through the Twelve-Step program of Alcoholics Anonymous, founded by William Wilson and Dr. Robert Smith (affectionately known in AA as Bill W. and Dr. Bob). The program of Alcoholics Anonymous originated in Akron, Ohio in 1935 with the meeting of William Wilson, a New York stock broker, and Dr. Robert Smith, a local surgeon. Wilson was in Akron on a business trip and, as a chronic alcoholic desperately trying to stay sober, he felt he might be helped by talking with another alcoholic. Through an Episcopal priest he contacted by way of a hotel directory, he was put in touch with Smith who, likewise, had a long history of alcoholic drinking. The AA movement resulted from their working with each other to keep themselves sober, and became perhaps the most influential self-help organization in the world with more than two million members worldwide. The Twelve Steps are laid out as follows (Alcoholics Anonymous World Services, 2006):

> We stood at the turning point. We asked His protection and care with complete abandon. Here are the steps we took, which are suggested as a program of recovery:
>
> 1. We admitted we were powerless over alcohol – that our lives had become unmanageable.
> 2. Came to believe that a Power greater than ourselves could restore us to sanity.
> 3. Made a decision to turn our will and our lives over to the care of God as we understood Him.
> 4. Made a searching and fearless moral inventory of ourselves.
> 5. Admitted to God, to ourselves, and to another human being the exact nature of our wrongs.
> 6. Were entirely ready to have God remove all these defects of character.
> 7. Humbly asked Him to remove our shortcomings.
> 8. Made a list of all persons we had harmed, and became willing to make amends to them all.
> 9. Made direct amends to such people wherever possible, except when to do so would injure them or others.
> 10. Continued to take personal inventory and when we were wrong promptly admitted it.
> 11. Sought through prayer and meditation to improve our conscious contact with God as we understood Him, praying only for knowledge of His will for us and the power to carry that out.

12. Having had a spiritual awakening as the result of these steps, we tried to carry this message to alcoholics, and to practice these principles in all our affairs. (pp. 59-60)

Participants of AA are expected to *work* the *Steps*. This means more than going through them once. The Steps are applied throughout one's life and some Steps, particularly three, four, and five, need to be undertaken with some regularity if one wishes to stay physically and emotionally healthy. Often the Steps are done with another recovering alcoholic who acts as a sponsor. Aspects of community and fellowship are strong within AA and sponsorship (member-to-member support) is depended upon to sustain sobriety.

Due to the prevalence of Christian culture in Western societies, the Christian undertones of the Twelve Steps of AA are familiar to many. Subject to personal interpretation, many of the steps of the program refer to God and hint at repentance and redemption. One is invited to conceive of a God of one's own understanding and atheists and agnostics might think of a Higher Power in a panentheistic way or regard their Higher Power as the other members of AA. However, because of the language used in the Steps, the AA program gives the appearance of being largely based on a Christian religious ideology.

The Christian emphasis in AA arose from the early days after the Akron meeting of Smith and Wilson (Alcoholics Anonymous World Services, 2004). Before the AA organization ever existed, alcoholics would attend meetings of the Oxford Groups, begun in 1921, which later became the Moral-Rearmament movement. The MRA movement was an international religious movement that, in 1938, grew out of Rev. Frank N. D. Buchman's Oxford Groups in the U.K; Buchman was an American Lutheran missionary stationed in Europe. The MRA was a response to the militarization of post-WWI Germany, claiming that the world did not need military re-armament but moral re-armament. Eventually, AA members realized that they could not co-exist with the mostly non-alcoholic and religious members of the Oxford Groups, as their objectives were so different, and at that time the alcoholic members split off and formed AA. The *four absolutes* that Oxford Group members worked to achieve in their personal lives – absolute honesty, absolute purity, absolute unselfishness, and absolute love – were eventually re-written and expanded into the Twelve Steps of AA, and some of the Christian religious language was preserved.

Currently, most AA members would insist that the program is *spiritual* rather than *religious*. Initially, members of AA are willing to overlook the language of the Steps and the Big Book because by the time they get to AA their alcoholic dilemma and problems are so severe that they are willing to accept any program which offers some hope of recovery. Eventually, members come to see that the AA belief system can be interpreted in a very liberal and non-theistic way.

The guiding text, *Alcoholics Anonymous*, was nicknamed the Big Book because the first edition in 1939 was printed on very thick paper to reduce cost, thus increasing the book's size considerably. It is now in its fourth edition, setting out the Twelve Steps and what are called the Twelve Traditions (Alcoholics Anonymous World Services, 2006). Throughout its long history, people affiliated with AA gained a great amount of experience with recovery from alcohol addiction. This experience has been abstracted into general guidelines known as the Twelve Traditions, first formulated in 1946. Primarily, these guidelines are meant to govern the functioning of AA and its groups around the world, to preserve its singleness of purpose in helping the active alcoholic recover. The Twelve Traditions are not compulsory for any participants or groups, but the majority of members have adopted them as the foundation for AA etiquette, which helps to assure the solidarity and survival of the group as a whole.

The structure of AA meetings is non-hierarchical. That is, each AA group is self-governing and cannot be compelled to action by a higher authority within AA. There are four main types of meetings: discussion, Step, Big Book study, and speaker. Each meeting is either open (anyone can attend) or closed (for alcoholics only). At meetings, members are invited to speak to the group about their experiences but are not required to do so. Most AA members believe that attendance at AA meetings is essential for their sobriety but those who live in remote locations might keep up communication by phone or email. Daily attendance at meetings in the first months of sobriety is recommended along with working through the Twelve Steps. The meetings and the Twelve Steps are offered as the path toward a healing spiritual experience.

Alcoholics Anonymous views alcoholism as a fourfold disease made up of physical, emotional, spiritual, and mental dynamics (Kassel & Wagner, 1993). Alcohol addiction is understood as the inability to drink without it inevitably leading to having more drinks, even if this happens days later. In other words, if a person is truly an alcoholic, the first drink will eventually lead to destructive drinking. Thus, first and foremost, recovery involves avoiding the first drink. Alcoholism is considered a disease, much like diabetes is a disease; therefore, AA members speak of themselves as *recovering*, but not *recovered*, from alcoholism. This disease requires a spiritual experience for recovery, not from alcoholism per se, but from the experience of helplessness. A *spiritual experience* is a psychic or personality change brought about by changing one's actions, leading to a life free from addiction. It can occur suddenly, but in most cases occurs gradually over a period of time.

Members who are successfully working the Steps are encouraged to become sponsors and to provide guidance and support for others. The concept of a *wounded healer* – someone who has been injured or ill, recovers, and returns to heal others – has been used by the AA program since the beginning (Kassel & Wagner, 1993). It is seen as a beneficial method for several reasons (Zemore,

Kaskutas, & Ammon, 2004). An important function of AA is that it creates a sense of community, a sense of support and family. Fellowship has been found to be a crucial aspect of recovery because this allows people at different stages to benefit. Those in the first Steps of recovering are given the opportunity to state and restate their dedication to sobriety, receiving support from those who are more experienced with sobriety. Those people in the role of experiential counselor provide support while strengthening their own abstinence position through encouraging others. No longer isolated, AA members find comfort and companionship, recognizing they can obtain their goals through their own strength and the strength of others (Green, Fullilove, & Fullilove, 1998). In this environment, trust is established and maintained, providing conditions for healing (Le, Ingvarson, & Page, 1995).

A CASE OF AA AND YOGA BELIEF SYSTEMS INTEGRATED

In 1981, Father Joe Pereira recognized a need and set out on a journey that would end in founding an organization called the Kripa Foundation. Today this organization has grown to thirty-one facilities throughout India. People suffering from substance use disorders are invited to join others at the Kripa facilities, inspired to release themselves from the discomfort of their current mental, physical, and spiritual states to awaken into a new state of personal awareness. Each participant is given guidance based on a modified AA program, the support of the Kripa community, and a basis for personal growth facilitated by traditional yoga practices.

Father Joe spoke in an interview about the principles of the program, its success, and the hopes the program creates. The interview was transcribed verbatim and then edited to facilitate ease of reading. The transcript was then reviewed by Father Joe for accuracy of meaning and further changes were made. The resulting text was analyzed using open, axial, and selective coding (Denzin & Lincoln, 2000). Open coding involves a microanalytic reading of the text, interpreting the meaning of passages, and staying close to the words of the interviewee. Axial coding analyzes the text by linking open codes to generate overarching themes. *The Caring Model* and its four thematic areas – "Complementary Medicines," "Existentialism," "The Clinics," and "Returning" – were developed using these grounded theory methods. Finally, selective coding identified portions of text that exemplified the meaning of the axial codes and a literature review was conducted to complement the analysis. What follows is a narrative organization of the grounded theory analysis that depicts Father Joe's story along with research that supports a holistic approach to the treatment of substance use disorder.

THE CARING MODEL

We were creating a very unique kind of healthcare, a caring model, where we recognized the value of a person in recovery. (Father Joe)

In all countries where alcohol is used, Alcohol use disorders also appear. In countries such as India, usually considered *dry*, alcohol use is rising. It is estimated that approximately 20 to 30 percent of men in India use alcohol (Benegal, Velayudhan, & Jain, 2000). Historically in India, primary preventative measures for alcohol use disorders have focused on the prohibition of alcohol, outlawing its production and consumption. However, prohibition in India led to economic and social disruption due to loss of jobs in brew factories and retail outlets, economic loss incurred by the state, along with an increase in bootlegging and smuggling (Patel, 1998). In spite of these loses, prohibition failed to eradicate alcohol use or alcohol use disorders (Benegal, 2005; Patel, 1998; Ranganathan, 1994).

Father Joe's story provides another option for managing alcohol use disorders. In the 1980s, he was working in India and attending to a vast number of alcoholics and drug addicts who were living on the streets and taking refuge in Mother Teresa's home. "Seeing a lot of helpless alcoholics and drug addicts," he says, "I felt they had to be given some very special understanding and so I took them in." Mother Teresa saw the impact Father Joe was having and gave him her centre in Calcutta to continue his efforts. As clients progressed, the program evolved, yet always in a way that is sensitive to the needs of India's people.

According to Patel (1998), the development and use of various non-government organizations that specialize in working with addictions in India is a crucial step toward addressing alcohol use disorders. Beyond simply organizing such programs, there are specific elements of the program and needs of the participants that must be considered when treatment begins. Price, Hand, Mahimananda, and Kriyamurti (2000) suggest three elements that should be addressed in treatment. The first is the development of an internal locus of control that coaches people to obtain and maintain control of their behaviors rather than allowing desires and cravings for external objects to rule. Second, there must be sustainable short-, medium-, and long-term goals used to gradually move away from addiction toward an internal locus of control and increased self-esteem. Last, specific patterns of thought and behavior need to be developed that will be a resource to help maintain a healthy addiction-free lifestyle (Price et al., 2000).

Father Joe refers to *The Caring Model* as "a deeply spiritual model, but it is a science and faith blend." Through yoga, one can find a fixed centre to one's being, providing a place from which to connect with others and define one's worth and purpose. Meditation enhances perception of this divine core, providing a clearer sense of self and giving an immutable centre to one's existence (Walsh, 1993). Addiction research has shown that developing or nurturing a sense of *purusa* – immutable awareness – is helpful in combating addiction and preventing relapse (Green et al., 1998; Leigh, Bowen, & Marlatt, 2005). Father Joe maintains that the restoration of self-worth and realizing the divinity, beauty and goodness at one's core is vital for recovering. Father Joe's teacher, Guruji Iyengar (2005), explains recovery in this way:

> People who are addicted to drugs or alcohol are encouraged not to do what is called "white knuckle self-control," as its egoic source will eventually be exhausted and a crash will follow. On the contrary, they are told to "hand over to a higher power," which means that their will is replenished every day through contact with the cosmic source of intelligent action." (p. 169)

However, what is not useful is the "encumbrance of original sin, which makes addicts run away from recovery" (Father Joe). A belief system that suggests addicts have sinned and must seek forgiveness is problematic because it can generate guilt that may lead to relapse (Le et al., 1995). Father Joe explains how "we have brought so much gloom through religion. We do not need that kind of gloom to come into the recovery program. You need spirituality, which will bring joy, celebration, and life."

COMPLEMENTARY MEDICINES

Based on interview data, *The Caring Model* is composed of several smaller elements that work together to heal a person and prepare him or her for a life free of substance abuse. The first of these smaller elements is "Complementary Medicines." Father Joe emphasizes the importance of allowing for unique interpretations of recovery, including personal interpretations of spirituality and addiction. Although many people believe in a personal God, both AA and yoga have a great understanding of those who do not and a strong willingness to accommodate them. The limbs of yoga need to be subject to personal reflection and interpreted according to each person's experience to develop a unique, personal system of liberation from attachments and suffering. For some people, interpreting spirituality within a religious context is most useful (Kassel & Wagner, 1993). However, others come to AA with a childhood background of churchgoing and, having rejected the church, experience AA as spiritual but not religious. The AA program would be difficult to accept if it were a religious instead of a spiritual organization.

Sharma (2001) proposes that by combining established practices of AA with the traditions of yoga psychology, addictions might be confronted with greater ease and success because people who do not follow a religious doctrine may resist the religious undertones in the wording of the AA steps. For example, in step six, recovering addicts declare they are ready to have God remove all defects of character and, in step seven, they humbly ask God to remove their shortcomings. Combining AA with yoga provides an alternative belief system by which to view addiction recovery as a path of spiritual development and not a religious affiliation. In yoga, a connection with the immutable consciousness of *purusa* emerges from natural processes, or *prakriti*. The practitioner's responsibility lies in developing and sustaining this connection with purusa, similar to maintaining a connection to a higher power, through disciplined practices in daily life (*yamas* and *niyamas*).

Father Joe sees a need in India for a program that is neither Christian nor Indian alone but, rather, a flexible hybrid of the best aspects of the two. Combining AA and yoga in one program, he believes, can provide a sense of community, foster spiritual awareness and personal competence, and help people to develop a physical and psychological practice that results in the healthy integration of body, mind, heart, and spirit. Furthermore, cross-cultural recovery programs could appeal to a more culturally diverse population (Sharma, 2001).

What makes the Kripa program different from most addiction treatment programs is its integration of two culturally distinct belief systems. The fluid integration of the self-help model (AA) and a holistic yogic interpretation of recovery has helped to make the program a success in India. In the Kripa program, yoga is used continuously and with specificity throughout the healing process. Both physical yogic exercises and meditative practices are incorporated at specific points in the treatment and are strongly encouraged throughout. Based on his experience, Father Joe asserts that: "the potential to change and to absorb this new lifestyle is so much more when you use the psychosomatics, the body and the breath . . . . I am one hundred percent sure that meditators fail to lapse."

Independent evidence supports Father Joe's conviction in the unlikelihood of relapse for people who meditate. Meditation is a process of calming the mind and becoming aware of physical, mental, and emotional processes. When Kavanagh et al. (2004) examined processes of substance-related desire and relapse, they found that suppressing substance related desires and urges was not productive. In place of thought suppression (i.e., not thinking about the craving or distracting oneself), recognizing and acknowledging the thought or the urge was found to be much more beneficial. Recognizing processes that underlie urges was a more successful way of handling compulsive desire. That is, when one is aware that a desire exists and can recognize it as a physical or mental reaction, and not the basis of one's whole self, then one is able to disconnect from the potentially overwhelming quality of a desire and manage the experience with greater freedom. In contrast, someone who is not able to recognize the distinction between the self and the desire may feel besieged by cravings and guilt.

Moreover, Lohman's (1999) research into the use of yoga in addiction treatment programs suggests that people with a history of addiction might be more responsive to yoga. The proposed reason for this openness is that people with addiction histories may be more familiar with altered states of consciousness, making it easier for them to accept and utilize the dimensions of consciousness experienced in yogic meditation. Calajoe (1986) also notes that substance-induced states of consciousness can be quite similar to altered states acquired through yoga practices. The feelings of freedom, total connectedness, detachment from particular objects, and relaxation are all sustained through the healthy and beneficial practices of yoga. Unlike substance-induced experiences, states acquired through yoga practices can provide a consistent sense of contentment and connection. The purpose of yoga practices rests in instilling a sense of clear awareness and a fluid ease of detachment from external events. This strengthens one's general sense of connection to a world and ability to generate a sense of sufficiency and contentment.

EXISTENTIALISM

> The most difficult obstacle is the ego. If one can really go past that, or just handle that, then everything is possible. The earth and the sky is the limit. (Father Joe)

What is common among addicts, in Father Joe's experience, is that "there has been some kind of existential void . . . . They're basically living in a world with a population of one, one self." In treatment, a person needs to gain a sense of meaning and mutuality through belonging. People with substance use disorders may feel alienated and disconnected from the world they live in. They may become focused on their addiction, only feeling a connection to the one thing that helps them disconnect from everything else. Substance use disorders are sometimes an example of the misguided attempts people make to avoid their existential needs. Grof and Grof (1993) characterize the existential struggle for connectedness:

> Many recovering people will talk about their restless search for some unknown missing piece in their lives and will describe their vain pursuit of a multitude of substances, foods, relationships, possessions, or powerful positions in an effort to fulfill their unrewarded craving. In retrospect, they acknowledge that there was a tragic confusion, a misperception that told them that the answers lay outside themselves. Some even describe the first drink or drug as their first spiritual experience, a state in which individual boundaries are melted and everyday pain disappears, taking them into a state of pseudo-unity. (p. 145)

Historically, existentialism can be traced back, somewhat indirectly, to the writings of Socrates and John Locke. The more contemporary and recognizable forms of Existentialism arise from the works of Nietzsche, Dostoevsky, Sartre, Kierkegaard, and Buber. Martin Buber (1923/1970) wrote about existentialism and the difference between an I-It and an I-You (or I-Thou) relationship. He stated that there are only two ways in which any human can attend to existence. The first and seemingly most common way is to address objects, subjects, or experiences as separate from oneself in an I-It relationship. The second, and fairly uncommon way, is when a relationship is experienced in terms of mutual existence, touching on the infinity of connectedness.

In this way, relating to our existence is two-fold: We may experience the world in terms of impersonal dealings or existence as a world of interpersonal relations. In an I-You relationship, one relates, whether with an object, a subject, a human being, or God such that there is no ultimate separation between oneself and another. Father Joe explains, "When you realize [the existential fullness at the centre of being] and restore an I-Thou relationship, you break that sense of alienation." Alienated from the experience of I-You relationships, Father Joe observes that people suffering addictions tend to have only I-It relationships, epitomized in relationships with substances. Yet he adds that "once you restore the I-Thou relationship, the I-It diminishes, or disappears" (Father Joe).

People may be unwilling or unable to engage in I-You relationships because such relationships are experienced as unpredictable, beyond personal control and, thus, too dangerous; they may have missed out on early I-You experiences and may be unskilled in forming such relationships; or they may be compulsively enacting only I-It relationships in an attempt to master earlier experiences where they were treated as an object. Nevertheless, being in an I-You relationship seems to be how one develops spiritual awareness and a sense of universal connection. Within the Kripa program, I-You connections are exhibited and nurtured in relations with family and significant others.

The Kripa program addresses physical and emotional needs by acting as an extended family. Once yoga practice begins, people tend to lose feelings of being isolated and begin to connect with others, not only in terms of being physically present but, also, psychospiritually in terms of sharing, loving and enjoying together. Recovery gives clients "the joy of living, the joy of loving, and the joy of saving" (Father Joe).

Father Joe warns that if meaningful connectedness is not maintained, relapse arises: "Over the years if not maintained, then there is a drop to as low as 35 percent after ten years, even 18 percent. But maintaining contact is a sure shot model. You can't go wrong." Quantitative researchers also find that maintenance, through such components as social support and exercise, is important to sobriety and relapse prevention (Brownell et al., 1986). Father Joe describes the community of Kripa not as a "typical therapeutic community" but, rather, a community wherein people connect with one another to rescript their lives. Because people are healing together, a consistent sense of community lessens the experience of loneliness. This approach differs significantly from a typical out-patient program where it is not always possible to contact others in times of need.

Closely following the tenets of existentialism, Viktor Frankl's (1962) *logotherapy* asserts that each human being has the ability to find and create meaning in life. He asserts that people have the capacity to find meaning under any circumstances, even in exceedingly difficult times. Frankl was a World War II holocaust survivor, yet he celebrates the human capacity to make life meaningful. According to logotherapy, when meaning is not developed a sense of wastefulness and behavioral problems may occur. Father Joe explains:

> Then there is logotherapy, finding meaning, starting with one's own self. Actually, as soon as you get rid of the existential void you begin to love yourself, you get in touch with the core of your being, and you start operating from that core of your being, rather than from the peripheral . . . one really lifts the person out of the realm of prakriti, in the Indian Samkya philosophy, getting out of the field of prakriti and bringing the person into the field of consciousness which is purusha.

THE CLINICS

The Kripa program has three clinics. The first clinic is part of the admission procedure and consists of preliminary interviews for assessing motivation. In this clinic, it is typical for close family, extended family (e.g., grandparents, siblings), a significant other, or friends to be involved. A sense of openness and honesty pervade over this phase. Recovery is not done in secret or looked at as shameful; rather, transparency and support is expected. McCrady (2004) reviewed the research on social networks and support systems in the treatment of alcohol use disorders and found that when social networks were thin (i.e., people living alone, having little contact with family or friends, participating in few social activities) and isolation was high, the prominence of alcohol use disorders was elevated. However, interaction with other people and receiving high levels of support from even just one person prior to treatment led to better treatment results (McCrady, 2004). McCrady also noted that the less supportive the family of the afflicted was, the less successful the participant tended to be.

The second clinic is primarily for detoxification, called the "de-addiction phase" (Father Joe). The client remains here for approximately twenty-seven days. There is not only physical cleansing, but emotional and spiritual detoxification as well. Father Joe emphasizes the importance of *asanas* and how "the restorative postures of Iyengar are suggested for detoxification." He explains: "getting in touch with their bodies in a manner that will help them see that they can love their bodies back to life is very vital. When they see that happening . . . that is an amazing lesson." Wood (1993) found that the application of yogic practices of pranayama and asana helped to increase the perception of vigour and enthusiasm in participants. As a result, these people felt more capable and willing to attend to a challenging task.

Read and Brown (2003) have suggested that acknowledging personal efficacy positively influences the patient's ability to overcome addiction problems and sustain sobriety. When people acquire a level of esteem that enables them to acknowledge their own abilities, they are more likely to reach and sustain sobriety. Read and Brown (2003) found that those who gain a sense of efficacy and esteem from their participation and success in physical exercises, are more positive about their recovery and more willing to maintain sobriety. In general, having a sense of self-efficacy plays an important role in the development and maintenance of health and well-being (Bandura, 1991).

Lohman (1999) found that centers that offered some type of yoga practice during detoxification were successful because yoga helped people to push past the initial withdrawal weakness. The purifying exercises of yoga seemed to resolve negative psychological and physical states. Improved breathing, posture, relaxation and meditation detoxified the body, fostered patience and increased attention span. When faced with frustration and the urge to turn to a substance, the practitioner was more prepared to acknowledge the situation honestly and use awareness to move through the urge and back to a preferred level of control (Lohman, 1999).

The third clinic handles aftercare, which tends to run two to three months. However, de-addiction and aftercare overlap: "There is the aftercare clinic, for the aftercare situation in the community. Even the de-addiction is lived in the community" (Father Joe). Due to the intensive live-in situation of the first two clinics, people are more prepared to face recovery on their own, with the tools of *ashtanga* (eight-limbed) yoga and the community support developed through the Kripa Foundation. Father Joe assures: "You see a transformation! There is a very high recovery rate of 60-65 plus. In some Centers even 75."

RETURNING

According to Father Joe: "The biggest problem in recovery . . . is playing God . . . . There is a God, but that is not you, and you just want to play God . . . . The grandiosity is sometimes amazing." He explains that this exists because of a basic sense of rejection and feeling that one is not loved, such that one exists in isolation. Consequently, people struggling with addiction feel little empathy or connectedness with their community. The *yamas* and *niyamas* are disciplines that can help people to live and interact in a community to "have a very meaningful productive life, you know, getting back to work, or doing something in service" (Father Joe).

According to Father Joe, the work of recovery is "a deepening of [the] experience of sharing one's 'brokenness' with others, the coming from poverty, rather than abundance." This poverty is not solely material or economic but it also represents a sparseness of emotional, spiritual, and interpersonal being such that healing must occur along all of these dimensions. Just as the last step of the AA program is to carry on the message of the group, Kripa Foundation participants are encouraged to support others and to work directly with the program in other communities.

The Kripa Foundation uses the wounded healer approach, wherein recovering addicts become experiential counselors to those who more recently have come into the program. With time, one is able to enhance his or her own sense of awareness and depend more on oneself. As this transformation unfolds, one begins to alternate positions from counselee to experiential counselor. This transition ensures that there are people to support those in need and help maintain the program in other areas of the country. In this way, not only does one person become healthier, there is also a community being developed and renewed.

Father Joe refers to the experiential counselor as a "vital component" that already exists in the medical and psychotherapeutic models. Experiential counselors are *returned* to a meaningful role within society and given the opportunity to heal while being a part of others' healing opportunities. In Father Joe's words, "the model . . . recycles an absolutely marginalized citizen into a very productive citizen."

Father Joe explained that "as people get well and want to spread this message to others, they get back in touch with the different parts of India from which they came." According to Father Joe, this is how the Kripa program spread throughout India, to locations as diverse as "Calcutta and Bombay, Delhi, Darjeeling, Shillong, and Mizoram." Without those who spiritually recovered, the program may not have spread so extensively, leaving the need for healing today much greater than it currently is.

Father Joe speaks fondly of all the people who have passed through the Kripa program: "They are always motivated to health and help. The last step of the program, the twelfth step, is all about reaching out, and they do that very well." He explains further: "We offer them opportunities to serve in the field, if they do not find a new profession outside." It is through this sense of community and connectedness that the Kripa Foundation has spread throughout India, with past participants supporting new participants, helping to pass on the healing powers of the integration of AA and yoga.

CONCLUSION

There are a number of striking parallels between the belief systems and practices of yoga and AA. Practitioners of yoga and members of AA seek to experience connection through a power greater than the egos of self and other; use meditation and reflection to move beyond the personal self; reflect on what is good, right, and honest; take spiritual experience as a central means for happiness and well-being; believe in the importance of community; and cultivate harmonious interpersonal connections. As such, these two belief systems seem to be compatible and complementary, with yoga providing physical practices absent in a strictly AA program of recovery. Although the AA program easily lends itself to a Christian sense of spiritual experience, yogic practices that cultivate spiritual experience – the realization of transcendental consciousness – tend to be more secular or psychological. By including this natural orientation, more diverse interpretations of psychospiritual healing may be made available.

The Kripa Foundation has integrated principles of AA and yoga to form a holistic treatment program. Detoxification and physical aspects of recovery are addressed through yogic practices within a recovering community that supports health. Beyond physical recovery, there is psychological, emotional, and spiritual recovery that complement the detoxification and sobriety of participants. A personal sense of efficacy develops that empowers participants to attend to their existential needs, to explore the meaning of their lives, and to cultivate self-awareness while developing a sense of community. This creates a safe and supportive environment for persons recovering from substance use disorders as they return to their communities. Success rates of participants in the program range from 60-75 percent; however, maintenance of community is an important aspect of the program and, when not attended to, success rates may drop (Kripa Foundation, n.d.).

Examination of interview material and the relevant research provided here suggest that, besides understanding addiction as a method of self-medication, a way of dissolving inhibitions and increasing tolerance and a sense of control, or acting as a substitute relationship, a psychospiritual dimension also exists in substance use and recovery. Addiction may be understood as disconnection from a source of joy and a dimension of consciousness that persists across situations and persons. Iyengar (2005), Father Joe's teacher, explains:

> By turning our minds inward (which automatically happens) in asana and pranayama and teaching us the art of constructive action in the present moment, yoga leads consciousness away from desires and toward the inner, undisturbable core. Here, it creates a new avenue by which reflexively to perceive, observe, and recognize the heart (*antarlaksa*). In this way, the meditative mind created by yoga is a powerful therapeutic tool for removing human ills. (p. 143)

Further investigation into applying yogic methods of substance use disorder treatment in Western communities would seem valuable. Additional inquiry into these areas could promote successful methods of addictions treatment and relapse prevention for individuals and families in diverse communities in North America.

Combining two traditions not only has the potential to appeal to a greater diversity of people, it also makes room for a fresh perspective. As long as there is enough common ground between them so that comparison is meaningful and goals can be shared, difference can renew understanding and increase meaning. One becomes distanced from AA philosophy by inhabiting the world of yoga and in turn distanced from yoga by immersing oneself in the world of AA. One belief system need not be imposed upon or absorbed by the other, but one can be seen as containing the other within it, as a variation on a theme. This play across difference can illuminate beliefs in a new light and enrich understanding.

NOTES

[1] The research for this chapter was supported by the Saskatchewan Health Research Foundation Research Establishment Grant and the University of Regina SSHRC General Research Grant Fund and The President's Fund.

References

Alcoholics Anonymous World Services (2004). *Alcoholics anonymous comes of age: A brief history of A.A.* (30th printing.). New York: Alcoholics Anonymous World Services. (Original work published 1957)

Alcoholics Anonymous World Services (2006). *The big book online fourth edition.* Retrieved December 7, 2006, from http://www.aa.org/bigbookonline/

Bandura, A. (1991). Self-efficacy mechanism in physiological activation and health-promoting behavior. In J. Madden (Ed.), *Neurobiology of learning, emotion and affect* (pp. 229-270). New York: Raven.

Benegal, V. (2005). *India: Alcohol and public health.* Retrieved June 22, 2006 from http://www.ias.org.uk/resources/publications/theglobe/globe200502/gl200502_p7.html

Benegal, V., Velayudhan, A., & Jain, S. (2000). Social costs of alcoholism: A Karnataka Perspective. *NIMHANS Journal, 18,* 67.

Brownell, K. D., Marlatt, G. A., Lichtenstein, E., & Wilson G. T. (1986). Understanding and preventing relapse. *American Psychologist, 41,* 765-782.

Buber, M. (1970). *I and thou.* (W. Kaufmann, Trans.) New York: Scribner. (Original work published 1923)

Calajoe, A. (1986). Yoga as a therapeutic component in treating chemical dependency. *Alcoholism Treatment Quarterly, 3,* 33-46.

Denzin, N. K., & Lincoln, Y. S. (2000). *Handbook of qualitative research* (2nd ed.). Thousand Oaks, CA: Sage.

Desikachar, T. K. V. (1999). *The heart of yoga.* Rochester, VT: Inner Traditions.

Eliade, M. (1958). *Yoga: Immortality and freedom.* Princeton, NJ: Princeton University Press.

Federn, P. (1952). *Ego psychology and the psychoses.* New York: Basic Books.

Fenichel, O. (1945). *The psychoanalytic theory of neurosis.* New York: Norton.

Feuerstein, G. (1989). *The yoga-sutras of Patanjali.* Rochester, VT: Inner Traditions.

Feuerstein, G. (1997). *The Shambhala encyclopedia of yoga.* Boston: Shambhala.

Frankl, V. E. (1962). *Man's search for meaning: An introduction to logotherapy.* Boston: Beacon.

Green, L. L., Fullilove, M. T., & Fullilove, R. E. (1998). Stories of spiritual awakening: The nature of spirituality in recovery. *Journal of Substance Abuse Treatment, 15,* 325-331.

Grof, C., & Grof, S. (1993). Addiction as spiritual emergency. In R. Walsh & F. Vaughan (Eds.), *Paths beyond ego: The transpersonal vision* (pp. 144-146). New York: Tarcher/Putnam.

Grossman, P., Niemann, L., Schmidt, S., & Walach, H. (2004). Mindfulness-based stress reduction and health benefits: A meta-analysis. *Journal of Psychosomatic Research, 57*, 35-43.

Hartranft, C. (2003). *The yoga-sutra of Patanjali.* Boston: Shambhala.

Heather, N., & Stockwell, T. (Eds.) (2003). *The essential handbook of treatment and prevention of alcohol problems.* Hoboken, NJ: John Wiley & Sons.

Iyengar, B. K. S. (2002). *Light on the yoga sutras of Patanjali.* Toronto: HarperCollins.

Iyengar, B. K. S. (2005). *Light on life: The yoga journey to wholeness, inner peace, ad ultimate freedom.* Vancouver, BC: Raincoast Books.

Kassel, J. D., & Wagner, E. F. (1993). Processes of change in Alcoholics Anonymous: A review of possible mechanisms. *Psychotherapy, 30*, 222-234.

Kavanagh, D. J., Andrade, J., & May, J. (2004). Beating the urge: Implications of research into substance-related desires. *Addictive Behaviors, 29*, 1359-1372.

Kernberg, O. F. (1980). *Internal world and external reality: Object relations theory applied.* New York: Jason Aronson.

Kripa Foundation (n.d.) Retrieved December 6, 2006 from Kripa Foundation Web site: http://www.kripafoundation.org/index.html

Le, C., Ingvarson, E. P., & Page, R. (1995). Alcoholics Anonymous and the counseling profession: Philosophies in conflict. *Journal of Counseling and Development, 73*, 603.

Leigh, J., Bowen, S., & Marlatt, G. A. (2005). Spirituality, mindfulness and substance abuse. *Addictive Behaviors, 30*, 1335-1341

Lohman, R. (1999). Yoga techniques applicable within drug and alcohol rehabilitation programmes. *Therapeutic Communities, 20*, 61-71

McCrady, B. S. (2004). To have but one true friend: Implications for practice of research on alcohol use disorders and social networks. *Psychology of Addictive Behaviors, 18*, 113-121.

Patel, V. (1998). Tackling alcoholism in India. *The Medical Council on Alcohol, 17*, 5. Retrieved June 20, 2006, from www.medicouncilalcol.demon.co.uk

Pilkington, K., Kirkwood, G., Rampes, H., & Richardson, J. (2005). Yoga for depression: The research evidence. *Journal of Affective Disorders, 89*, 13-24.

Price, M., Hand, G., Mahimananda, S., & Kriyamurti, S. (2000). Addiction – A systems approach: Issues for Yoga teachers. *Yoga Magazine.* Retrieved June 14, 2006, from http://www.yogamag.net/archives/2000/6nov00/yogasys.shtml

Ranganathan, S. (1994, September). The most sensible thing is not to drink. Alcohol in the third world, excerpted from the World Health Forum. *World Health Organization* Retrieved July 5, 2006 from www.unhooked.com/sep/thirdworl.htm

Read, J. P., & Brown, R. A. (2003). The role of physical exercise in alcoholism treatment and recovery. *Professional Psychology: Research and Practice, 34*, 49-56.

Read, J. P., Brown, R. A., Marcus, B. H., Kahler, W., Ramsey, S. E., Dubreuil, M. E., Jakicic, J. M., & Francione, C. (2001). Exercise attitudes and behaviors among persons in treatment for alcohol use disorders. *Journal of Substance Abuse Treatment*, *21*, 199-206.

Saraswati, N. (2000). Yoga and addiction. *Yoga Magazine*. Retrieved September 5, 2006, from http://www.yogamag.net/archives/2000/6nov00/yogandad.shtml

Sharma, G. (2001, July/August). The alcohol trap. *Hinduism Today*, 58-59. Retrieved November 22, 2005, from http://www.hinduismtoday.com/archives/2001/7-8/58-59_addiction.shtml

Shetty, R. C. (2005). Meditation and its implications in nonpharmacological management of stress related emotions and cognitions. *Medical Hypotheses*, *65*, 1198-1199.

Volkan, K. (1994). *Dancing among the maenads: The psychology of compulsive drug use.* New York: Peter Lang.

Walsh, R. (1993). Mapping and comparing states. In R. Walsh & F. Vaughan (Eds.), *Paths beyond ego: The transpersonal vision* (pp. 38-46). New York: Tarcher/Putnam.

Winnicott, D. W. (1989). *Psycho-analytic explorations.* Cambridge, MA: Harvard University Press.

Wood, C. (1993). Mood change and perceptions of vitality: A comparison of the effects of relaxation, visualization and yoga. *Journal of the Royal Society of Medicine*, *86*, 254-258.

Zemore, S. E., Kaskutas, L. A., & Ammon, L. N. (2004). In 12-step groups, helping helps the helper. *Addiction*, *99*, 1015-1023.